CW01214160

Early Praise for Regression Hypnotherapy

"Randal Churchill has done it again! His first book, *Become the Dream*, received the ACHE Founder's Award for 'Excellence in Professional Literature' and his latest text, *Regression Hypnotherapy*, is certain to contend for another award. Memorable clinical examples, in the form of case transcripts, fix techniques in the reader's mind. The theoretical sections include insights about key concepts of Gestalt Therapy as modified and incorporated into Analytic Hypnotherapy. The methodology is presented with great clarity for practical integration into modern hypnotherapy practice. The process comments accompanying the therapy transcripts are invaluable. Randal Churchill's merging of Gestalt Therapy concepts into regression, reeducation and integration processes of Clinical Hypnotherapy is a major advance in the teaching literature of Hypnotherapy. A brilliant blending of theory and practice, *Regression Hypnotherapy* is a must read and study for practitioners and students of hypnotherapy."
Gil Boyne, Executive Director, A.C.H.E., author of *Transforming Therapy*

"*Regression Hypnotherapy*, by Randal Churchill, is destined to become an instant classic and will be used by hypnotherapists for decades to come. This ultimate teaching text is highly recommended for all in the field."
Ormond McGill, *The Dean of American Hypnotists*

"Randal Churchill has written a rich and stimulating book on the complex and ever sensitive topic of regression hypnotherapy. I recommend it highly for its lucid text, steeped in his many years of practice and his masterful training of hypnotherapists. The depth of Randal's experience and his thorough sense of care and compassion for his clients shine through again and again. *Regression Hypnotherapy* is a superb contribution to the field."
Kenneth Kelser, LCSW, author of *Deep Journeys*

"*Regression Hypnotherapy*, written by one of the most insightful and innovative regression therapists in the field, is the most important book about regression to be published in many years. Randal Churchill's unique style and gifted insight give clarity to the rich potential for transformation existing in the deeper intelligence of our own minds. With expert guidance and sensitivity, he leads individuals into the inner world of subconscious memories and emotions - assisting them through powerful emotional clearing and the access of their own inner wisdom for understanding and reeducation - transforming past traumas and emerging with triumphant clarity and peace. Churchill's skilled direction in actual sessions is an art form as well as powerful therapy."
Cheryl Canfield, CHT, author of *Steps Toward Profound Healing*

About the Author

RANDAL CHURCHILL is President of the American Council of Hypnotist Examiners, the largest and oldest Hypnotherapy Certification agency with over 10,000 members in 40 countries. Founder and Director of the Hypnotherapy Training Institute, one of the first state-licensed hypnotherapy schools in the world, he is known as "Teacher of the Teachers"™, having trained many of the state-approved hypnotherapy instructors in the United States. HTI draws students from many countries to the San Francisco area, graduating more Certified Hypnotherapists annually than any other school. It's alumni of thousands of graduates spanning three decades is the largest of any licensed hypnotherapy school.

A clinical hypnotherapist since 1969, Randal has completed over 30,000 hours of hypnotherapy sessions. He is a graduate of Sonoma State University, receiving his degree in Psychology with Honors. He has taught hypnotherapy to psychiatrists at Napa State Hospital, has taught at various other institutions, and has been a featured speaker at many International Hypnotherapy Conferences.

Randal Churchill has received international acclaim for his skill, creativity, sensitivity, and comprehensive approach to a wide range of challenging issues. An intuitive, supportive therapist, he is originator of Hypnotic Dreamwork™ and has been a pioneering leader for over 30 years in Gestalt therapy, regression therapy and advanced ideomotor methods.

Randal is the author of numerous published books and articles, including the award-winning text, *Become the Dream: The Transforming Power of Hypnotic Dreamwork,* which is the first book about the integration of dreamwork and hypnotherapy. His work has been the subject of a television documentary, and he has been interviewed for various television documentaries, including by PBS, the BBC and Japanese television. He has been interviewed on many radio talk shows.

Regression Hypnotherapy

Regression Hypnotherapy

Transcripts of Transformation

Volume I

Randal Churchill

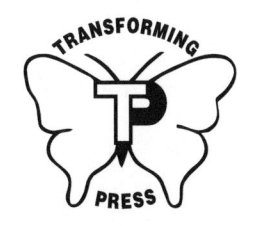

Transforming Press

REGRESSION HYPNOTHERAPY: *Transcripts of Transformation* is printed on acid free, natural recycled paper with soy-based ink.

Copyright © 2002 by Randal Churchill

All rights reserved

No part of this book may be reproduced in any form, with the exception of brief excerpts in reviews, without the written permission of the publisher.

Some names have been changed in certain transcripts included herein.

Cover photo by David Cavagnaro

Cover design by Nadise Whiteside

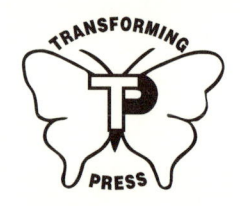

Transforming Press
P.O. Box 9369 Santa Rosa, CA 95405
Phone and Fax: 209/962-6403
email: info@transformingpress.com
www.transformingpress.com

ISBN 0-9656218-1-2
1. Psychology 2. Regression 3. Hypnotism - Therapeutic use
4. Recovered Memories

Library of Congress Catalog Card Number 2002103462

FIRST EDITION. Printed in the United States of America

10 9 8 7 6 5 4 3 2 1

To my mother and father
With love and profound gratitude

And to Gil Boyne
Thank you for transforming the world
Thank you for transforming my world

Contents

acknowledgments	xiii
preface to volume I	xv
1. Regression Hypnotherapy and Its Profound Potential	19
The Power of Regression	19
The Relevance of Regression to the Practice of Hypnotherapy	20
Transformation and the Mind-Body Connection	24
Churchill's Recipe for Outstanding Therapy	25
In Perspective	25
2.. Uses of Regression to Non-Traumatic Experiences	27
Self-Discovery	27
Finding Lost Valuables	28
Remembering Important Details	29
Exploring Wish Fulfillment Dreams	30
Keith's Life-Saving Dream	30
3. Uses of Regression to Traumatic Experiences	35
Checking for Subconscious Permission	35
Regression without Consciously Recalling Memories	37
Recall of Memories with Emotional Detachment	38
Working with Memories and Emotions	40
Summary of Major Steps in Emotional Clearing Regression	44
4. Accessing Gestalt Methods	47
Establishing Dialogue	48

Concept of Maturation	50
Gestalt Strategies in the Context of Hypnosis and Regression	51
Creating Ideal Parents	52
Mistakes to Avoid and Directions to Take with Gestalt	53

5. Utilizing Ideomotor Signals in Regression — 57
   Establishing Ideomotor Responses — 58
   Examples of Eliciting Responses — 59

6. Direct vs Indirect Suggestion — 63
   Understanding the Broad Context of Suggestion — 63
   The Myth of the Inherent Superiority of Indirect Suggestion — 64
   Toward an Accurate Representation of Erickson and the Field of Hypnotherapy — 67

7. Mary's Fear of Public Speaking
   Humiliated in Grade School — 73

8. Sophie's Grief
   Saying Goodbye to Grandma — 95

9. Ericka's Difficulty with Boundaries
   The Little Girl Who Had to be Grown-Up — 107

10. Kenn's Terror of Further Neck Surgery
   The Former Gambler Stooped with Shame — 127

11. Questions and Answers — 153

12. Beneath Janine's Sabotage of Her Success
   The Real Issue Explored — 161

13. Jacquie's Attraction of Unhealthy Relationships
   Nary a Sensitive, Successful Man to be Found — 193

14. Recovered Memories
   Reclaiming Logic on Both Sides of the Controversy — 225
      The Recovery of Memories — 225
      The Controversy — 226
      The Power of Suggestion — 230
      Some Therapists in Denial — 232

Toward a Balanced Perspective ... 235
Effective Procedures for Recovering, Revivifying and Enhancing Accurate Memories ... 236
The Purpose of Therapy ... 240

15. Christine's Overwhelming Responsibilities
The Breech Birth: "I Can't Do It" ... 241

16. Ron's Mysterious Heartache
Discovering the Source of His Sadness ... 263

17. Pat's Struggles from Abuse
The Baby Who Didn't Dare Cry ... 281
Follow-up Session ... 303

18. Lynette's Lack of Confidence
The Teenager Who Couldn't Stand Up For Herself ... 319

19. Craig's Lingering Resentment
The Absent Father ... 337
Follow-Up Session ... 353

20. Gerrie's Fear of Abandonment
A Year in a Drawer ... 375

21. Hypnotic Dreamwork as Regression
The Integration of Gestalt Dreamwork and Hypnotherapy ... 395
The Gestalt Perspective on Dreamwork ... 396
Accessing the Subconscious with Gestalt Dreamwork Methods ... 398
Combining Additional Hypnotic Processes with Gestalt Dreamwork ... 400
Common Steps in Hypnotic Dreamwork ... 402

22. Marilyn's Dream
The Crumbling Mountain ... 405

references ... 422

annotated bibliography ... 424

Acknowledgments

My gratitude goes to the many people whose support has led to the publication of this book; what I give here is not a complete list. First, I wish to express my appreciation for Gestalt therapy founder Frederick Perls' profound contribution to the healing arts.

I am most grateful for the visionary initial trainings and generous encouragement I received from Gil Boyne in the late sixties. I also appreciate his frequent exceptional support and insights since, and the great leadership and priceless contributions he has given to the profession of hypnotherapy.

I deeply appreciate Marleen Mulder's many years of inspired work as Co-Director of the Hypnotherapy Training Institute. The quality of the HTI sessions, including those transcribed in these two volumes, is partly a result of the tremendous dedication of her exceptional teaching and many other responsibilities, and her brilliant, heartfelt hypnotherapy demonstrations and sessions.

I am grateful for all of my students and clients. In particular, the volunteers for therapy in class who, in baring their souls, have given so much to the classes through their trust and courage.

I wish to thank Pat Stone for her many skills and great dedication to the Hypnotherapy Training Institute over nearly a quarter century. My gratitude also goes to Jan Shade for her valuable book production support, Leslie Curchack for proof-reading some of the chapters, Nadise Whiteside for her excellent cover design, and David Cavagnaro for his marvelous untouched butterfly slides and inspiring prolific work for the Earth. I am grateful and honored for each of the endorsements.

Many thanks to Kenneth Kelzer for his very generous time and important insights regarding Gestalt therapy. I thank the many graduates who have sent me articles, emails or videotapes over the years regarding recovered memories, especially the inspiring dedication of Dennis Alsop's numerous valuable contributions over many years, including his most generous help during the final production of this book.

I cannot give enough appreciation for the enormous amount of excellent work done on all phases of this book by my editor, Cheryl Canfield. From her initial transcriptions to her organizational work, editing, book production, cover ideas, proof-reading and fine-tuning of the final product, her beneficial influence is found from cover to cover. In particular, I am extremely fortunate to have a good friend who is an irreplaceable editor, with such an exceptional combination of extraordinary skills of hypnotherapist, writer and editor.

Preface to Volume 1

Both volumes of the *Transcripts of Transformation* set are designed as regression teaching texts for beginning and experienced practitioners of hypnotherapy. Some of the techniques used in these books often bring forth strong emotions, as is demonstrated in many of the sessions of this volume. The forthcoming second volume, *Catharsis in Regression Hypnotherapy*, continues where this one leaves off, including guidance and in-depth explorations of sessions that include various forms of cathartic abreaction.

There has been a strong need for more comprehensive literature in the extremely important field of regression therapy. Guidance and details regarding therapeutic options is severely limited in most books. Almost all books on the topic provide little or no information on certain powerful forms of the work, with few even touching on the profoundly significant integration of Gestalt and hypnotherapy, which was first published in Gil Boyne's groundbreaking *Transforming Therapy*. Another of many limitations in this area is the practice of automatically steering clients to either avoid feelings during regression, which often excludes profoundly effective options, or to always confront memories and related feelings, which is not always a wise and safe choice. And many books do not give crucial information to help achieve accurate memory retrieval, or worse, encourage ideas, techniques and expectancies which can lead to inaccurate recall.

This current volume fills significant gaps and adds details that are missing from other books, making this first volume alone, I believe, the most comprehensive text published to date about how to use regression for powerful therapy. It is important to note that certain modalities in this book will necessitate working, at times, with the exceptionally strong expression of emotions from clients, so for practitioners doing this work, Volume II will provide essential additional guidance.

These are not beginners' texts for the subject of hypnosis. The professional without previous hypnosis education is urged to get qualified eclectic training from a state-licensed hypnotherapy school before using the regression interventions in these books as an adjunctive therapeutic modality. It is not recommended for professionals or nonprofessionals to attempt hypnotic regression work to a traumatic experience alone in self-hypnosis. It is important to have the support of a well-trained and skilled professional under such circumstances.

Two of the sessions transcribed in the second volume were done in private work, while all of the other sessions in this series are of actual demonstrations during my Hypnotherapy Training classes. The transcriptions are from videotape (in most cases) or audiotape. Selected questions and answers from the transcripts in class have been retained as one of the forms of commentary.

It would seem a reasonable assumption that many clients would be more forthcoming about intimate issues during private sessions, as opposed to being taped and in a group. However, the transcripts of this series show a tremendous openness during these class demonstrations. This is partly because of the bonding that occurs in the 200-300 class hour trainings at the Hypnotherapy Training Institute, where we strive to maintain a very supportive atmosphere. In fact, there can be potential advantages to the client inherent in such demonstrational therapy in contrast to private session work, including in some cases an added intensity and focus. Also significant is possible feedback from class members at the conclusion of some sessions, as well as the intrinsic value of a supportive group presence for which the client and I can be most grateful.

That said, I've found a consistency in the profound effectiveness of comprehensive regression strategies, like those in this series, in private and in other groups as well. My private clients for decades have gotten very powerful results from a single session or two of regression work (which is usually done in the context of a brief series of sessions), and so have volunteers for demonstrations I have given at other schools and at International Hypnotherapy Conferences. In fact, a few of the sessions in these volumes were at such conferences.

There are many therapists interested in the subject of past life regression, in fact many who specialize in this area. I've noticed a particularly strong interest from those coming for training from various cultures around the world, as well as with many individuals from our Western culture. Even from the viewpoint that this form of regression is, at most, merely symbolic or metaphorical, work in the realm of alleged past lives can be very effective, when selectively proceeding with the comprehensive regression strategies outlined in this series. This would be within the context of a client who is receptive to the subject and an operator who is not religiously or philosophically opposed to it.

While the subject matter of this volume is ostensibly about age regression, this entire two volume set (with the possible exception of the Hypnotic Dreamwork™ material at the end of the book) is relevant to past life regression therapy. And there is much important material herein that has not been included in any books on this subject. In addition, this form of regression will be specifically explored, including with full transcripts, in a section of Volume II.

CHAPTER 1

Regression Hypnotherapy and Its Profound Potential

Hypnosis is a bridge to the subconscious mind. The subconscious is the seat of the emotions, imagination, memories, habits and intuition. It also regulates our autonomic body functions, is the part of the mind that dreams, and is the pathway to the superconscious. It is the very essence and core of how we experience ourselves and the world. To attain powerful and lasting results in therapy, it is essential that the methods employed reach and affect the subconscious mind. The best results in therapy always come from a hypnotic state, whether or not the state was achieved intentionally, and whether or not the therapist uses or understands hypnotic theory and semantics.

The Power of Regression

A hypnotic regression is a process in which a person in hypnosis recalls a memory or series of memories from the subconscious mind. While in hypnosis a person's awareness is heightened and memories can become much more vivid. Also, there is easier access to the emotions, barring suggestions for detachment. And because of the heightened suggestibility that occurs as the subconscious mind is accessed, insights can have a much greater impact than they would normally have.

Major events from childhood and infancy, both positive and negative in nature, can have a tremendous impact, and expectancies that result from these experiences continue to affect us in our lives. Events in extreme cases can serve as an imprint, a powerful single-impact learning experience that greatly influences our ways of experiencing ourselves and the world. Much hypnotherapy is about de-hypnotizing ourselves from the limiting influences of significant negative experiences from the past. In many cases, a potent aspect of effective hypnotherapy can be regression to facilitate more thorough and lasting results.

An irony of regression work is that what makes a past event important is the way we frame it and manifest it in the here and now. We carry traumas from the past with us into the present and filter our experience of ourselves and the world through the lenses of those past experiences. The form of regression hypnotherapy emphasized in these volumes, including returning to an initiating sensitizing event(s) and working with Gestalt, hypnoanalysis and reeducation, sometimes has the effect of an imprint. The work can be so powerful that major changes from a session or two of regression are typically immediate and yield long-term transformation.

Regression strategies, as described and demonstrated in this series, are options highly recommended for appropriate use by hypnotherapists and by clinicians using hypnosis as an adjunct to their therapeutic specialties. The great value documented in the sessions of this *Transcripts of Transformation* series is not because they were exceptional in my work, as a kind of "greatest hits" collection. The majority of sessions that I have taped over the years, in the demonstration of exploratory hypnosis using regression and ideomotor methods, have been transcribed for insertion into a book. In the late 1990's, for example, a string of 16 consecutive taped sessions are all being included in full in texts. That's remarkable, considering there are many very effective taped sessions over the years that were not selected because the theme, presenting issue, or some elements of the therapy were too similar to another session already transcribed for inclusion.

The Relevance of Regression to the Practice of Hypnotherapy

Within the field of hypnotherapy there are many potential benefits in harnessing the power of the subconscious mind to affect change. Hypnosis is used in a wide variety of ways for chronic and acute pain relief; it can be effective to improve confidence, communication, relationships, motivation, achievement, concentration, recall, health and stress management; it can help overcome addictions, habits, eating disorders, insomnia, fears, phobias, procrastination, and negative thought, emotional and behavior patterns; it can help utilize one's full potential in endeavors such as work, sports, writing, performance, art, public speaking and creative expression.

The potential use of regression within a series of hypnotherapy sessions for these and other issues will be individually evaluated. Considerations include many factors about the presenting issues that begin to get explored in the initial intake interview, the kind and severity of difficulties that the individual is working on, underlying reasons, associations and history regarding these difficulties, the stage of the therapy, and the purpose and kind of regression techniques being considered.

As described in the next two chapters, there are many forms of regression. In fact, a hypnotic regression can be as simple as encouraging your client to focus for a moment on a positive memory that's relevant to the presenting issue. For example, almost anyone working on confidence can recall a context in which he or she felt confident about something. Such a basic use of regression could be done at some appropriate point in almost any hypnotherapy session. What is more pertinent to the transformative emphasis of these two volumes is the context of making a decision to reserve a session or more to do deeper regression work to help overcome major effects of trauma.

As enthusiastic as I am about the therapeutic regression options to help with substantial unresolved issues, a regression is selectively relevant on a case by case basis. Comprehensive regression strategies will be of great benefit in many cases in a wide variety of issues for which people seek therapy.

In my private practice an initial session has typically been a 50 or 55 minute interview that does not include a formal hypnotic induction (although I will endeavor in many ways to work with subconscious rapport and expectancy factors). During that session I have the opportunity to gather significant details about the presenting issue(s). This will include any known underlying factors regarding behaviors and symptoms, the possibility of secondary gains, causes of current problems as well as relevant traumas at the time of initiation or the development of similar significant ongoing or recurring problems, historical attempts to overcome the difficulties and the positive and negative results and side effects of those attempts, relevant personal and professional lifestyle issues, medications, stress factors, etc.

A regression is often called for if the initiation of some experience is still tied in directly with one's current experience in a major way. A severe problem that has been difficult to overcome over years, in many cases will be pointing to doing regression work. An unexplainable compulsion, reaction, emotion or behavior would be a signal to reserve a session for exploratory ideomotor questioning which would typically lead to regression in that session or a subsequent one. There are many obvious developments in the above-described initial session that could encourage at least one planned comprehensive regression. Sometimes it's a judgment call, and a decision one way or the other could be a close call, to be determined as the sessions progress. Initially there may not seem to be a need for regression but something unexpected could occur in the course of the therapy, signaling otherwise. For example, someone may reach a new stage of success and have a strong adverse reaction signaling surprising subconscious resistance, which can encourage an exploratory ideomotor and/or regression intervention.

When doing major regression work in private practice, I have found that commonly a single session or two, out of a brief series of perhaps five to ten sessions, is needed to work on a particular issue. However, in at least one prior session (typically the initial session) there will be significant preparation for the regression, and there is usually at least one subsequent session involving hypnotic work that is strongly associated with the results of the regression, even if it's not a regression per se. It's difficult to generalize because there are any number of possible presenting issues and each individual, situation, and experience in regression is different.

To give a specific example, some significant regression strategies will often be included in helping overcome most kinds of addictions. But in my experience, about 85 percent of the time regression does not need to be included for smoking cessation. This is partly because the reasons why most people start smoking don't have much to do with why they are still smoking. Most commonly, people started smoking in teenage years to be adult, to be part of the group, to feel sophisticated or cool, those kinds of things. Years later they're smoking because they're addicted and they have the habit pattern, the psychological need and oral fixation that most of them didn't initially have, or that was not significant at the time. However, there are circumstances when regression is appropriate for smoking cessation. For example, sometimes there is trauma around the initiation of smoking that is still having an effect, such as the example described early in Chapter 3, which in that exceptional case led to an unusual form of regression set up to avoid conscious recall. Another example is discussed in Chapter 17 when the client, preparing to quit smoking, develops an overwhelming fear that is a signal that these deeper emotions need to be faced and cleared.

When addictions are of substances that create altered states, as is true for most substance addiction, this adds a complexity that is not usually relevant to those who seek smoking cessation. Including regression is more often of major value in cases that developed from being drawn to or escaping from certain feelings via an altered state, and/or there is a continuing struggle with breaking the addiction partly for difficulties regarding such feelings. Some substance abuse problems are serious enough that I will only work with the individual at the conclusion of completing a detox program, and our work would very likely include regression. On the other hand, a regression may be irrelevant for someone who wants to break the habit of needing a glass of wine late each evening to help fall asleep.

In the case of working with a client on something as simple as increasing reading speed while maintaining comprehension, such an issue would normally entail a brief series of sessions, perhaps weekly, working with direct and indirect suggestions, metaphors, etc. Such a scenario would not usually call for major regression work. However, every situation is unique. In an exceptional case, even this simple sole presenting issue could have a complication relating to a lack of confidence or a significant trauma associated with studying or concentrating, that might necessitate something along the lines of an in-depth regression.

A somewhat similar presenting issue of desired increased concentration and recall for studies typically will not need significant exploratory work beyond questioning during the first session, unless exceptional resistance develops as the sessions progress. But besides the sample of possible complications of the above paragraph, proper initial questioning will sometimes yield additional factors that may signal the appropriateness of digging deeper. The concentration-recall could be tied in with preparation for exams, for example, and this in some cases will be associated with a phobic reaction. To give another example, I had a client who had always had great resistance to studying because his father had often bragged that he had done well in college without ever studying, and insisted studying wasn't needed. My client had managed to get through school until now avoiding studying, but even with his deteriorating grades in Chiropractic School he had not been able to overcome his aversion. We included a regression in one of the first sessions, and his resistance cleared right up.

Transformation and the Mind-Body Connection

Many scientific studies have surfaced documenting the mind/body connection - that is, the thoughts we think do significantly affect our bodies and the environment around us. A recent study that has come to my attention is the work of Japanese researcher, Masaru Emotos. Using water as his medium, Emotos used special photographic equipment to show the power of thought to effect the molecular structure of water (the element that we ourselves are overwhelmingly comprised of).

Emotos first discovered that the crystalline structure of water is different under various conditions and in different parts of the world. Pure, pristine water from natural resources formed beautiful, geometric designs, while polluted water from industrial wastes and populated areas formed distorted and random crystalline structures. His experiments with music and thoughts also changed the form of water. Praying over polluted water, for example, altered the molecular structure to form more organized geometric designs.

Hypnotherapist Hal Isen, co-author of *The Genesis Principle* and originator of transformational Core Wisdom® workshops, writes of Emotos' research: "Perhaps the tradition that exists in so many cultures of saying a prayer or grace before meals is not mere ritual, but actually alters the energy of the food itself.... The remarkable photos validate that what we think, feel, and most of all, who we are being, shapes our reality all the time."

The evidence overwhelmingly conveys that our thoughts affect everything in and around us, as practitioners of hypnotherapy and other modalities that tap into the vast power of our subconscious minds have long been witness to. We can positively tap into our profound potential to heal and transform ourselves and our planet by directing our thoughts and moving them into action. The techniques and examples in these volumes present tools that allow us to work deeply with the memories, emotions and expectations of the subconscious mind, and reeducate and integrate the power of suggestion to transform trauma into lasting positive change.

From many years of practice and teaching, I've outlined the following combination of factors as likely to yield great success, usually within a relatively brief time span.

Churchill's Recipe for Outstanding Therapy

1. *Client*: motivated. Good work can always be done no matter how challenging the issues, when the client is highly motivated, in the circumstances outlined here.

2. *Therapist*: compassionate and centered. The Buddhist concept of detached compassion fits well here. The therapist cares and does his/her best possible work, but does not try to do the client's work. The therapist does not get caught up in the drama, but is totally present and supportive - flexible, intuitive and creative, rather than rigidly adhering to a system of techniques.

3. *Together*: good rapport, enthusiasm, and positive yet realistic mental expectancy. Therapy includes working comprehensively with the whole person, including underlying issues.

4. *Therapist training/experience*: a solid foundation that includes a wide variety of methods to reach and affect the subconscious (i.e., hypnosis).

In Perspective

In spite of my enthusiasm for certain regression modalities, I must emphasize that learning a comprehensive set of techniques is just one aspect of becoming a good therapist. "The most important thing you bring to your client is yourself," states Sidney Jourard. "Your methodology is additional." We bring to our work our education, professional and life experience, creativity, intuition, dedication, compassion, inspiration and love. With each session of each client we can be receptive to learning, being present in the moment and continuing to fine tune our skills. Also, subconscious personality and rapport factors can strongly influence the speed, ease, and thoroughness of therapy.

Jack Schwartz said, "There are at least 21 paths to the top of the mountain. If somebody tells you he's on *the* path, he's not even on the mountain." There are so many ways to heal. Each person must discover and rediscover what works for her or him. The awareness, wisdom, creativity, and power of our subconscious minds is astounding. We may not fully understand how people can be deeply healed by various forms of prayer, faith healing, touch, spirituality, work, devotion to family, shamanistic rituals, or positive mental expectancy. But with the right people, under the right circumstances, any of this and much more can produce extraordinary results. Also, recognition of the power of the placebo, as described in Chapter 14, is relevant to understanding the potential for dramatic physical and mental shifts resulting from mental expectancy.

The potential we hold for change is awe inspiring. A new client once described to me how he had been scheduled for triple bypass heart surgery but then just before the surgery he suddenly felt better. He went to his doctor and the doctor was shocked to discover that his patient had grown an entire new artery. His heart was now in good condition. Visualizations can work wonders, but he had not as yet consciously tried to visualize anything, and certainly did not expect or consciously imagine that such a thing could occur. He came to see me because he wanted to shape up, improve his eating habits, and take responsibility for himself. He felt that God had given him a new heart and a whole new lease on life. This is a sample of the profound potential of the subconscious mind, which in the forms of regression demonstrated in these two volumes is consistently harnessed with even greater power than the dramatically increased access normally associated with hypnosis.

CHAPTER 2

Uses of Regression to Non-Traumatic Experiences

This book is primarily about the powerful affect regression can have in overcoming the continuing effects of unresolved traumatic experiences. While some therapists associate regression exclusively with past trauma, it is important to keep in perspective that there are many valuable uses of regression to experiences that are not associated with major difficulties. The following are examples of the many opportunities available for such regressions.

Self-Discovery

Even simple forms of regression to positive memories can potentially be very effective. Much can be accomplished by having a person relive and integrate past pleasant experiences. Such explorations can help individuals to re–own aspects of themselves or to deepen the value of an experience. Regression to positive memories can even lead to peak experiences. But to give a less dramatic example, during a group hypnosis I experienced at age 17 we were instructed to go back to a happy childhood experience, and what I recalled was playing. As a result of this I realized how much I longed for more physical activity and I became much more active, including through P.E. classes in college over the next few years.

A person can even do a regression to remember details of a memory just to satisfy a curiosity. For example, there are some individuals who had a generally positive childhood but recall few or no memories from their early years. Such a person might be curious to go back and recall details of positive or neutral memories from very early years. Because the subconscious is the seat of our memories, we can frequently help people to recall very early memories, and that in itself can be quite a joy. If someone with few early memories seems to be a candidate for this exploration, it is important to use ideomotor methods to check with the subconscious to confirm that it is good to do that (e.g., that the lack of memory is not because of protective blocking of unknown traumas from that period).

When I have worked with clients in my private practice who had some kind of ongoing difficulty as a result of childhood trauma, I would often feel called to move right into regression in our initial hypnosis work. If such a client has not experienced prior hypnotherapy I may not want the first hypnotic experience to be regression to a terrible experience. In such a case I might use the first hypnosis to have the person go exclusively to positive childhood experiences, to re-own and gain value from them. An example of one way to do that is to have the person tap into some positive emotion and use an affect bridge to bring the person back to explore one or more positive early experiences when that emotion was felt. The affect bridge will be discussed in the next chapter, and will be demonstrated in many of the transcripts of this book.

Finding Lost Valuables

Another function of regression is to find a lost item of value. This can be quite useful for someone who has lost a wedding ring or other jewelry, a valuable book or article of clothing, important papers, or a container of family heirlooms, etc. I've helped people living in rural areas who buried gold or other valuables on their land and then couldn't remember where they were hidden.

Ideomotor finger signals are so valuable in this kind of work. Nothing, including finger signals, can be certain to be completely accurate, but proper questioning techniques have a tendency to get effective results. Even when the recall is detailed and accurate, a lost item may have been moved or stolen subsequent to the client's last experience of having or seeing it. But when that hasn't occurred, memories of details can frequently lead to the recovery of lost objects.

The essence of this work may appear to be the use of hypnosis without therapy, although I normally take the opportunity to integrate positive suggestions late in the session. Also, at times there may be a hidden agenda that isn't initially apparent to the client. Questioning during the intake interview, and ideomotor questioning early in the hypnosis, can determine whether there is a subconscious ulterior motive or secondary gain for losing the item. One of my clients was trying to find the retainer (removable braces) for her teeth. Ideomotor questioning revealed that she had subconsciously lost the retainer because of her great difficulty in getting her former boyfriend to move out. Her subconscious had come up with this as a means of attempting to appear less attractive.

Helping people find lost objects is also a useful way for a new hypnotherapist to develop skills for being neutral in preparation for working with clients involving the possibility of recovered traumatic memories. My forthcoming book, *Ideomotor Magic*, will explore finding lost valuables in greater detail, including a transcript of a sample session.

Remembering Important Details

A similar use for non-trauma regression to finding a lost object would be to recall details of a lost memory of some kind. It might be a name, address or phone number, a combination lock, directions to a particular location, or some other information that is needed. When some important information is lost or not currently available, hypnotic modalities may be able to retrieve it.

Forensic hypnosis also fits into this category in cases in which a witness to a crime, someone who was not traumatized by it, is trying to remember details such as a description of the suspect or the letters and numbers on a license plate. Regressions can bring much greater details of important memories.

Since the focus of this chapter is regression to neutral or positive experiences, additional methods that will be described in the next chapter (such as protective ideomotor methods, detachment techniques and emotional clearing skills) are not applicable here. Therefore, in many cases the structure of sessions to non-traumatic memories may be simpler in the sense of often involving fewer steps and having the likelihood of fewer possible directions of developments. (However, recall of lost objects or memories in some cases can become a very long questioning process, even though the overall structure of the work may be simpler.) Much of the work in recovering lost valuables or memories does not necessitate therapy per se, although some relevant positive post-hypnotic suggestions by the conclusion of almost any session is a good addition.

Exploring Wish Fulfillment Dreams

Hypnotic recall of dreams can be considered regression, since the dream is a form of reality to the existential subconscious mind as it occurs. Hence, Hypnotic Dreamwork™ with wish fulfillment dreams is another valuable form of regression to positive experiences. Hypnotic Dreamwork is covered in the final two chapters of this book and presented in detail (including the transcripts and commentary of dreams and a hypno-dream that are of the wish-fulfillment variety) in my book, *Become the Dream: The Transforming Power of Hypnotic Dreamwork.*

To illustrate the use of regression to non-traumatic experiences, the following summary of a dream session is given as an example of a decision to explore an exceptional positive experience with regression. Every session is unique, and this one develops with some unusual results. It happens to involve an apparent dream, but the purpose (rediscovery of the memory) and resultant direction of the brief regression is different from the form of therapy called Hypnotic Dreamwork.

Keith's Life-Saving Dream

Keith, a Christian minister, came to take the hypnotherapy training from Japan, where he had spent the past five years working in the ministry. He wanted to use regression to explore in greater depth one of two exceptional childhood experiences that still intrigued him. One was an experience in which some unexplainable phenomena had protected him and his family from a potentially fatal collision. In that experience, he had been in a car with his parents as a young boy and they were driving along on a highway when he was suddenly struck by a feeling like a pin digging into his side. He was is such distress that his parents pulled over to the side of the road to see what was the matter. Nothing could be found but immediately after they pulled over a catastrophic accident occurred on the highway just ahead in which many people were killed. His brief mysterious affliction (or premonition) got them off of the road and they were saved.

The other experience had occurred around the time of his third birthday. He had strept throat and was in bed sleeping. When he woke up he went to his mother and told her he had had a dream in which he had been picking flowers in a field with someone named Jesus. He hadn't remembered the dream as he grew up, but his mother recalled it and told him about it fifteen years later.

They were a non-Christian family and it scared her that her sick little boy would have such a dream. She took him to the doctor, who immediately saw a hemorrhage in Keith's eye and had him hospitalized. Keith remembered his parents telling him that he had terrible nosebleeds and almost died in the hospital with a heart infection. His mother's fear of the dream had gotten him to the hospital where he was put on strong antibiotics that saved his life.

Keith was interested in regressing to either or both of the exceptional life saving experiences and I chose the dream because it had such a dramatic impact on his life - it was learning about the "dream" he had at three years old that influenced him to become a minister, as well as having saved his life.

Before the induction I asked Keith to describe a pleasant scene, which might be put to use as part of the deepening process. Keith told about a vacation he had taken in Viet Nam in which he had been driving down into a valley through the fog. As he came into a clearing it was so incredibly beautiful that it was like a peak experience. The scene was very spiritual in essence and I felt that because Keith was going into a regression to a spiritual experience, he could use this scene as part of a pathway. Also, during the pre-induction interview Keith had stated that he was concerned about not being able to go deep in hypnosis. I felt the regression to the Viet Nam scene would be an exceptional multi-purpose deepening process at the conclusion of the induction. The more he not only recalled but re-experienced the peak experience, the deeper he would go.

When we moved to ideomotor questions I asked Keith's subconscious mind if it was safe and appropriate to recall the experience he had had before the age of three. Keith signaled "no" to that question. Then before I even finished the next question, in which I was asking for instructions from Keith's subconscious mind as to what would be a good direction to go in, Keith's "yes" finger signaled. I checked it out and discovered that Keith's subconscious, for whatever reason, had now accepted that it was safe and appropriate to go ahead and recall the early incident. He had apparently made some kind of a shift to get himself ready to do that, and it seemed to be helped by my communication as I was leading up to the question. Some statement, perhaps the encouragement that he could go wherever he wanted to go, had made it appropriate for him to move ahead.

I asked the question, "Is this an experience that you had in a dream?" because even though the three year old described it as a dream, the language of a three year old is inadequate to assess what it was that he had experienced. Keith's signal was, "I don't know." I took him back in regression and there were several excellent signs of hypnotic depth, including the rolling back of his eyes and a great slackening of his jaw. As he regressed back Keith began crying and gasping, and his body began shaking. I periodically gave him key suggestions such as, "Whatever you're experiencing, you don't have to explain it, just stay with it and feel it." Later I asked if there was anything he would like to say and Keith stated that he was recalling seeing Jesus as a glowing child about his own age. He was surprised because he had expected to see Jesus as a man, not as a child like himself. He said that he wanted to touch him but he couldn't. As a child of three, Keith tried to explain what he saw but it was very difficult. Was it a dream or a vision or what?

Toward the end of the session I gave suggestions for the value of continuing to integrate this experience into his life and to have a greater awareness than he had before. When Keith was brought out of the hypnosis he sat up and sobbed. Then he described that he had experienced such a bolt of energy when the memory came back that it was a shock to his body. He was still feeling the energy and it was too much for him even yet. I did a brief re-induction and gave suggestions to encourage the dissipation of the feeling of that energy and then brought him out of the hypnosis again.

In describing his experience later Keith said that he had wanted to look for Christ and expected to find himself in a field picking flowers with a man named Jesus, as he imagined in the dream his mother had described. Instead, the image he came to was of himself as a child with another glowing child. He was looking at it from the perspective of a third person and was so taken by the glowing child that he didn't necessarily notice what he, as the little boy, was doing.

"I was watching and when that child came close to the other child, I felt it through my body. But those two children never changed reaction. They never changed facial expression. This body felt a bolt like electricity and it was hard to accept at times. I was partially conscious because I thought to myself, 'Quit or do something!' but part of me wanted to see what was going to happen at the end. The main thing was that touch and when that happened I got a jolt! Even as the child I thought, 'This is a spiritual being.' At the conscious level I was just a little afraid...I'm sure someday I'll know what it is but right now I have no idea exactly what happened or how it happened."

Keith also said he wasn't certain this experience was definitely a recall of the dream or vision he had as a child. There is no way to actually know for certain, even with ideomotor methods. Chapter thirteen gives insight and information on the important topic of recovered memories.

Keith sent an enthusiastic email three months after his session. He discussed his meditations on the session, which had caused him to wonder if he was spared for a specific reason. "I've now come to the conclusion that my special purpose is actually no different than anyone else. I'm here to do my best and help whenever possible. I must thank you for your training, as I'm sure it is one of the ways I will be able to help others."

CHAPTER 3

Uses of Regression to Traumatic Experiences

Regression is often a vital component of hypnotherapy when there is an ongoing or recurring difficulty that is partly a result of past experiences. As we have seen in the previous chapter, the potential uses of regression are not limited to trauma issues, but the proper use of regression for overcoming the lingering or returning effects of trauma can frequently lead to powerful, lasting results. This is the use of regression that will be demonstrated in the examples of individual sessions transcribed in these two volumes. In this extremely important area we have many valuable tools at our disposal.

The range of potential directions given for regression in this chapter are for practitioners who have received a thorough hypnotherapy education. Hypnotherapy for those with major psychological disturbances, such as schizophrenia, psychosis or severe personality disorders should be limited to hypnotherapists who are licensed psychotherapists, and in select cases only, by referral and supervision from such psychotherapists. In addition, working with the emotions in regression is not recommended under any circumstances for those with severe psychological disorders. The chapter in Volume II, *Grounding and Centering for the Therapist*, will be of further assistance in working with the emotional clearing strategies described in the final section of this chapter.

Checking for Subconscious Permission

When I'm working with an individual who has experienced significant difficulty in the past that is still causing him or her to not be fully actualized in the present, regression is usually one of the directions to explore within a series of hypnotherapy sessions. After the hypnotic induction I will normally check with the subconscious mind through the use of ideomotor methods to get guidance and permission before proceeding. Not everyone is ready to be open to their emotions, and in some cases individuals aren't even ready to be open to recalling or revivifying key memories. This checking in can be very important. The subconscious mind, the seat of memories and emotions, knows what is buried and what the individual is ready to recall on a conscious level, and can intuit whether to be open to associated emotions.

The first ideomotor question I ask has to do with consciously recalling the significant experiences that were causal or reinforcing events regarding the issue we're working with. For example, the question may be framed, "Is it safe and appropriate for you to remember any and all experiences you have had that have to do with your fear of failure?" If the signal is affirmative, commonly a single additional question can be asked, such as, "Is it safe and appropriate for you to be open to your emotions during the recall of these experiences?" However, the particulars of an individual's issues may yield additional questions, even when the above answers are affirmative. For example, during regression to a trauma involving severe physical pain, someone may not need to re-experience the physical sensations, but may be receptive to recalling emotions to some degree.

A person may have memories or information on the subconscious level that is not necessarily remembered as yet consciously. That is particularly common if he or she doesn't fully understand a fear or reaction to certain situations. Even when the client begins with a seemingly good understanding of the apparent event or events that are unresolved, there may be further significant unconscious memories or related issues.

When asking these questions it is very important for the hypnotherapist to be completely neutral. The practitioner must communicate clearly the unequivocal intention of finding out the true choice of the subconscious mind. Because of the heightened suggestibility and desire to please that tends to occur in hypnosis, it is very easy to pick up and be influenced by subtle hints of an expectancy, preference, or seeming preference, of the therapist.

Regression without Consciously Recalling Memories

In my experience, the vast majority of people will signal that it is safe and appropriate to be consciously open to their memories. When a client signals that an experience is still so traumatic that he or she is not ready to receive this information, then I'm going to assume that emotional receptivity to the trauma is not an option. But even when a negative response to the initial question leads the practitioner to carefully avoid bringing up memories and emotions, good work can still be accomplished.

I'll give an example of a particular session with a man in his early fifties who came to see me over 20 years ago for smoking cessation. He was a heavy smoker who had never been able to quit smoking for a full day in spite of his many attempts. I remember the details because the associated issues and therapeutic direction were exceptional.

Early in my initial interview of the first session I found out that he was thirteen years old when he began smoking. When I asked the man what the circumstances were when he started smoking, he said, "I was in a concentration camp." Obviously there were horrible difficulties during that time so I told him I would need to check with his subconscious mind to find out whether residual effects associated with the initiation or early development of his smoking were preventing him from quitting. He responded, "I really don't want to deal with that." I said, "I certainly understand. We can work with you in such a way that you don't have to remember any experiences but we can still clear away any remaining issues, if there are any, that are keeping you from achieving your goal of smoking cessation."

After the hypnotic induction and setting up of ideomotor signals, I used different phrasing than usual to keep rapport while exploring our options. "As we proceed, would it be good for you to avoid consciously recalling memories related to the initiation or early development of your smoking?" He signaled that recall was inappropriate, as he had already verbally indicated. I used a variety of detachment techniques, along with suggestions and instructions that only his subconscious mind would be engaged in gathering the data that was relevant to any decisions he may have made at that time that were still affecting him in regard to smoking. I narrowed it down to smoking because that was the issue he had come to work on. It was especially important to keep that focus, to respect his wishes to avoid those experiences.

I did a series of questioning methods with him that included having his subconscious mind recall the first several times he smoked. Questioning included, "Were there any decisions that were made then that are still affecting you now?" After using ideomotor methods to help him retrieve and communicate selected information while emotionally detached and protecting the conscious mind from memories, we eventually reached a point where I could have him verbalize. The message from his subconscious was that he had made an association that he needed cigarettes for his survival. That was a misconception I could work with to help his subconscious mind fully understand that he did not need to continue to have that idea. He could recognize that it was a misconception, he could certainly forgive himself for having developed that misconception, and he could let go of it and quit smoking. His smoking cessation was successful and he quit smoking with no weight gain or other negative side effects.

Recall of Memories with Emotional Detachment

Another possible set of ideomotor responses to the question of exploring memories and emotions is a signal that it's fine to remember an experience consciously, but it's not okay to be open to emotions. There are various ways to help detach. Prior to initiating regression in such a case, I will give suggestions of protection, such as being surrounded by radiant, protective healing light.

An example of creating detachment (dissociation) is to create a whole scenario of the client going downstairs in an old theater to look through rows of old-fashion reel-to-reel films for a specific one, or more than one, that relates to whatever issue it is that is being worked on. Such imagery can help add to the impression of going back in time. The person imagines bringing it back up to the projectionist who adjusts the film and gets ready to show it in the theater. I suggest being alone except for the projectionist in the theater, and may give further dissociation by having her imagine being the projectionist watching herself observe the movie. Two of the transcripts of this book use similar theater imagery. (Various grounding and centering techniques that can help with detachment will be explored in detail in Volume II, *Catharsis in Regression Hypnotherapy*.)

Here is an example of the work that can be done while the client is detached. Suggestions can be given to return to the initial sensitizing event as "the hidden observer" to use Ernest Hilgard's term. The hidden observer is able to watch the experience from this detached position, almost as if being a spirit in the room quietly observing what's happening with someone else. You can instruct the conscious mind to study and report the scenario, then remove the client from this memory to discuss what misconceptions developed as a result of that experience. You can also encourage some self-hypnoanalysis to help increase recognition that certain decisions made were indeed misconceptions that can be eliminated. The hypnosis can be completed with post-hypnotic suggestions.

Often, just remembering something with greater detail with dissociation can be a therapeutic step in itself. It gives a separation from the experience, and the client may or may not need to go through emotional clearing at a later time. Every individual and every situation is different.

Additional work in clearing emotions may be indicated if emotional triggers from the past continue to be activated in the present. For example, someone is working on an issue of not being able to express himself, and signals not to be open to his emotions. He does good work in session, going through details of early childhood experiences in a detached way, of having to stifle his emotions as a child. He is able to see how he learned to shut off his feelings, especially during times of conflict between his parents. Suppose he reports in his next session that he has made some progress, but continues to find it difficult to communicate with his wife, especially during any kind of disagreement or argument. He still finds himself shutting off or shutting down and he wants to do further work in this area.

A regression is usually best done as part of a series of sessions that include some that emphasize post-hypnotic suggestions for integration. However, the scenario of this, shall we say, "hypnothetical" session indicates immediate further exploratory work. After a hypnotic induction the question regarding being open to emotions can be asked again, to indicate if his subconscious mind wants to give permission to be open to emotions at this time. It is common for the subconscious mind to be receptive this time around, especially with supportive suggestions, such as about only proceeding as far as his subconscious mind is comfortable going.

If he still signals to avoid being in touch with his emotions, detachment can be encouraged in explorations that might include ideomotor questions to uncover blocks or to gain further insights. The establishment of ideal parents and the development of dialogue with the inner child (or continuing encouragement if already done) can be given, along with the suggestion of ongoing visualizations in self-hypnosis between the inner child and the ideal parents.

Working with Memories and Emotions

Another form of direction can result from green light signals for full memory recall and emotional receptivity regarding regression for trauma. This gives us the greatest range in working with regression, allowing for the tremendous potential that emotional clearing work can have. Samples of synergistic options available to us are summarized below, and occur in myriad ways throughout the transcripts of this two volume set.

Prepare for the first regression session with a thorough interview, which may be a session in itself. The therapist wants to get much pertinent information, although not necessarily every detail or aspect of every single thing that the person can think of regarding the presenting issue. Get to the essence of the most important aspects of the presenting problem, including history and known related issues, and then get into the hypnotherapy.

Of course the therapist will take into account whether a client is just starting out with his first hypnosis or has had some experience. If the subject has had little or no experience in hypnotherapy, the therapist will want to discuss the field, particularly as it is relevant to the client. An interview regarding previous hypnotic experiences and an explanation of hypnosis when necessary, plus an overview of the work to be done and expected potential directions for upcoming sessions, may conclude a first fifty minute session. Then when I expect to do a regression in an upcoming session, I will schedule a time slot of up to two hours. In some cases, especially with a student or former client I have already spent considerable time with, the initial interview may move more quickly and leave room to go right into a hypnotic induction, perhaps even a regression, if enough time is reserved.

The initial interviews transcribed in this book tend to be brief because all but one of the case studies were students who had spent many hours in class with me, and had done much self-hypnosis and hetero-hypnosis practice in and out of class. Some of them also had substantial experience in therapy.

After initiating a hypnotic induction for a regression, I will ask questions as previously described to determine whether there is subconscious approval to bring up memories and emotions. If the ideomotor signals give permission, I will typically use the affect bridge to take the individual back to an initiating experience. In this context an affect bridge is begun by tapping the person into the feeling that is currently causing difficulty and then regressing the person to a major incident that brought up the feeling, perhaps to the initial sensitizing event in which the negative response first occurred. In some cases the client may regress to a series of secondary reinforcing events before we reach a key initiating event. In other cases there may not be one or two major initial events but rather an ongoing struggle, such as years of similar ongoing difficulties in childhood, of which a few major examples can be explored.

Working on the initial event, or perhaps a series of events, and doing the emotional clearing work around that is frequently effective in cutting the cord that has brought the associations of the event(s) into the essence of the client's deep-seated subconscious mental expectancy, world view and apparent character. Usually this work helps significantly to break up the pattern that has been established.

Even though there is subconscious permission for the client to be open emotionally, that doesn't mean there has to be some big catharsis. The degree of emotional expression that develops depends upon the situation. One client in hypnosis may be very quiet and another may abreact. An abreaction is a release of psychic tension through a highly emotionalized, expressive reliving of a repressed traumatic experience, processing through to a resolution. Some people feel emotions very strongly without much outward expression of them and others may be fairly detached throughout. There is no goal of a particular amount of emotional expression, but any significant emotions that are being suppressed need to be released or expressed. The affect bridge, Gestalt, and other potential avenues such as bioenergetics, frequently bring up strong emotions.

Once we get to significant memories the individual can be guided into a thorough Gestalt dialogue, including expression of feelings and communication that could not or did not occur at the time of the initial incident. I often move into that fairly quickly, after getting some details of a regression scene. The Gestalt dialogue between the different parts of a person and/or characters in conflict, moves the person toward a healing and integration of the splits within them. This also includes aspects of the inner child. Some therapists use transactional analysis to work with the adult, the child and the parent parts of the client, which has some similarities to Gestalt dialogue. Psychosynthesis and various forms of parts therapy are also examples of techniques that may work effectively with internal splits.

Gestalt frequently becomes one of my key methods when the subject signals receptivity to emotions in regression. The integration of regression and Gestalt methods is described in the next chapter and Chapter 21, as well as being demonstrated in most of the regression transcripts of both volumes.

As we move through to the integration and healing that frequently occurs in Gestalt, the therapist can then direct the client to discover misconceptions developed as a result of the initial trauma that have been continuing to affect the person up to the present. Typically I do this by progressing the person to the present to tap into the adult reasoning mind, while staying in touch with the part that has just worked through the healing to this point. Then I have the adult analyze the effects of the explored incidents and similar ones, and any resulting misconceptions. This phase of therapy may yield a dialogue between the part sharing the insight and the part being healed, in a process that includes reframing and sometimes reinterpretation of cognitive errors that became entrenched in the subconscious. Whether the explored memories were entirely previously remembered or not, they need to be integrated within a wise and accepting understanding that releases unnecessary and inappropriate blame, especially self-blame.

Sometimes, to support this process, I will suggest connecting to an apparent vast source of wisdom and compassion. The therapist can use whatever language seems to fit for the client's character and belief system. The subconscious mind can be incredibly wise and knowing and powerful, and may be regarded exactly in that way. Some clients might get further inspired insights by suggestions for tapping into God's wisdom, or for getting in touch with the superconscious or the collective unconscious. Some might relate to communication with the higher self or angels. However the client may identify, the bottom line is that within the subconscious there is access to great wisdom and compassion.

Some subjects will work with parental issues that may go rather far under the circumstances, but are limited in Gestalt dialogue to some degree by the character or lack of consciousness of the parent. In such cases, the potential for inner wisdom and compassion may lend itself to further healing by the imagining of an ideal father and/or mother. This can lead to a dialogue between this parent and the inner child, as described in the next chapter.

Once misconceptions have been identified and understood as such, they can be released, which could be confirmed with ideomotor signals. Then we can move into acknowledgments by the therapist for the client's fine work, and positive post–hypnotic suggestions for further integration and healing. In addition, the client may be encouraged to come up with his or her own self-appreciation and visualizations as well.

As the hypnosis begins coming to completion, the therapist can check in to see if the client has anything further to say or ask. You may also ask your client if you remind him or her of anyone. This is done in case there is some transference, such as being identified as a mother or father figure. In such a case, projections will need to be cleared. If there seems to be completion, the therapist can bring the subject out of hypnosis and then have a post-hypnotic interview.

Regression work is usually done within the context of a series of sessions, even if the regression itself is just one session. There is so much work that can be accomplished and although you don't have to get everything done in that one session, it is important to allow for plenty of time. A strong abreaction or some Gestalt dialogues, for example, can get very involved, and it's crucial not to let time pressure get in the way of the full benefits of the many steps available in this work. There can be various stages of completion, but we do want to allow for a first regression to be thorough.

We have all had traumas from the past that affected us so strongly that we continued for years to respond to that trauma through our attitudes, expectations, and feelings about ourselves, others, and our environment. We cannot take away our memories of what happened, but we can release the trauma, misunderstandings and negative expectancies associated with those memories. Thus we reintegrate the memories, creating new associations and feelings. We can transform the relevance of the experience to our lives. If the client is ready to conclude the process one of the final steps is often the liberating experience of forgiving others and oneself. By the time all is truly forgiven regarding the initial incidents, current related issues in a person's life begin dramatic transformation as well. Usually, however, additional sessions of post-hypnotic suggestions and/or training and practice of self-hypnosis is best to further establish positive new habits.

Most of the sessions explored in the transcripts of this book did not have follow-up sessions. But almost all were with hypnotherapy students or hypnotherapists who had substantial experience in self-hypnosis and group hypnosis processes, and in many cases had experienced more in-depth private hypnotherapy. Subjects were consistently encouraged to follow up their session or two of regression with ongoing auto-suggestions and/or healing imagery in self-hypnosis.

Summary of Major Steps in Emotional Clearing Regression

The following are steps I frequently use when the ideomotor signals are affirmative. Depending upon our training and expertise, we can also integrate many other modalities as appropriate, such as transactional analysis, psychosynthesis, parts therapy, bioenergetics, NLP, Reiki, Lomi work, various forms of massage, etc.

1. A comprehensive interview regarding the presenting issue.
2. Relevant explanation and discussion of hypnosis and hypnotherapy, as necessary. Discussion of client's significant previous hypnosis experiences. (In some cases these first two steps will be a separate initial session.)
3. Induction of hypnosis.
4. The use of ideomotor responses to check the safety of facing the memory and feelings of causal events related to a current life problem.
5. Strongly connecting a feeling that is currently related to the presenting problems in a person's life.

6. Regression to the initial event(s) in which the negative response first occurred. (When #5 and #6 are in this order, this is called the affect bridge.) Often an expression and release of emotions begins to occur now or in the process of the Gestalt dialogue.

7. Thorough Gestalt dialogues, including expression of feelings and communication that could not or did not occur in the initial incident(s). This usually develops into healing and integration of splits of the person (including aspects of the inner child).

8. Progression to the present, keeping conscious awareness of the hypnotic work done to this point.

9. Brief self-hypnoanalysis via subconscious wisdom. Discovery of misconceptions developed as a result of the initial trauma(s) that had been continuing to affect the person until now.

10. Discussion and release of misconceptions. Further accessing of the wisdom and compassion of the subconscious, including forgiveness of oneself and others, and the release of blame, when applicable. When the session has involved parental issues that could reach more full resolution if not for significant parental limitations, the creation of an ideal parent and dialogue with the inner child is an option.

11. Positive post-hypnotic suggestions for further integration and healing.

12. Checking in for possible questions, requests or comments, to help facilitate completion.

13. Arousal from hypnosis.

14. Post-hypnotic interview.

15. Usually some follow-up sessions. (When the client has a background of substantial self-exploration including through self-hypnosis and therapy, extensive follow-up self-hypnosis will in some cases be sufficient.)

CHAPTER 4

Accessing Gestalt Methods

The word "Gestalt" is a German word for which there is no exact English equivalent. A gestalt is a configuration or organization of parts that make up the whole, and the basic premise of Gestalt in psychology has to do with the whole (of human psyche) being greater than the sum of the parts. An analogy would be to look at a triangle, made up of three sides. If the sides are separated the configuration disappears. Think of how much more useful and powerful a working computer is as opposed to the various parts sitting next to each other on the table. Gestalt therapy is about integrating various parts of ourselves that have been disowned to some degree, or that we've lost touch with, back into wholeness by helping conflicting parts communicate with each other and eventually find common ground, appreciation and integration.

Gestalt developed into a powerful phenomenological-existential therapy during the middle of the twentieth century, through the work of founder Frederick "Fritz" Perls and others. Rather than analysis, interpretation and explanation, the focus is on awareness, feeling and acting. The goal for clients is authenticity and self-actualization, which is accomplished by becoming aware of what they are doing, how they are doing it, how to make changes, and how to accept and value themselves. Word spread rapidly during the human potential movement of the 1960's, in particular of the dramatic work of Perls at Esalen Institute. The publication in 1969 of his most famous book, *Gestalt Therapy Verbatim*, rapidly expanded further interest among the general public.

A striking quality of this work was the uncanny way that it plunged participants into widely divergent aspects and emotions within the individual's own personality. Gestalt sometimes encourages the individual to release repressed emotions, which may be a step in the comprehensive healing of emotional clearing.

There are very few books that integrate Gestalt into regression methodologies. Many therapists, in fact, are taught to automatically avoid eliciting emotions via methods that help detach the client during regression. There is much that can be done without Gestalt, but using this process when appropriate can greatly expand the potential value of regression and can often help yield more complete resolution. Gestalt can often be a vital component to help facilitate powerful and rapid growth.

Establishing Dialogue

Intent on finding and evoking opposition, Perls created dialogues between different parts of the personality such as controller and rebel, bully and victim, parent and child, or as became his special interest, between different parts in a dream. Dialogues can also evolve between parts of a part, or between different body parts or internal feelings.

As dialogues developed what would frequently emerge, in Gestalt terminology, was a topdog and underdog. Perls, who had been trained as a psychologist and medical doctor in Germany, often criticized Freud's work, and in *Gestalt Therapy Verbatim* he said, "If there is a superego, there must also be an infra ego. Again, Freud did half the job. He saw the topdog, the superego, but he left out the uderdog, which is just as much a personality as the topdog." He enhanced the differences in the parts dialoguing by using two chairs and having the person switch between the chairs as he or she "became" each part and dialogued with the other, as symbolized by the empty chair.

As at other times during Gestalt, while two parts dialogue the therapist encourages the client to become aware of and stay in touch with his or her feelings. Each side is given the opportunity to express itself and the therapist supports each side in doing that. Switching between two characters or parts and becoming first one and then the other, gives the person an opportunity to work through struggles between conflicting parts (and/or increase communication and appreciation between complementary, harmonious parts), integrating characteristics of each part into a more balanced whole.

It is the therapist's role not to help the person along or take sides, but to help the individual get in touch with, own and express each part.

Perls said, "Lose your mind and come to your senses." It is a matter of not trying to figure it out, but of experiencing these different parts. The client plays one side and then the other, working through a conflict in a supportive environment. By playing the part and becoming it, the person is owning that part that may have been internalized, yet projected onto the world.

During the process of dialoguing between parts in Gestalt, frustration can become an important tool in mobilizing the inner resources of the client. Without frustration there is no motivation to move beyond the impasse or stuck place. The idea is not to give answers, but to empower individuals to expand their own awareness and tap into the inner potential that is there. Questions between characters are to be avoided or turned into statements. In this respect, questions are seen as an attempt to manipulate the environment or not take responsibility. It is also a request for an intellectual explanation, which can tend to diminish the hypnotic state.

Gestalt dialogue can be very effective in some cases even if the hypnotized client speaks softly in a monotone and doesn't express much emotion. One possibility is to check to see if the individual is being clear physically. You do that by having the person periodically get in touch with internal awareness, which is a classic Gestalt method. "Go inside. What do you feel?" He or she might respond with something that sounds strained, like, "My throat feels closed." That's a sign that feelings are being repressed. Or the person might respond, "I feel fine. I'm aware of breathing down into my stomach and I'm feeling relaxed." In that case you can go on, unless there is some apparent tension or movement ignored by the client that is getting your attention.

In the case that there is a significant physical repression you can use the golden rule of Gestalt, which is to do unto others as you do unto yourself. If, for example, there is restriction in your client's throat while doing a Gestalt dialogue with an intimidating person, you might help put your client's hands around a pillow and, using the pillow as a symbol, put that choking feeling into that character. Just doing that to a sufficient extent usually moves the energy and clears that feeling from the throat. Sometimes there can even be powerful breakthroughs, such as freeing energy that the person may have been holding back in certain ways for many years. The value here is not to be construed that such a feeling is now released so it won't ever have to return. Rather, the client is learning to get unstuck, to integrate, to mobilize his or her potential, which can develop over time in various ways internally and through self-expression into processes of greater self-actualization.

Concept of Maturation

Perls described maturation as "the transcendence from environmental support to self-support," which first begins at birth. While in the womb a developing fetus gets all of its support from the mother and then immediately upon birth is faced with an impasse, what Perls calls a crucial point in therapy and growth. "The impasse is the position where environmental support or obsolete inner support is not forthcoming anymore, and authentic self-support has not yet been achieved." The infant has to learn to breathe on its own or die. Environmental support may be given (hopefully more welcoming than being suddenly turned upside down and/or slapped and setting up a possible birth trauma neurosis) as the infant makes its entrance and begins the process of growth, increasingly discovering and utilizing more and more of its inner resources and potential. Following the idea of self-support, the intention of therapy is to help the individual move away from a dependency on others and to discover the deep resources and potential that lie within.

An example of this comes from the maturation process itself. When children get frustrated the two possible responses are that they learn how to overcome the frustration, or they manipulate the outer environment to have it done - such as the child cries and the parent jumps in and takes over. With the frustration removed there is no motivation to learn or grow. In therapy, an individual may become frustrated and say to an opposing part something like, "Why are you doing this?" You can begin to redirect the person to face the frustration by saying to turn the question into a statement. Perhaps the statement will be about the client's feeling toward the opposing part regarding its previous communication. This encourages individuals to mobilize their own resources, expanding awareness of their inner potential and taking responsibility.

Gestalt Strategies in the Context of Hypnosis and Regression

In the 1960's Gil Boyne trained with Perls. Already a pioneering leader in the emerging profession of hypnotherapy, Boyne was the first person to integrate Gestalt into hypnotic regression and into the overall practice of hypnotherapy. Boyne has demonstrated the tremendous synergy between Gestalt and hypnotherapy, in particular with comprehensive regression strategies which are at the heart of much of his Transforming Therapy™ work, and prominent in his landmark text, *Transforming Therapy: A New Approach to Hypnotherapy*.

The intention of Gestalt therapy is not to interpret events from the past, but to experience how we are in the present. A seeming irony of this process is the power it brings to regression work. Gestalt in its very essence is about being in the here and now. For that reason, some therapists at first glance might consider regression work to be incongruous with the existentialism of Gestalt. However, although it may seem that the nature of regression work is to return to the past, it is only that part of the past which is being brought into and affecting the present - blocking inner resources and potential - that is important to work with. Those stuck places in the present.

The relevance of Gestalt to regression becomes even more obvious when we consider Gestalt dreamwork, which became Perls' favorite use of Gestalt. He recognized that a dream is absolute reality to the person as it originally occurs. The basis of a regression is to recall a distant or recent past experience in hypnosis. Therefore, Gestalt dreamwork, which is about vividly recalling a dream and bringing it into the present, is a form of regression.

In my book, *Become the Dream*, and in my classes, I have pointed out what has not been generally recognized, that the use of Gestalt methods are so powerful partly because many of the processes tend to induce or maintain a hypnotic state. The relevance of many Gestalt methods to hypnosis will be explored in detail in Chapter 21.

During a hypnotic regression dialogue takes place between the person at whatever age he has regressed to, and the individual(s) or representative or thing that he is in conflict with. Unlike traditional Gestalt, when using Gestalt in regression the chair switching technique is not used. Hypnosis has already been induced and the switch between characters can be encouraged by telling the person to switch, and perhaps simultaneously tapping the shoulder or the arm. Just as in dreamwork, where individuals are encouraged to relate the dream in the present tense as though it is currently happening, in regression each character is reminded to dialogue in the present tense.

Becoming the different parts or characters in a regression opens the potential for integration. The client can become the mother or the father or the aching heart or the fear or whatever, and act this out. Various aspects of memories can be experienced for the purpose of owning parts of oneself and deepening self-awareness. While emotional release may also take place in varying degrees, that is only part of the process in the resolving of associated issues that leads to important emotional clearing.

Emotional clearing involves healing the splits between different parts, which can be accomplished in traditional Gestalt or through a combination of methods such as described in Chapter 3. The expression of emotions may be a major element in that process, especially when emotions have been stifled. Someone who has not thoroughly grieved the death of a loved one, for example, may experience deep emotional clearing in part by getting in touch with that grief and shedding long held back tears, as occurs in two of the sessions in this book.

For those practitioners who do not yet have substantial experience in Gestalt, doing Gestalt dreamwork and then Hypnotic Dreamwork™ as described in Chapter 21, can be a good way to develop skills as part of the preparation for doing Gestalt in regression. This is the way I introduce the experiential practicing of Gestalt in my classes. Gestalt dreamwork, and even Hypnotic Dreamwork, is less likely to develop into as many complexities of steps and directions as the 15 step process for emotional clearing regression described in Chapter 3. Also, experience for the therapist, and a stage of completion and value for the client, can often be achieved in dreamwork in early practice sessions while keeping a relatively narrow focus and more limited time frame.

Creating Ideal Parents

As you do Gestalt with these splits during regression, say with a parent who is neglectful or abusive in some way, or a teacher who is being very hard on the child, that in itself often heals those splits so that integration can take place. But there is more that you can do, if necessary, to take it a step further. For example, often both parent and child will make dramatic breakthroughs in relating to each other during a dialogue in regression. But occasionally the client works through a dialogue to as much completion as possible while the parent, who in reality had major issues or limitations, may only be able to go so far.

You can help the subject create an idealized mother or father to be with the inner child. This would take place after the Gestalt dialogue, and usually after progression to the present, hypnoanalysis, and reeducation including discovery and release of misconceptions. I may ask for a description of the appearance of an ideal mother or father. The ideal parent may look like somebody she knows, or a famous person, or maybe somebody she's never seen. Ideal parents might look like the individual's own mother or father but with the qualities of an ideal parent.

Value comes from encouraging the individual to experience this relationship from the child's perspective, and also from the parent's perspective of experiencing the joy of appreciating and nurturing the child. Both sides can gain from everything the other side has to offer. Such processes can further contribute to the healing of the inner splits. From a transactional analysis viewpoint, the therapist works with the adult, the parent and the child parts of the client.

Mistakes to Avoid and Directions to Take With Gestalt

Some therapists attempting to do Gestalt work make the mistake of often taking sides in a dialogue between two parts. One problem with this is that it can get in the way of the part of the client that is mobilizing his or her resources. Also, more often than not, when a person during regression is dealing with a difficult character, he or she has internalized certain qualities of that character. If a 40 year old is regressing back to an issue at four years of age with an excessively critical parent, the reason it remains an issue after so many years is because that critical parent is still there inside. If the therapist takes sides, saying, "Oh, she's being a terrible mommy!" that's not doing the therapy. (The reference to "mommy" here is in talking to a four year old child, who may now be called Johnny instead of John.) That mommy is a part of him that needs to be integrated.

The internalized critical parent may not necessarily express itself outwardly to others as the parent did, but is all too present within, excessively finding fault and projecting itself onto expectancies of what others will think. And whenever you have one extreme, such as an insensitive, excessively critical parent, then on the other side you have a helpless child who feels victimized and is terrified of judgment. Among other things, the child needs to become stronger and more confident, and the parent needs to become more accepting and flexible, and they need to and can find their own way to accomplish such steps. Both sides, the boy and the mommy, need to be able to totally express what they're feeling, respond to the other, and eventually come to a better understanding and appreciation of each other, with both sides communicating with greater respect and maturity.

Although it is usually a mistake to take sides, there are some exceptions. Gestalt during regression is not always the same as a here and now process of internal awareness or a dreamwork session, as is evident by the option of sometimes creating an ideal parent. An abused child may need some protection from the energy of the abuser. In some cases the purpose is not to identify with the perpetrator, but to create some protection and detachment that allows the person to feel safe to proceed. Dialogue can still take place but the subject can "hear" what the other side is saying. The normal Gestalt dialogue may be replaced by a dialogue in which the therapist asks, "And what is his response?" rather than having the client become the abuser in the dialogue. If the child is afraid to communicate, you can suggest various kinds of protection. "I'm here to help you and there is a powerful invisible barrier between you. He (She) is never going to hurt you again. You can say whatever you want." The therapist can make various suggestions of this kind to encourage the person to get his or her feelings out. You still support each side in saying what it wants to say.

The therapist needs to be careful to avoid helping too much. The dialogue needs to take place, as much as possible, from the individual. It can be a temptation, when you clearly see that a person isn't getting a realization, to want to help out. But part of the power of this therapy is in allowing individuals to work through their confusion and come to realizations on their own. Remember, we're encouraging transcending environmental support with self-support.

That said, Gestalt gets the best results in a supportive atmosphere. Avoid giving answers, if possible, but it is good to provide some guidance in increasing the client's self-awareness and directions to proceed. A validating, nurturing presence provides the most powerful environment for healing and growth.

Perls was a very judgmental practitioner at times, and some of the other early Gestalt therapists followed the example of his tough demeanor. Gary Yontef states, "As experience in doing Gestalt therapy has grown, earlier therapeutic practices have been altered. For example, earlier Gestalt therapy practice often stressed the clinical use of frustration, a confusion of self-sufficiency with self-support, and an abrasive attitude if the patient was interpreted by the therapist as manipulative. This approach tended to enhance the shame of shame-oriented patients. There has been a movement toward more softness in Gestalt therapy practice, more direct self-expression by the therapist.... Thus a patient is more likely to encounter...an emphasis on self-acceptance, a softer demeanor by the therapist, more trust of the patient's phenomenology, and more explicit work with psychodynamic themes."

The therapeutic process can get stifled in a non-supportive setting, and criticism can be reframed. To give a client an environment of acceptance is to allow that much more potential for Gestalt to develop into its full capacity to do great work. Dialogues in these volumes demonstrate that there are many ways to communicate in a non-judgmental manner. Within the Gestalt process itself, for example, a client can be supportively encouraged to continue a dialogue that has become frustrating so that they may become more aware of what they are doing that is causing that frustration. If a client is confused, he or she can be helped to come to a better understanding more effectively through patience than through criticism.

Even without a formal induction, most Gestalt processes tend to initiate or further a hypnotic state. Persons in hypnosis are extremely receptive and suggestible. I do not consider it appropriate to ever criticize someone in hypnosis.

CHAPTER 5

Utilizing Ideomotor Signals in Regression

The word ideomotor refers to mind and movement. It describes an involuntary, subconsciously produced movement of the body in response to a particular thought, feeling or idea. The broad usage of ideomotor methods in hypnotic work would encompass spontaneous unconscious movements as well as hypnotic testing, but in general usage the term typically refers to signals requested by the hypnotist to elicit information from the subject. They are utilized in part as a valuable means of obtaining information that is in the subconscious, but not necessarily available to the conscious mind.

Common ideomotor methods employed for this purpose are finger signals and pendulums. Automatic writing is another form of ideomotor communication. As shown in this book, my preferred method is usually finger signals, which for the most part is very effective in eliciting information. On those rare occasions when an individual is not able to respond or is resistant to finger signals, a pendulum can often be successfully employed.

Finger signals are often valuable in bringing up information from a deeper part of the mind than is reached by verbal responses. Sometimes a client may even be surprised and perplexed by an answer at first, until the reason for it is uncovered. Or the person may verbalize one answer, and give an ideomotor signal of another. Suggestions for nodding or shaking the head can sometimes bring true ideomotor responses, but the subconscious mind can create a message more easily, with much less muscular work, via the subtle movements of fingers. Also, direct information from the subconscious is sometimes more easily and accurately attained by finger or pendulum signals than head movements, which in some cases are more influenced by conscious thought processes.

This important tool has been in use for many years but is unfortunately too often neglected or not even known by many hypnotherapists. It is not mentioned in most hypnotherapy books and barely touched upon, if at all, in many hypnotherapy trainings. The first book to explore the use of ideomotor methods was Cheek and LeCron's 1968 classic, *Clinical Hypnotherapy*. Various uses and values of this technique can be seen throughout the sessions of this two volume set, and will be thoroughly explored in my forthcoming hypnotherapy training text, *Ideomotor Magic*.

Establishing Ideomotor Responses

After the hypnotic induction, a subject may be asked to focus the attention on one or both hands, imagining the word "yes" until a certain finger begins to rise. During the initial establishment of ideomotor signals it may be helpful to continue coaxing the subject to keep visualizing, sensing and feeling "yes," until a finger lifts up. Eventually a finger will usually begin to move. The process is repeated for the selection of a "no" finger, and I usually ask for an "I don't know" finger, and a finger for an alternative such as, "I don't know how to properly answer the question." Questions are then carefully formulated with the intention of being able to be answered by a simple yes or no, and directed to the knowledge and insights of the subconscious mind.

One hand is used in some cases to avoid confusion. It's easier for the hypnotherapist to look for movement from one hand rather than shifting attention back and forth, and the use of one hand avoids the possibility of cross-over in the signals. Cheek and LeCron observed during early research that with some individuals when both hands were used the "yes" signal, which might be the right index finger, could cross over to the left index finger even though that finger had been designated as a "no" signal.

It is also important to note that it is not unusual for a client to want to please or to be overly cooperative. Without necessarily realizing it, there are times when an individual may signal with the conscious mind. With experience and close observation, the hypnotherapist can learn to usually differentiate finger responses that are consciously made or influenced. In many cases, a subconscious response will come slowly and with a somewhat jerky or repetitive movement. A conscious response, which can be slight or dramatic, will sometimes come quickly and with one movement. The subconscious needs at least a little time to take in the question and process. An immediate "I don't know" signal is a sign of conscious response. If conscious involvement in the signals is suspected, the client can be encouraged to take time and just keep focusing on the question until a certain finger begins to respond, seemingly on its own.

When giving ideomotor responses, the subject may or may not be aware of the signal. There are even times when a finger will move in response to some statement being made by the hypnotist, confirming the accuracy or affirming the statements being made, at a time when no ideomotor signal was sought. For these reasons, it is a good practice for the hypnotherapist to get into the habit of verbally confirming whatever signals are coming from finger movements.

Neutrality is very important throughout - in setting up the signals, asking the questions, and announcing the answers. This is not a time to express surprise or to have judgment about an answer. In fact, it is always important be supportive. There is never an appropriate time to be critical of a person who is in this very sensitive state. However, if answers appear to be contradictory to each other, the hypnotist may proceed carefully and supportively to solve any apparent contradictions. Some answers may be incorrect, perhaps as a result of confusion, a conscious response, or a literal answer that may be correct on one level but not on another. Keep an open mind for discovering unexpected possibilities and creative solutions from the client's subconscious that may solve the mystery of an apparent contradiction.

Examples of Eliciting Responses

In the transcripts of this book, ideomotor signals will be elicited in a variety of ways that demonstrate its usefulness in working with regression. As described in Chapter 3, after induction and the setting up of ideomotor responses, at least two questions are generally asked to determine whether the subconscious feels it would be a good idea to face the memories and feelings associated with the relevant traumas. The answers to these important questions determine whether or not, or to what degree, the individual may need to be detached, or in what direction it might be appropriate to proceed.

Uses of ideomotor questions include drawing out more information or getting details from the subconscious that the conscious mind is not yet aware of. For example, if a significant initiating event has been uncovered a question might be asked such as, "Is there any other information that would be valuable for you to focus on regarding this issue?" If the answer is affirmative, you may ask, "Is your conscious mind aware of what that information is?" Depending on the answer, the hypnotherapist can continue questioning for ideomotor responses from the subconscious or move on to verbal communications and processing.

Another example is the use of this technique to uncover subconscious reasons for emotional and physical symptoms. One area to check is that of "secondary gains." An individual may be subconsciously holding onto some symptom because of an underlying benefit. It may be that chronic pain produces unemployment benefits and avoidance of a job that the person has resistance to, or a benefit might be in the form of getting attention or affection. Another subconscious reason might have to do with fear, expectancy or association to a parent or family member with similar symptoms at the same age, and so on.

Frequently, information elicited from the subconscious mind is more accurate or detailed than what is consciously known. There are times when an individual might answer verbally in one way while subconsciously signaling something different. Milton Erickson was one of the first to write about noticing ideomotor responses. He began the occasional use of ideomotor responses as an induction technique after observing some patients shaking their heads or nodding in opposition to their actual verbal responses. He concluded that such movements indicated subconscious communication.

Ideomotor questions can also be used throughout a session to check in at various points. If giving directions for visualization, for example, you can ask for an ideomotor signal to give you information about the process. "Let the correct finger signal whether or not it would be a good idea to do that." Or, "Signal with your 'yes' finger when you get an image or a feeling of succeeding in this way." Verbalizing takes more energy and uses more complex thought processes. Ideomotor signals do not require effort, and in some cases could allow your client to stay more deeply in hypnosis.

There are a wide range of possibilities in which ideomotor methods can support regression work. In Chapter 16, for example, Ron's session begins with ideomotor exploration that leads into regression, which has a similarity to an affect bridge using emotions to link a person to a past experience.

In a few of the examples of actual sessions it is interesting to note that a "no" answer is sometimes given as a kind of emotionally protective response, which in some cases changes to "yes" after additional clarifying questions or more information is given, including reassurances that we will only go as far as is determined by the wisdom of the subconscious.

The utilization of ideomotor methods in regression work gives us the opportunity to access information regarding experiences from long ago, sometimes consciously forgotten, that may still be affecting an individual as an adult. The value of regression is not in working out the past, but in working with information from the past that is still affecting an individual in the present. With a combination of tools that include ideomotor methods, Gestalt dialogue, self-hypnoanalysis, reeducation and post-hypnotic suggestions, regression therapy offers profound opportunities for personal growth and healing.

CHAPTER 6

Direct vs Indirect Suggestion

Understanding the Broad Context of Suggestion

Virtually all writings comparing and contrasting the use of direct and indirect suggestions in hypnosis refer to the structure of language. But there is much beyond the way we word suggestions that can have a major suggestive impact. These impacts are something we need to be keenly aware of in order to give maximum benefit to the influence of suggestions. Body language, facial expressions, tone and volume of voice, gestures, timing, eye contact, physical contact such as a handshake, gender, age, bearing and appearance, including health, body type and clothing can all be major indirect suggestions that affect the meaning of our language. The meaning of language will also affect and be understood by each individual uniquely because of the various personal meanings and connotations each of us associates to words and phrases, and by the emotional state, mood and expectancies of your client.

Further indirect suggestions are given by colors, harmony of styles, cleanliness, temperature, aromas or odors, condition of the office, reception area, facilities and office building, and by the function, form, style and quality of furniture. Various additional aspects of location include the size and prestige of the city or town, neighboring offices and adjacent buildings, section of city or town and immediate neighborhood, people one may encounter in the vicinity of your office, and noise levels. Cultural and semantic factors also influence the meaning of suggestions, including the culture and language in which you and your client meet and converse, and each of your backgrounds and life experience. Time of day or night, current events and seasonal factors, including holiday periods, can be indirect suggestions that affect the way language influences people at a particular time.

There are many indirect influences in the written word as well as the spoken word. When seeing a suggestion or opinion in writing we are influenced by the venue, be it a book, magazine, newspaper article, advertisement, letter, email or billboard, and whether it be from a friend, a relative, an organization we belong to, a government agency, or spam email. When reading a book the quality of writing, the book's quality and size, the cover, the background and additional writings of the author, etc., all add a context that affects the meaning and attention given to suggestions.

There is no such thing as a simple, independent direct suggestion. The context of a so-called "direct suggestion" always has a great many indirect surrounding influences. In fact the distinction of such influences becomes blurred, and some of the influences may be considered direct rather than indirect, depending on the situation and moment in time.

The Myth of the Inherent Superiority of Indirect Suggestions

As shown above, the degree of directness or indirectness of suggestion is far more complex and individualized than generally considered. I feel it is important to address the topic of direct and indirect suggestions because of the tremendous extent to which significant misconceptions about direct suggestion have been disseminated for the past quarter century by many influential people in the field of hypnotherapy, including teachers, therapists and major authors.

The misconception that direct suggestions are inferior comes mainly through individuals among those who identify themselves as Ericksonian hypnotherapists. For example, Stephen and Carol Langton claim, "Direct suggestion will only bring temporary relief, will intensify the transference relationship toward authority, and will increase repression of the conflict which led to the symptomatology." They add, "An Ericksonian hypnotist strives to be artfully indirect in all suggestions and interventions."

Working only indirectly makes no sense in certain forms of hypnotherapy, such as when working with Gestalt or ideomotor methods. For example, there are times when a Gestalt dialogue will go back and forth, progressing quickly and effectively, with each character saying a sentence or two. Following the Langtons' admonition, instead of the therapist saying, "Switch," each time the side appears to be done, with every completion the therapist would be required to say anything and everything indirectly, which would become awkward and plain silly. "I wonder if you might feel drawn to expressing another side. Perhaps the one you were just talking to?" Or, "Perhaps you may be ready to say something. You might be pleased to notice yourself communicating from the other perspective. Or you might prefer first saying something further?" Or, "I wonder if you'll be surprised at how easy it may be to imagine a response. Maybe or maybe not, it doesn't really matter."

Erickson, Hershman and Sector claimed that directive hypnotherapy will be successful in only a small minority of cases because direct methods do not address the natural defenses of the client. It is interesting that Milton Erickson would make such an extreme statement. He used both highly directive and even authoritarian suggestions with some patients, and indirect suggestions with others. Jay Haley has been particularly fascinated in *Uncommon Therapy*, and in some of his other books and articles, about Erickson's use of authoritarian, sometimes extremely authoritarian, methods.

According to Erickson, Rossi and Rossi, direct methods ensure that any response to a suggestion may be due to the demands of the situation or to the prestige of the hypnotist, rather than in response to the suggestion. It allegedly follows that since an indirect suggestion cannot be mediated by conscious awareness because of its covert nature, that, as Robert Meyer puts it, "any response to an indirect suggestion will be due to the intervention and not to situational or prestige factors." Taking into consideration the power of suggestion in placebo studies as described in Chapter 14, as well as many broader aspects of suggestion discussed in the beginning of this chapter, I find it hard to comprehend how an expert in hypnosis could even entertain the thought that prestige is not a factor in response to suggestion if you structure your wording indirectly.

Many scientific studies have been done to compare the efficacy of direct and indirect suggestions. In some cases the studies clearly surprised the researchers, who had set out to prove the superiority of indirect suggestions. The preponderance of evidence of scientific research to date clearly documents that direct suggestions are as good as or better than indirect suggestions. While a few studies have concluded the superiority of indirect suggestion, some of those have been seriously flawed. For example, Joseph Barber's claim of superior results with indirect suggestion have repeatedly failed in attempts to replicate, and the indirect condition used by Matthews, Bennett, Bean and Gallagher, was substantially longer than the direct condition. Hammond states, "The furor of the past decade over the belief that 'indirect is always better' is rather reminiscent of the extensive research literature that has now failed to replicate the creative, but nonetheless unfounded tenets of NLP. As mental health professionals we may stand too ready to adopt unproven theories as truth."

Many who use indirect suggestions describe a wonderful multitude of forms of varying complexity. However, the vast array of possible uses of direct suggestions are sometimes summarized in a simplistic generalization, such as the statement by Meyer, "Direct techniques are those that directly attack a problem or symptom by suppressing them with orders (suggestions)...." To the contrary, direct suggestions are commonly used in comprehensive ways in which the underlying issues are taken into account. It is rare to find a hypnotherapist trained through a licensed school who does not attempt to work holistically with clients.

If I'm helping someone with smoking cessation, for example, even when regression modalities are also used, some of our work will be in direct (and indirect) suggestion. I can give individualized direct suggestions that include increased confidence, tapping into motivation, constructive activities for the hands and mouth, healthy eating habits, good habits of attention, self-expression, breathing techniques and awareness, exercise, hobbies, self-acceptance and appreciation, good relationships, good focus at work, encouraging emotional stability and healthy channeling of energy. All this is tied in as part of the overall process of tapping into one's full potential to reach a stated objective. Initial cravings for tobacco and associations of habit patterns can be transformed and redirected in a myriad of constructive ways, that for many clients helps them succeed in ways that go far beyond their presenting goals.

To give another example, if I am inducing hypnosis with directive techniques, that doesn't mean I'm attacking a problem by suppression. If I am developing ideomotor responses I might say, "Keep thinking of the word, 'yes,' until a finger begins to rise." This is a direct suggestion. Even if I gave the direct suggestion, "Imagine the middle finger is your yes finger, and imagine it lifting and rising," that is certainly not attacking a problem by suppressing it with orders. If I'm doing a Gestalt process in hypnosis and I say, "Now become four-year-old Mary," or "Focus on your breathing," or "Become aware of your hands," these are direct suggestions. These are just samples of the countless possibilities of using direct suggestions in positive, effective ways.

There are many circumstances in which I feel indirect suggestions may be the most appropriate choice. For example, when far along in therapy and a client is doing well, I may move mostly indirectly for one or more sessions. It also tends to be my preferred method when working with various forms of pain relief. I usually prefer being indirect on the occasions when I give amnesia suggestions. At various points in many types of sessions, I may use indirect language. However, I will normally stick primarily with a particular style throughout a session, from the pre-hypnotic interview to the post-hypnotic discussion, whether the style is very directive, moderately directive, permissive or indirect.

There are times when predominantly indirect suggestions may be more effective, and times when predominantly direct suggestions tends to be preferable. As D. Corydon Hammond states, "Hypnosis - like so much of psychotherapy - is still more art than science." Some individuals tend to respond better to one type of suggestion than another, but the majority of people tend to respond well to the skillful use of a range of styles. What is often more important is what a person is working on as well as related issues, the primary emphasis of hypnotic work being done in that session (e.g., suggestion, regression, exploratory ideomotor, dreamwork, or systematic desensitization), and the stage of therapy. For example, in my experience in helping most individuals break an addiction, the session in which the person is to cease the substance abuse is usually best done in a firmly directive motivational style, and typically in the next session a few days later as well. The style of those sessions that are primarily suggestion-oriented will tend to gradually shift, and by the time we're moving on to suggestions for long-term results, a session with an indirect style may be particularly appealing.

Some therapists claim as a broadly generalized truism that the way to overcome resistance, or potential resistance, is to use indirect suggestions. There are many reasons for and forms of resistance, but I do many things over the series of sessions to help lessen the possibility or transform it. As part of a first session, I will do my best to build rapport and positive yet realistic mental expectancy. I check for significant motivation, get details of reasons for the goal, history of successes and failures including important situational factors in the presenting issue and other related issues in a person's life, begin checking for possible secondary gains, find out about various past experiences with hypnosis or lack of experience, discuss the importance of the client's commitment and cooperation, and, if necessary, give a detailed explanation of hypnosis and hypnotherapy including the removal of misconceptions. I endeavor to work comprehensively, taking account of underlying issues, personality factors, fears, strengths, other issues that may be beneath the conscious awareness, and so forth.

I work with exploratory ideomotor methods and various regression strategies as applicable, as part of the strive for long-term success. In utilizing the strengths of the client and the vast potential of the subconscious, potential areas of resistance can be turned into strengths. For example, the rebel part of the client can be encouraged to rebel against the old patterns of negative behavior and thought processes. And in many ways, including during interactive hypnosis, what might appear to be resistance can often be reframed into opportunities and cooperation. For that matter, within a Gestalt process, nothing needs to be considered resistance; anything that comes up for the client is a valuable part of the process that can be worked with. In the context of all of this, if something I would consider to be resistance arises, how I work with it will depend upon the form and context of the resistance. If some aspects of the resistance seem best to approach via a form of suggestion, either very a directive or indirect style will be best, as opposed to mildly directive or permissive.

Certain techniques emphasized in these volumes, such as the affect bridge, Gestalt and ideomotor methods, call for a primarily directive manner, so that is the principal style in this series and my forthcoming *Ideomotor Magic*. Also, *Become the Dream*, in combining Gestalt dreamwork with hypnotherapy, demonstrates the primarily directive style that is appropriate for that form of therapy.

Toward An Accurate Representation of Erickson and the Field of Hypnotherapy

The wild distortions communicated regarding direct vs indirect suggestion are part of a bigger picture. While I have great respect for Erickson's genius, history is being dramatically altered by a significant number of Ericksonian therapists, including many prominent leaders, who have had an alarming level of ignorance about vitally important realms of hypnosis history, theory and application. Many talk about Erickson as "The Father of Hypnotherapy." The brochure of a hypnosis school brushed off great ranges of long-established modalities of non-Ericksonian hypnosis with a single sentence about how grateful we can be to Erickson for lifting the field of hypnosis out of the domain of stage hypnosis.

In his contribution to *Hypnosis: Questions and Answers,* and again in *Trancework: An Introduction to the Practice of Clinical Hypnosis,* Michael Yapko says there are three major models of hypnosis: Traditional, Standardized and Ericksonian. According to Yapko, the Traditional hypnotherapist has an authoritarian demeanor, demands a high degree of compliance, knows only direct styles of suggestion, does not have an individualized approach to different clients, reacts to resistance through confrontation or interpretation, gives low value to insights, does not recognize the possibility of secondary gains, and has a negative characterization of the subconscious. Yapko's portrayal of the Standardized category is the same kind of caricature given above, except that the demeanor may be permissive.

A writer in *Recovering* magazine contrasted Ericksonian hypnosis with "standard clinical hypnosis" in which the therapist allegedly merely repeats a series of commands. This "authoritarian hypnotherapist," who "often uses a technical aide," is assumed to have the answers, and in hypnosis "communication is a one-way street."

Such caricatures did not fit the profession decades ago, and do not fit now. I have taught thousands of hypnotherapists and have discussed hypnotic procedures with hundreds of other hypnotherapists from around the world over several decades. I don't know if I've ever met this "standard clinical hypnotist." Hypnotherapists I've talked with are consistently holistic (doing their best to work comprehensively, including underlying issues), are familiar with various interactive processes, and the majority use a variety of directive, permissive and indirect styles. Especially considering the recent proliferation of non-licensed schools, I'm sure there are some incompetent non-Ericksonians in practice, just as there are some incompetent Ericksonians.

I have often heard absurd generalizations made by a minority of zealous promoters of technique packages, including claims about the limits of "traditional" hypnotherapy. First, whatever was done decades ago by some stage hypnotists and amateurs is not relevant to the history or traditions of the field of clinical hypnotherapy, a field which had plenty of scientific documentation and many intelligent and creative clinical practitioners before Erickson began influencing the field. Secondly, there will always be inept or irresponsible practitioners of any form of therapy, and we need to be careful what generalities and conclusions we draw from what we hear. Also, we need to be aware of potential limits and pitfalls of the techniques we do use, recognizing that any system of therapy has its place and its limitations, and needs to be balanced by our sensitivity, creativity, intuition, life experience and knowledge of other forms of therapy.

Milton Erickson is described in the *Recovering* article as having single-handedly "revived serious scholarly and pragmatic interest in hypnosis in the 1940's." I've repeatedly heard similar kinds of dramatic claims, which consist of two fallacies. First, serious scholarly and pragmatic interest had been continuing prior to that. Second, Erickson was no more influential than some other important hypnotherapists of his time, until after Jay Haley's *Uncommon Therapy* was published in 1973. (For example, the word "Ericksonian" did not exist prior to 1974.) During the middle third of the 20th century, hypnotherapists were influenced by a very broad array of hypnotic procedures, including major insights and discoveries of LeCron, Watkins, Kroger, Elman, Weitzenhoffer, Cheek, Boyne, Crasilneck, Wolpe, Wolberg and Hilgard.

Contrary to the article and many other claims I've heard and read, many options of established clinical hypnosis procedures are far more complex than merely giving commands, and various forms are interactive. Here are a few influential examples, which developed from foundations set by interactive processes of the late nineteenth and early twentieth centuries: Elman's pioneering breakthroughs in hypnoanalysis in the 1940's; various uses of ideomotor methods, first developed by LeCron in the '50's; Wolpe's systematic desensitization techniques, developed in the '50's; comprehensive emotional clearing strategies, including the integration of Gestalt and other modalities with hypnosis, developed first by Boyne in the '60's. Traditional texts such as Kroger's *Clinical and Experimental Hypnosis* (1963) and Cheek and LeCron's *Clinical Hypnotherapy* (1968), each emphasizing working with underlying and associated issues to presenting problems via a wealth of interactive exploratory, regression and insight oriented interventions, were classic training texts for years before Haley's own classic began the explosion of interest that would soon make Erickson a demigod in some circles.

Many practitioners of named hypnotic styles greatly exaggerate their uniqueness. For example, many "Ericksonian" techniques were used prior to Erickson, and independently by his contemporaries, including various forms of indirect suggestions, metaphors, truisms, encouraging resistance, seeding ideas, double binds, use of space and position, implying a deviation, amnesia, emphasizing the positive, and uncommon homework assignments. The masterful Erickson developed some of his methods in his own way or with greater complexity than they had been used before. But regarding the huge gray area of defining Ericksonian hypnosis, I accept the assertions of those who use such techniques but are adamant that they are not doing "Ericksonian" hypnosis. Those methods and styles Erickson used that were also used independently by contemporaries or earlier practitioners do not have to be considered "Ericksonian."

I am not criticizing Ericksonian-oriented practitioners as a whole. They have fine tools at their disposal, and there are many who have a broad appreciation of non-Ericksonian modalities. I teach a wide variety of techniques in my classes that could be associated with Erickson. It's fine for therapists to emphasize a particular set of methods, but I would like to encourage all hypnotherapists to not limit their training to one or more packages of techniques or styles. For example, most Ericksonian teachers and texts are limited in regression modalities, and unfamiliar with some powerful emotional clearing methods and most of the treasures of ideomotor methods.

I am concerned about the substantial number of hypnotherapists who claim the superiority of their package of techniques, often creating a whipping boy out of the mythical "standard clinical hypnotist." This is not limited to some Ericksonians. For example, such chauvinism has been communicated by some NLP Practitioners. Contrary to the claim that therapists who use a particular brand of hypnosis have a wider range of techniques than others, the opposite is true. If you want to have a truly broad range of options at your disposal, don't limit yourself to one or a few hypnotic orientations. Include tools that are associated with Erickson and others, whether or not your source is directly from such a named system, and study therapeutic modalities not generally associated with hypnosis. There is plenty of evidence that relying on a limited range of methods and one approach is usually associated with inexperience as a therapist. In fact, research has found that the most highly experienced therapists ascribe to an eclectic approach, refusing to be limited by adherence to only one orientation.

I have refrained from giving a sampling of disturbing stories from some videos I have seen and information told to me by former clients of Ericksonian therapists. The purpose of such a sampling would have been to emphasize my point about not making generalizations from stories of incompetent or insensitive therapists. But my intention is not to be confrontive. My intention is to help lessen the dissemination of demeaning misinformation, and encourage hypnotherapists from a wide range of backgrounds and interests to unite in appreciation of the magnificent diversity, range, capabilities and complexities of our great profession.

CHAPTER 7

Mary's Fear of Public Speaking
Humiliated in Grade School

RANDAL: I want to do a demonstration on regression. Does anybody have an ongoing issue you would like to work on? You don't even have to know if it's something that occurred in the past because ongoing current issues usually relate to past events. Mary?

MARY: There is something that I think falls into this realm. I'm not sure though.

RANDAL: Why don't you come up here and talk about what you're considering working on and we'll see if it fits. (Mary sits on a chair next to Randal)

MARY: Well, although I've done a lot of public speaking in my life, I seem to be having a little trouble with it lately. More so. I mean, it pops up when I least expect it.

RANDAL: This is an example, by the way, of what I was asking for. This is an ongoing current issue in your life. Are there some forms of public speaking that are fine for you and others that are difficult?

MARY: (big sigh) Well, it seems to be just at different times. And I never know when the problem is going to come up so I never know if I can speak.

RANDAL: When you say you've done a lot of public speaking, can you give examples of public speaking you've done in recent years?

MARY: Well, recently I haven't done too much because I'm concerned about this.

RANDAL: So you've been avoiding doing public speaking recently?

MARY: Yes.

RANDAL: Okay. When you have done a lot of public speaking are you referring to at work or when you were in school or what?

MARY: At work.

RANDAL: Teaching people?

MARY: Yes, I'm an instructor and I've given speeches and taught classes without difficulties. It's no problem to stand up in front of several hundred people and make announcements or talk to them or do whatever I need to do. But sometimes I start getting nervous and I won't even be looking at anybody. I'll just be making an announcement, a normal thing that I've done a thousand times.

RANDAL: It sounds like it didn't used to be a problem and then over the years it's popped up more and more often. Would that be accurate?

MARY: Right.

RANDAL: So it seems to be coming out of nowhere. Have you had any experience of difficulty beyond nervousness when you were in front of people? Was there a time when you actually felt severely embarrassed by something? Can you recall anything like that at the time this started happening or the immediate years before that?

MARY: No. The first time it happened I was instructing a class and everything was going fine. Then I looked down and saw the little sister of a very close friend of mine. The next thing I knew I just went to pieces. I couldn't do... (Mary starts to stutter and lose her words) I was...

RANDAL: This was a sister of a friend of yours?

MARY: Yes, a new trainee in the airline training class. She was a friend.

RANDAL: So you had positive feelings for her.

MARY: Oh, yes.

RANDAL: And yet somehow seeing her was distracting in some way. Did it make you nervous or make you forget what you were going to say, or what?

MARY: Well, I got this nervousness just looking at her, and there was no reason because she was just sitting there waiting for me to start teaching. The next thing I knew I was feeling very much like I am right now. (laughing nervously) And it comes up here in class sometimes and sometimes it doesn't.

RANDAL: It comes up in class if you're going to be asking a question or if you're going to be practicing in front of a small group?

MARY: I never know.

RANDAL: When you say you never know, do you feel nervous about public speaking when you're in class even if you're just considering asking a question? Or are you saying that if you're talking in class, sometimes it comes up and sometimes it doesn't?

MARY: Well, recently it caught me by surprise. Marleen was teaching and I went to tell her about something and in the middle of talking about it, all of a sudden I had this awful feeling and I had to cut it short and stop.

RANDAL: Have you felt nervousness at any other time in class?

MARY: There was only one other time and that was when we were doing a three person practice. But the thing is I don't know when it's going to happen. I don't have any warning, it just starts all of a sudden.

RANDAL: Let me feed this back to you and tell me if it's accurate. You find that you've been really comfortable with public speaking in our classes almost all of the time and there have only been a couple of instances when you didn't. Is that correct?

MARY: Yes.

RANDAL: Even though you felt comfortable most of the time, were you feeling nervous about whether this might happen? Like worrying, "What happens if I ask a question and I get nervous?"

MARY: Well, it is an issue because there are times I would like to speak, like to share something or ask a question, but I don't know if right in the middle of it this is going to happen.

RANDAL: That makes this issue much more major. Even if it only happens once in awhile you are often afraid because you never know when it's going to happen.

MARY: Yes.

RANDAL: A phrase that comes to me, and I don't know if it fits for you at all, is panic attack. Does that fit in the worst cases of this? Would you consider it to be a feeling of panic or would you use another word such as nervousness or fear?

MARY: (sigh) I never thought of it that way before.

RANDAL: I just made up some words. Forget the words I made up. What would you call it?

MARY: Well, to tell you the truth, when I thought I was going to do therapy up here in front of the class before, that was a panic attack. (laughing nervously)

RANDAL: So maybe that does fit sometimes. I think maybe a sudden feeling of panic might be the more extreme feeling, but it's basically a feeling of sudden fear regarding public speaking.

MARY: It's a nervousness that...it's not panic. It's just a feeling of nervousness that I'll lose the effectiveness of what I want to say or do or the point I want to make.

RANDAL: Okay, just nervousness but sometimes extreme nervousness.

MARY: Right.

RANDAL: Approximately how many years ago was it that you suddenly saw the sister of your friend?

MARY: Oh, maybe fifteen years ago.

RANDAL: Can you recall, either as a teenager or as a child, ever feeling a sudden extreme nervousness or fear about something having to do with performance or doing something challenging in front of a group? An exam or anything at all?

MARY: No.

RANDAL: When it first happened, then, did it seem to be clear out of the blue? That not only had you always felt fine about public speaking until then, but you also had not really had that kind of experience?

MARY: That's right.

RANDAL: This is quite an interesting mystery. One of the things we might do in our session, Mary, is to go back and ask you some ideomotor questions about that incident to try to get a sense of what it was about. Usually when someone has a sudden strong feeling like that it can be associated with one thing or another.

MARY: There is one thing. I was reading something in a book that took me back to an experience in first grade which...(Mary's voice becomes almost inaudible) was a horrible experience.

RANDAL: What happened?

MARY: A horrible experience. And I really hadn't thought of it before until I was reading this. I don't know if that's what this current issue stems from or what that was.

RANDAL: Can you talk about that experience now, about what happened in first grade?

MARY: Sure. I got hauled up to the front of the class and...(Mary sighs and stops)

RANDAL: (joking) I don't see that this has to do with anything here. I got hauled up to the front of the class! (Mary and the audience laugh) Please go on.

MARY: And got my mouth taped up shut.

RANDAL: (Randal and several people in the audience moan) That's too bad. Because you were talking in the class or something?

MARY: Yes, I was talking.

RANDAL: You were in the first grade. Did the teacher sit you in front of the class then or send you back to your seat or what?

MARY: I sat up in front of the class for the entire day with my mouth taped.

RANDAL: The whole rest of the morning or the afternoon or what?

MARY: Well, we took a break and we took lunch and both times I came back and got taped up again. (the audience and Randal moan again) I sat there for the whole day. I guess I felt that if I had been guilty and I was getting punished, you know, getting what I deserved, it wouldn't have been so bad. But I felt I was unjustly charged.

RANDAL: That certainly can make such a trauma even worse.

MARY: Well, I thought I had gotten over it but now I'm kind of wondering.

RANDAL: Uh huh. Are there any other memories you can think of or anything about the feeling you get that you would like to add before we do the hypnosis?

MARY: I don't think so.

RANDAL: We have plenty here to work with. Let's lay this blanket down and you can get comfortable. (Mary gets comfortably settled on the blanket with a pillow under her knees and Randal sits beside her) Perhaps you'll be surprised at how comfortable you can feel even with bright lights overhead. In fact you can use that as part of your induction, okay?

MARY: Okay.

RANDAL: I want to assure you, Mary, that I'm only going to take you where your subconscious mind signals it's okay to go. I know how difficult it has been for you to deal with this. I'll help you in a way that will be safe and will work out fine for you.

Now I'd like you to look at that bright light over there. Stare at that light and take a deep breath. That's right, exhale slowly and relax now. Take a second deep breath, staring at that light. Exhale slowly and relax now. Take a third deep breath and this time I want you to look at my fingers as they move toward your face. (Randal moves his hand slowly toward Mary's eyes) Look at my finger tips as I move my hand down and it will cause your eyelids to close down. (Mary's eyes follow Randal's fingers and close down)

Continuing to breath slowly, comfortably and deeply as I count from three to one. At the count of one feel your eyelids lock tightly closed. You will try to open them but the harder you try the tighter they lock together and the deeper into hypnosis you go. Three, stuck tightly. Two, sealed together. One, go ahead and try but they're stuck together. When I touch your left shoulder stop trying and go deeper. (Randal touches Mary on her shoulder)

All right, let your breathing be slow, steady, rhythmic and continuous. I'm going to lift up your left hand. Let your hand hang loosely and limply in my hand. I'd like you to take a nice, comfortable, deep breath and fill up your lungs. On the exhale, as I drop your hand, send a wave of relaxation down your body and go much deeper. (Randal drops the hand as she exhales) That's good. Now another nice deep breath (Randal picks up the right hand) and on the exhale send another wave of relaxation down your body and feel yourself go much deeper. (Randal drops the hand) Much deeper.

I'm going to put the tips of your left thumb and left forefinger together. I'd like you to imagine that I'm placing epoxy glue on the finger tips. (Randal squeezes the fingertips together) The glue is hardening, hardening, hardening, until they're stuck tightly together. I'm going to count from three to one. At the count of one try to pull your finger and thumb apart. The harder you try the tighter they squeeze together and the deeper into hypnosis you go. (Randal moves his fingers away) Three, stuck tighter and tighter. Two, sealed together. One, go ahead and try to pull them apart but they're stuck together. (Mary's fingers strain to pull apart but stay stuck) That's good. When I snap my fingers you'll be able to separate your fingers just as if the glue instantly dissolves and you'll go much deeper. (Randal snaps his fingers and Mary's finger and thumb fall apart) As I adjust your hand you go much deeper and let go of any remaining sensation of the glue.

This time I'm going to count from three down to one. At the count of one only your eyelids open. When your eyelids open I'll snap my fingers like this (Randal snaps his fingers) in front of your face. When I snap my fingers your eyelids instantly close and you go much deeper. Getting ready now, three, two, one, opening, opening, opening. (Mary's eyes open) Sleep now (Randal snaps his fingers and Mary's eyes close down), close your eyes and go deeper. We'll do that again. Three, two, one, opening. (Mary's eyes open, Randal snaps his fingers and they close down again) Sleep now, close your eyes and go deeper. One more time. Three, two, one (Mary's eyes open, Randal snaps his fingers and they close down again), close your eyes and go deeper. Whenever I snap my fingers and say the words "sleep now" you close your eyes and go deeper.

Mary, I'm going to be asking you some questions about the subject we've been discussing, a feeling of nervousness that you sometimes get regarding public speaking. Before I ask you questions about that I'm going to have you practice putting attention on your right hand. There is a certain finger that is your "yes" finger. I'd like you to see the word "yes" in your mind's eye. Hear the word "yes." Think the word "yes" until a certain finger begins to rise and to lift. That's right, keep thinking the word "yes." (Mary's right index finger rises) That's good. You can rest that finger now. Your index finger is your "yes" finger. (Randal taps the finger)

Now I would like you to visualize the word "no." There is a certain finger that is your "no" finger. Just think, hear, see the word "no" in your mind's eye until a certain finger begins to lift and to rise. (Mary's middle finger rises) Good, your middle finger is your "no" finger. (Randal taps the finger)

Now, there is a certain finger, your thumb or your little finger or perhaps your ring finger, that can signal "I don't know." If even your subconscious mind doesn't know the answer, then imagine a gray question mark and the proper finger begins to lift and to rise. (Mary's thumb begins to rise) There we go. You can rest the thumb back down. This is your "I don't know" signal. Usually your subconscious mind will know the answer but if it doesn't then you can signal with your thumb. And if there is some reason you can't answer the question, maybe the question is structured in such a way that it's not answerable in a yes or a no way, then you can signal with the little finger of your right hand.

I'm asking your subconscious mind now, Mary, and your subconscious can respond with the appropriate finger signal. The question I'm about to ask you has to do with the feelings of nervousness that you sometimes get regarding public speaking. Is it safe and appropriate for you to become consciously aware of any and all memories that have to do with your fear of public speaking? (Mary's index finger moves) The answer to the question is yes. Fine. The next question, Mary, is it safe and appropriate for you to be open to your emotions as you recall any and all memories that have to do with your fear of public speaking? (Mary's index finger moves) And the answer is yes. All right.

I'm going to help you get in touch with some uncomfortable feelings so that you can go through them and be very successful in getting beyond them. This will be a safe place for you to do this. I want to assure you that even though you're going to be moving soon into an uncomfortable place, that it'll be for the purpose of being able to get to the other side. To not have this be a part of you any more, to have it rapidly diminish until it fades away as a memory. You have many experiences of being a very talented and comfortable public speaker and you'll have all of that background to work from as well.

Here we go now. I'm going to count from one to ten and with each number that I count you're going to be more and more aware of that feeling of nervousness that you sometimes get. That feeling of nervousness about speaking. Number one, two, becoming aware of that feeling. Three, four, you're standing there or you're sitting there and you're getting nervous about something. Maybe it'll be difficult to get the words out. Five, perhaps your throat is tightening. Six, perhaps your knees are feeling weak. Seven, perhaps you're breathing quickly. Eight, perhaps you're feeling some other kind of uncomfortable sensation. Number nine, feeling the feelings more and more intensely. The feeling of extreme nervousness. Number ten.

Stay with the feeling you're feeling right now. I'm going to count quickly from ten down to one. You're going to go back to an earlier time when you had the same feeling of nervousness. Where it was hard for you to talk, hard for you to think. You were really feeling nervous and scared. Ten, nine, going back in time. That's good. Stay with the feeling. Eight, seven, six, going back to an earlier time in your life where you felt that same feeling. Wherever you go is fine, there is no set place. Five, four, three, some place where you felt

Mary's Fear of Public Speaking 81

that feeling of nervousness. Two, when you felt that feeling of nervousness. On the next number I count you're right there. One. You're right there now. You can verbalize and respond to me. Mary, are you inside or outside? Pick one.

MARY: Inside.

RANDAL: Is it nighttime or daytime?

MARY: Daytime.

RANDAL: Are you alone or with others?

MARY: With others.

RANDAL: Are you under thirty years old? Yes or no. (Mary sighs) Are you a fairly young adult?

MARY: No. About thirty.

RANDAL: You're about thirty years old. I picked a number at random and it happens to have hit it. You're thirty years old, Mary, and you're inside. Describe where you are when you say inside. Is this a building or something else?

MARY: It's a classroom.

RANDAL: Are you taking a class or are you teaching a class?

MARY: I'm a teacher.

RANDAL: Okay, you're in a classroom and you're a teacher. Are you in the process of teaching at this moment?

MARY: Yes.

RANDAL: So this is the situation. What are you feeling right now as you teach?

MARY: I'm feeling nervous.

RANDAL: Did this nervousness suddenly happen or did it happen gradually?

MARY: Just happened.

RANDAL: Just happened. Suddenly felt nervous. Have you felt nervous as a teacher in front of a class before?

MARY: No.

RANDAL: All right. Now you suddenly feel nervous. Is there something you were doing or saying or something that happened that suddenly made you feel nervous? Be there now. Suddenly you feel nervous. What is causing you to feel nervous?

MARY: I look at the class and see that one girl.

RANDAL: Is this the girl you referred to before, the sister of your friend, or is this someone else?

MARY: No, it's her.

RANDAL: Is there something about looking at this young woman, some association you have, that causes you to feel nervous?

MARY: I don't understand what's causing it.

RANDAL: So you just know that you're looking at her and you start feeling nervous. Is that it or is it something different?

MARY: (Mary sighs) I feel like I'm not going to be clear enough. Like I'm not going to be able to present the material as well as I should.

RANDAL: Is there a time in the past when you didn't present the material as well as you should?

MARY: No.

RANDAL: In general you've been a very good teacher, haven't you?

MARY: Yes.

RANDAL: All right. Stay with this feeling of nervousness. In fact, give me a report. Physically, what do you feel right now in your body?

MARY: I feel all shaky.

RANDAL: Do you notice anything else?

MARY: I'm short of breath.

RANDAL: Is there anything else that you notice?

MARY: I'm tight.

RANDAL: Where do you feel tight?

MARY: My eyes.

RANDAL: Your eyes.

MARY: My mouth.

RANDAL: Your mouth. Uh huh. Stay with those feelings. Feeling shaky, shortness of breath, tightness in your eyes and mouth. You're going to go back to an earlier time when you felt these same feelings. Something about being in public and being afraid of the situation. I'm going to count from five down to one. At the count of one you'll be there. Five, feeling shaky, shortness of breath, tight eyes, tight mouth, that tension, that nervousness. Four, feel those feelings. Three, you're going back to an earlier time when you had those same feelings. Two. One. Going back to the earlier time now. You're starting to see the scene. All right, this time is it nighttime or daytime? Pick one.

MARY: Daytime.

RANDAL: Are you inside or outside?

MARY: Inside.

RANDAL: Are you alone or with others?
MARY: With others.
RANDAL: Your age, are you under twenty years old?
MARY: Under.
RANDAL: Are you a child?
MARY: Yes.
RANDAL: How old are you?
MARY: (Mary sighs) Six.
RANDAL: Six. All right, you're six years old. What's the situation? Stay with your feelings.
MARY: I'm in the classroom.
RANDAL: You're in the classroom. What's happening?
MARY: (sigh) I'm sitting in the chair in front of the class.
RANDAL: Uh huh. Is this the incident you were talking about before or is this a different incident?
MARY: It's the same one.
RANDAL: And how do you feel as you're there in the chair in front of the class?
MARY: Not very good.
RANDAL: No, I'll bet you don't. Are you feeling nervous or are you feeling something different?
MARY: Mad.
RANDAL: Mad, yes. Get inside your body right now and feel that. What does your body feel like?
MARY: I'm angry.
RANDAL: Who are you angry at?
MARY: That damn teacher.
RANDAL: That's right. What do you want to tell the teacher?
MARY: She should be a little more fair.
RANDAL: Put her in front here. She's right here and I'm helping you. You've got my support and you can tell her off. Talk to her now. "You should be more fair." What do you want to say to her?
MARY: Well, you should have a better understanding of what's going on in your class.
RANDAL: Right! Tell her some more.
MARY: If you were taking care of your class the way you should be I wouldn't be here.
RANDAL: Good! Now be her. What does she say?
MARY: Oh, you kids. Little brats. You need to be quiet when I'm talking.

RANDAL: Uh huh. Switch and be Mary. Is that what you're called when you're six years old? (Mary nods) Okay, Mary, tell the teacher off. She's just called you a bunch of brats and she said you should be quiet when she's talking. What do you want to say to her?

MARY: That little boy pulled my hair. It's kind of hard to be quiet when you're getting your hair yanked.

RANDAL: Good. What does she say in response to that?

MARY: You shouldn't have such a problem.

RANDAL: What do you want to say to that?

MARY: Well, it's not my problem.

RANDAL: Uh huh. Good. Get inside your body. What do you feel in your body right now?

MARY: Still mad. (Mary's hands are clenched into fists)

RANDAL: Mad. Okay, I want you to imagine the teacher being here right now. (Randal gets a pillow and holds it in front of Mary and puts her hands on it) And I want you to squeeze her or punch her or whatever you want to do. (Mary punches the pillow several times) Good. Punch her. Punch her again. Use both hands now. (Mary delivers several blows) That's good, hit her hard now. (Mary punches the pillow hard) Say, "I hate you." (no response from Mary) "I hate you." (no response again but Mary punches the pillow) That's good. Hit her. Tell her, "You're wrong!"

MARY: You're wrong!

RANDAL: That's right! Say it again!

MARY: (shouting) You're wrong. You're wrong.

RANDAL: Good. Relax. Breathe into your stomach. That's very good. You're doing something that you couldn't do at the time but you're doing it now and that's so good for you because you've been carrying around that teacher for a long time. What do you feel now?

MARY: Okay now.

RANDAL: Good. What do you want to tell the teacher now? Do you want to elaborate or have you pretty much said what you need to say for the moment?

MARY: I'd just like to ask her if she wouldn't be a little more observant.

RANDAL: Okay, now turn that around and tell her "I want you to be more observant." Put her right here and tell her that.

MARY: I want you to be more observant and fair to each one of the kids. And treat each one individually.

RANDAL: Yes, good. Now switch and what does the teacher say in response to that?
MARY: It's probably a good idea. I hadn't thought about it.
RANDAL: Good. You're getting through to her. Now switch. What else would you like to say to her?
MARY: Just treat me fairly and let me learn.
RANDAL: What does the teacher say to that?
MARY: All right. We'll work something out.
RANDAL: Switch and be Mary. What do you want to say to the teacher? Is there anything else you want from her?
MARY: No, I just want her to promise..
RANDAL: Say, "I want you to promise."
MARY: I want you to promise that you'll be fair.
RANDAL: What does the teacher say now?
MARY: Okay, sweetie.
RANDAL: Good, now be Mary. What else do you want to say? What else do you want from her?
MARY: That's all.
RANDAL: All right. Teacher, do you have anything else to say or to ask of Mary?
MARY: No, that's all.
RANDAL: All right, switch and be Mary again. Go inside your body. Breathe down to your stomach, slowly and deeply. What do you feel in your body?
MARY: Relaxed.
RANDAL: Good. Is there anything you notice in particular in any part of your body?
MARY: No.
RANDAL: You feel good?
MARY: Uh huh.
RANDAL: Great. You sure look good. Good job. (to the audience) It's all there in the body. Her body feels clear. Sometimes a person will need to continue to release feelings or make further communication. It just depends upon the individual. There was so much going on in Mary's body. The golden rule in Gestalt is to do unto others as you do unto yourself. She had been forced in that situation to hold back all that tension and all that anger. Now she was able to get it out by hitting the pillow and communicating as she did and she's feeling really clear.

(to Mary) You've just expunged that experience and I want you to feel that in your body. Feel the joy in your body. Feel how clear your body feels now from your head to your toes. Feel the energy in your body and the aliveness there. Feel the clarity, like clean, warm water flowing through your body. You're completely loose and limp and relaxed from your head to your toes.

At this point in a session, Mary, I will often have a person analyze what happened and how it had an effect on their life. My intuition is that I don't feel that needs to be done now. I'd like you to just stay in touch with your experience. Your body feels so clear. You know what happened. You're aware that there was a certain experience you had that still affected you and you've just released the tension from that experience. It no longer needs to have a hold on you. You can be yourself now. You can be relaxed and express yourself clearly. You can have a memory of something that happened that was difficult at the time but you've released the tension and it's just a memory.

You've got many pleasant experiences of speaking clearly and expressing the thoughts you wish to convey. In fact, you are an outstanding public speaker. You've done that many times. You are also a very good teacher. You teach clearly and with confidence. Your mouth is moist and gestures flow spontaneously from you. If you are standing when you speak in public, you stand with good posture. If you are sitting, you sit with good posture. Your head is held high, your eyes see the beauty of the world around you and you pick out people in the audience. A smile automatically comes to your lips at the proper time and there are many such proper times. You are eloquent. You are knowledgeable.

People appreciate what you have to say and are interested in you. They like you. They respect you as a good, decent, talented, skillful, intelligent, warm, loving human being. As the best comes out from you only the best is returned. As you give your caring, your knowledge, your love, your enthusiasm, your insights and your wisdom, as you give of all of these parts of yourself, only the best is returned to you. You deserve the best.

You are finding now in class that if you have a question to ask and it's an appropriate time, you enjoy asking it. And if it's time for you to teach you enjoy being a teacher. You like being in such a position of authority and responsibility. People appreciate you in those positions. You are an excellent teacher, an excellent communicator. In fact you always have been an excellent communicator and there was just a little part of you that needed to get clear. You just let go of something that is rapidly moving into the distant past.

(Note: The purpose of post-hypnotic suggestions is not to proclaim or guarantee that everything is now perfect. The suggestions are given in hypnosis as positive visualizations for the individual to imagine as true, helping to set up the possibility and tendency for that to happen.)

Is there anything that you would like to say now about your experience or is there anything you would like to ask me at this point?

MARY: No.

RANDAL: Are you still feeling clear in your body?

MARY: Yes.

RANDAL: Very good. I'm going to stop talking for a couple of minutes, Mary. I want you take some time to just enjoy this feeling of being clear. You may even get a time distortion because you're so aware right now. You have such a heightened awareness that this two minutes is going to seem much longer. It'll be a perfect length of time for you to just be with your experience. Be in your body. Breathe down into your belly and feel yourself feeling clear. Feel yourself being totally free, strong, healthy and joyful, and I'll begin talking again in a couple of minutes. (after two minutes) Okay, Mary, are you looking forward to public speaking under the appropriate circumstances? Looking forward to speaking up in class when you have an inkling to do that?

MARY: Yes.

RANDAL: Are you looking forward to doing some more teaching at work?

MARY: Yes.

RANDAL: Are you looking forward to teaching as a talented self-hypnosis instructor in self-hypnosis classes?

MARY: Absolutely.

RANDAL: Great. Are you looking forward to speaking in front of hundreds of people on how they can get value from hypnotherapy, as a very well known and talented and well respected hypnosis instructor?

MARY: Yes.

RANDAL: So whether you're doing hypnosis work in private sessions and self-hypnosis classes, or perhaps leading seminars for large numbers of people as a very talented instructor, the world is out there for you, Mary. You can go wherever you want to go and you deserve to have all the success. Let your joy shine through.

I want you to know that since the beginning of the class I have found you a joy to be around. You've been so enthusiastic and positive. You've been commuting 6,000 miles roundtrip each weekend to class for four months and I really appreciate that. I don't know how anyone could not really like you.

MARY: Thank you.

RANDAL: You're welcome. You're a beautiful person. I thank you for being in this class and for everything you've given. And I thank you for the courage you have to deal with your greatest fear during this process. That says a lot for this class and it says a lot for you. I appreciate that you can trust me and yourself and this group. You were feeling so concerned about having this experience and I'd like you to notice how well it works to face your deepest fears and know that you can trust yourself. You've come through to the other side and come through just brilliantly and freely.

In the days ahead you're going to be feeling a tremendous feeling of joy and relief and lightness. You've always had so many positive aspects within yourself, Mary, and I don't know exactly how it's going to take place, but you're going to find even more self-discovery in the days and weeks ahead. Even more ways of enjoying your life and feeling your happiness and your friendships and your enthusiasm. You're just feeling that much more alive and aware in appreciating the many wonderful things you have in your life.

I'm going to count from one to five. With each number that I count you become more and more alert, awake and aware. At the count of five you open your eyes and you are then fully alert, rested, refreshed and feeling good. You'll notice that colors and sights and sounds are beautiful. It's a tremendous feeling of awareness. Before we count I'd like to do something, Mary. Just stay in hypnosis. Is there anybody in the class who would like to say something to Mary?

ANN: Thank you for your courage.

LOUISE: I'd like to speak for the children who witnessed what happened to you, Mary. I'm sure they felt bad, too, because I witnessed a boy who had to hold a towel in front of his face and I cried for weeks. I still think of him. So even in your agony there were probably a lot of other kids who were feeling your pain.

KAY: I'm really happy for you that you had the courage today to do this by yourself. I know you really wanted to and I'm glad you had a chance.

SUSAN: I hope you could feel our energy but if you could have seen it – we were so behind you. Just right there with you. We're so proud. You were doing exactly what we all wanted to do and we thank you for that.

RANDAL: All right, thank you all. Counting from one to five, coming back to your full, conscious awareness. Number one, getting ready. Number two, hey, this coming back to full consciousness has never been so good, has it? Number three, more and more alert, awake and aware with each number. Number four, getting ready to open your eyes. On the next number I count you open your eyes and are then fully alert, awake and aware. Coming back, number five. Open your eyes, wide awake. (Randal and Mary hold each other for about two minutes and talk quietly) Are you ready to sit up now? Look around you. Take a look at these beautiful people. Take a look at everybody in the class, at all the love that is there for you. (Mary looks around)

MARY: Thank you. Thank you all.

RANDAL: Let's hear it for Mary! (applause)

RANDAL: (after a break Randal and Mary come back and sit in front of the class) Is there anything you would like to say to the class about your experience or anything you've thought of since you came out of the hypnosis?

MARY: It was such a calming experience and I felt so clear and so good. I got rid of all that nervous worrisome feeling I had and it happened so quickly. I mean all of a sudden it disappeared. It was great.

RANDAL: Usually I would have a person do some hypnoanalysis but I skipped that process because your body was so clear and you were so peaceful. It was obvious that you had been holding this stuff in and then you released it and it was gone. It's really a compliment to you that you were able to do it just like that, fairly simply and easily, with no resistance. You did well with hitting the pillow and doing some dialogue. It was very pleasing to see the teacher coming around and finally listening to you. Once you start hitting a teacher they start waking up. That's not something for you to do to me - you can talk to me! (laughter)

I got several comments during the break and I've been waiting to acknowledge what some people said about how simple and powerful this process is. This was a relatively easy version in the sense that there wasn't any resistance and it went like clockwork. These catastrophic expectations had been such a difficult thing for Mary, then imagine dealing with these public speaking fears as therapy in front of the class. Some of you have already done therapy in class and you know it's not easy. Realistically you might think, "Well, this is a very supportive group, a good teacher, I'm ready to work on this," but it still can be quite a challenge. At the time, just before the breakthrough, it can feel very scary.

(to Mary) When you were talking with me during the break you communicated how the process of just being up here was difficult for you but you were confronting it. You were hitting it head on. (she nods)

Once you've done this process for awhile it becomes obvious what to do next. It goes step by step, Gestalting it and expressing it and going back. And notice that I didn't tell Mary to go back to that incident when she saw the sister of her friend or when she was six years old. I just told her to go back to an earlier incident. It's not surprising that she went back to the time when she was about thirty years old.

By the way, it's not necessary to know what exactly that girl reminded her of. What's important is that something about that triggered the extreme nervousness and the next step is returning to the initial sensitizing event. Mary was really ready for it and her subconscious mind came up with it. The two places she went were the obvious ones from our pre-induction interview but I was careful to be neutral in coaxing the memories in case there was another significant memory that needed to surface.

You could feel Mary's energy when she was in front of the class and the tension that was rising in her body. (to Mary) Your hands were in fists. I knew you needed to get something out, and I suggested that you do something with the pillow. Punching was what you ended up doing. Then I came up with a spontaneous comment that seemed to fit, which was to tell the teacher, "I hate you." If a suggested comment doesn't fit it's of course fine for someone to change it. You didn't respond to that so I came up with another one, saying, "You're wrong," and you responded to that. I want to check that out with you, Mary. Did the first comment seem too strong or what? What was your feeling?

MARY: It felt inappropriate.

RANDAL: (to the class) So that is a perfect example of someone being highly suggestible, highly responsive to direction at a particularly emotional time, but being her own person. She was saying "no" to me, that she was not going to do that, so I quickly dropped it. On the other hand, there are times when a person might be holding back because of fear of the response. It's important to know the difference. If Mary had said earlier, "I really hate you," then I may have encouraged it more vigorously or discussed it with her. In this case she was doing well with hitting the pillow, so I sensed the first suggested statement wasn't good and came up with an alternative that worked.

During Gestalt, I sometimes suggest words to say that I feel fit the situation because I want to keep clients in their feelings or bring them even more into their feelings, so they don't have to think what to say. If you say something that doesn't quite fit, the person will usually let you know in one way or another and you can go in a different direction. But another option would be to say, "What do you want to say to the teacher? Tell the teacher how you feel."

Now we'll open up for questions. Janet?

JANET: I liked the way you kept saying to her, "Give me a report on what's happening in your body," because when a person is going through those heavy emotions I think it's really good to verbalize that. It takes them back to that place.

RANDAL: There are actually several things that are accomplished by that. The report is valuable for the therapist and valuable for the client as well. It lets the therapist know what the person is feeling. Some things can be sensed, especially when it's physically obvious because the person is shaking or the throat or hands are tense, but there are other things that might not be as obvious. So it tells the therapist about the person and it is also a way for the person to get in touch with her own experience and feel it without running away from it.

On top of that, the therapist can get a sense about which feelings seem to be the prominent ones. The one that jumps out at me is intuitively the one to go with. Is it the tension, is it the shaking, is it the fiery ball inside of someone? Whatever they describe, I look at how I can help them to express that. When that energy is held inside the body it's unhealthy. The energy needs to be released. How can this be done? By becoming the fiery ball in the stomach, or becoming that pounding sensation in the heart. If there is a tight sensation then you ask the person to intensify the tightening or squeeze a pillow. It's so natural how this works. To take whatever the feeling is and find a symbolic way of expressing it.

There were several possibilities for Mary. Her hands were clenched in fists and she was announcing that she was feeling angry. Hitting was a natural direction to develop from that. It doesn't always have to become a physical thing. If the person is having that sensation you can encourage a dialogue with another part to communicate that sensation. It can be done verbally as well as physically.

JANET: If you don't see those signs but you know they're struggling with all those emotions could you have just said, "Describe that feeling of pain?"

RANDAL: Within the hypnosis I try not to give it a name unless it's really obvious or the client has used the word. If Mary hadn't used the word angry and had just said, "I feel my hands are clenched," then there may be other feelings, too. By the way, there is no one feeling a person should feel. Instead of anger she might have felt horror or fear or grief or shame, etc. Whatever the feeling is, that's the one to get in touch with. You can be aware that beneath fear there may be anger or something else and you want to help her express her fear to get it out of her system. Then you can discover if something else is there. That communication of long-repressed feelings is so healthy for people to be able to do within a safe Gestalt context.

ROBERT: When you regress someone to an earlier age like that, is it necessary to bring them back to the present before you bring them out of hypnosis? To unregress them, so to speak.

RANDAL: That depends. When Mary became very clear I sensed she had released that experience so much that she had spontaneously come back, and intuitively I didn't feel I needed to do that. So I don't automatically feel that it has to be done every time. But more often than not, I will give a suggestion to bring the person back just to make sure. As a habit, once any dialogues are completed and all other aspects of a regression are finished, I will usually do a counting method. I frequently do that progression during the hypnoanalysis which we skipped over with Mary, but in her case it was accomplished indirectly by acknowledging how Mary had let go of this experience.

If I had done the hypnoanalysis at that point what I would typically say is, "I'm going to count from one to ten. As I count forward you will remember this experience but you will be able to get in touch with your adult self now and look back on that experience and see what effect it has been having on you until now. When you get a realization about how that has been affecting your behavior you can signal with your 'yes' finger and then we'll talk about it." With Mary what it was about was so obvious that I didn't feel any need to do that and a progression could have possibly distracted her from the essence of her experience, which was her powerful presence and feeling of being completely clear in her body.

MARY: You were asking me how I was feeling in my body afterwards, when I began to feel good. I didn't really realize it until you asked, that all of a sudden I didn't have any tightness. It was all gone, but I hadn't consciously realized it before you asked.

RANDAL: You were feeling clear and good but you weren't aware of that lack of tightness because you were paying attention to the process as it was happening and not comparing it to the recent past. That's another reason for having you go within and describe your internal experience. It's so healthy for us to keep getting in touch with ourselves. Until you became aware of it you couldn't fully appreciate it, and once you fully appreciate it, your experience becomes even more terrific.

MARY: Yes, really.

RANDAL: It's amazing how the physical, mental, emotional and spiritual are all tied in. One part will affect the other parts so profoundly. If she is feeling clear emotionally then her body will feel clear. It's so simple and beautiful. What an honor to be able to be with someone that has just done such profound regression work and is so wide open. It's like being a newborn baby in some ways. The subconscious is so receptive during hypnosis. We're able to reach someone in such a deep state of inner awareness and to work with and shift the subconscious tremendously. Thank you again, Mary. (applause)

MARY: Randal, your love of your work is contagious. I caught it.

RANDAL: Thank you. That's great. (Randal and Mary hug)

Mary Writes Six Years Later

After reading the copy of my session, I discovered that I've received many more benefits than I had realized at the time - over and above, eliminating the fear of public speaking.

What was remarkable to me was, that for the first time, I had confirmation of having reached a level that I had striven for all of my life (and felt that I was living) but was a little hazy about. When I didn't respond to the suggestion to the teacher that: "I hate you!" I now know that I have truly learned from early parental guidance NEVER to hate anyone, say it, or even think it. The fact that I didn't respond in that manner in spite of the emotion that wracked my heart and body is proof to me. Being able to punch that pillow as hard as I could was an enormous release - although I would never have chosen that method if you hadn't suggested it, it felt perfectly right. I felt completely safe in expressing and releasing that powerful anger, *feeling* it "washing out of my body" as you suggested. On reflection I now feel immeasurably stronger from knowing myself better.

Yet another lesson learned - even six years later!

I know that your intuition when working with a client is incredible, having observed it in class so many times. And I know that there is a reason for everything you say and suggest, whether it's apparent at the moment or not.

In addition to your openness, enabling intuition and telepathy to serve you on whatever level you require, there is another element - that of creating a feeling of safety, a sanctuary extending around and enfolding the person with whom you are working.

I would like to add that I have had opportunity to "test" my public speaking skills since that magnificent session with you, and I am happy to report that public speaking is not only possible now, but it is a pure joy! There is an entirely different feeling about conveying my thoughts to a group - a feeling of excitement and fun - a feeling of setting the mood, being in charge, and communicating like I've never felt before - a feeling that I am in the process of learning as I'm teaching. This last awareness keeps subject matter alive, fresh, and open, no matter how many times it's taught.

Once again, Randal, Thank you!

CHAPTER 8

Sophie's Grief
Saying Goodbye to Grandma

SOPHIE: You led a guided meditation during class in which we met a loved one, and I met my French Canadian grandmother, who raised me in Quebec. She started to raise me, actually, when I was two months old because my mother went back to work and she lived with us. Then she died in a very sudden way when I was thirteen. I came home from school one day and found out she had died during the night. She was just gone. I realize there is a lot of sadness attached to her memory instead of feeling all the love that was there between us. For me, when someone talks about unconditional love, she is automatically the one I think about. We were so close and I know I was all she had in the world and she would have died for me. I always said that.

RANDAL: Were you an only child?

SOPHIE: I was the oldest. For five years I was alone and then my sister was born. During the guided visualization I realized how deeply I feel a sense of loss inside and there was that experience of, "I love you so much. Where are you now?" It was painful. I've been trying to process the whole thing by myself but it's too big to do alone. It's not a huge issue but it's something I really want to work on.

RANDAL: Actually, it sounds like something that is very important to you.

SOPHIE: Yes.

RANDAL: Often a problem is the solution to a previous problem, but in this case you've got a problem that is in large part the result of a great deal of good fortune in having had such a special grandmother. Are you ready for some hypnosis?

SOPHIE: Yes.

RANDAL: I'm really getting quick at this pre-induction interview. (laughter) All right. (Sophie lies down on a mat) Do you feel comfortable?

SOPHIE: Uh huh.

RANDAL: Look at my little finger. Keep watching my little finger and feel your eyelids growing heavy. (Randal is moving his hand back and forth toward Sophie's forehead, then down in front of her eyes) Follow my finger down until your eyelids close. (Sophie's eyes close) Relax your eyelids completely. Now imagine them becoming so heavy that they are locking more and more tightly closed. Sealing tightly together. When I snap my fingers you can go ahead and try to open them but the harder you try the more tightly they lock and seal. (Randal snaps his fingers and Sophie tries to open her eyes) When I snap my fingers again relax, stop trying and go deeper. (Randal snaps his fingers) That's good, deeper relaxed. You can let any sensation of heaviness or feeling of your eyes being stuck together fade away. You could open your eyes if you wanted to, but letting them stay relaxed and closed helps you go deeper and deeper into hypnotic relaxation.

Focus on your breathing now. Let your breathing be slow and steady and deep and continuous. Breathe down deep into your stomach. I'm going to push down on your shoulders and when I do let that be a signal for you to go much deeper. Take a nice deep breath and fill up your lungs. On the exhale send a wave of relaxation down your body. (Randal pushes down as Sophie exhales) That's good. Now another deep breath and on the exhale feel yourself go deeper still. Way down. (Randal pushes down again as she exhales) That's good. And another deep breath. On the exhale this time feel yourself go five times deeper. Way down.

Now I'm going to lift up your left leg. Let your leg hang loosely and limply in my hand. When I drop it send another wave of relaxation all the way down your body and feel yourself go much deeper. (Randal drops her leg) That's fine. Now your right leg. Another nice, deep breath. This time on the exhale feel yourself go much deeper. Way down. (Randal drops her leg) I'm going to gently rock you at your ankles and that will cause your whole body to feel a wave like motion that is taking you deeper and deeper relaxed. (Randal rocks her by her ankles)

Now I'm going to touch your forehead with my finger like this. (Randal taps Sophie on the forehead) The next time I tap your forehead I'd like you to count downward silently and slowly from ten to one, and feel yourself going deeper with each number. Going down to a good, safe place where you can get deeply in touch with your own inner self. Okay, getting ready. Focus on your breathing. As I touch your forehead begin counting silently to yourself. (Randal taps Sophie on the forehead and stops talking for a couple of minutes) That's fine. Going deeper and deeper. If you're continuing to count just keep counting as you listen to me now.

I'd like you to imagine a brilliant star of white light shining down on your head, your neck, your shoulders, your chest. (Randal's voice temporarily slows down) Shining down on your arms, your stomach, your hands, your pelvis. All the way down your legs, all the way down to your feet. Any tension, any negativity, is draining out of your body through the palms of your hands and the soles of your feet as you continue to be bathed in this white light. Something very special is about to happen. You're going to get a chance to meet with your grandmother. I'm going to count from five down to one and when I reach the count of one you'll be able to speak and describe the scene. Five, four, three, two, one. What's the scene?

SOPHIE: She's in the hospital.

RANDAL: Is this at a time just before she passed away?

SOPHIE: No. It would be a year or two before that. She had an operation and we all thought she would die. I'm just entering the room. She sits up in her bed when she sees me and puts her arms out so she can hold me. (pause) The emotion there is very strong. She's holding me so tightly that it's hard for me to breathe. And she says, "It's so good to see you." (Sophie's voice is trembling) It was so touching.

RANDAL: This is something that actually happened, right? (Sophie nods) Good, be right there. Are you about eleven or twelve years old at this time?

SOPHIE: About that.

RANDAL: Just stay there with it. Feel all that love she has for you and how thrilled she is to be there with you and how thrilled you are to be there with her.

SOPHIE: (in a tearful voice) But there is something else there. I feel that she was afraid of dying.

RANDAL: Turn it into the present tense. You're there now with her and you can sense that she is afraid of dying. At this time the part of you that has lived through that knows she is going to live a while longer, but you can be back there now and feel that she's afraid to die.

SOPHIE: She's holding onto me and it's very powerful. It's hard to describe what I feel. I'm a little bit afraid but I also love her so much and I say that. I hold her back.

RANDAL: You say you hold her back. Is that the way you feel you can be most supportive of her?

SOPHIE: Yes.

RANDAL: Imagine being there as if it's really happening right now and if you could tell her something about your feelings, what would you like to say? She's here in the hospital and she's been holding onto you and you really love her.

SOPHIE: I want to answer you but something else is going on.

RANDAL: Yes?

SOPHIE: I got kind of an insight. On a deep level, I don't know how to express it, but maybe in a way I feel responsible that she's dead.

RANDAL: Let's go with that. (Sophie breaks into sobs) Keep breathing down into your stomach. It's okay to cry. Feel your feelings. Become that part of you that feels responsible for her dying. (Sophie cries louder) You don't have to say anything. It's good to cry.

SOPHIE: (halting and sobbing) She was trying so hard to...when I was a child it was very difficult...my relationship with both of my parents was very difficult and she was always the one accepting me and loving me. She was always there between my parents and me, taking my side.

RANDAL: Can you make that present tense? "She's always here taking my side."

SOPHIE: Yes, she's always here for me. She understands me and she protects me, but at eleven years old I became rebellious and I'm afraid she couldn't deal with that. She couldn't maintain the role of protecting me and she just had to go away. ((breaking into sobs) She couldn't love me anymore the way she wanted to.

RANDAL: Let's bring her here and find out. I'm going to count from five down to one. At the count of one she is right here. We're going to go forward to a time just before she died, so you're thirteen years old. She may be close to death now but she's able to speak. At the count of one you're right there with her. Five, four, three, two, one. She has been listening to you and she has heard what you just said. I'd like you to tell her what you're afraid of.

SOPHIE: She wasn't sick when she died. It was a sudden heart attack during the night. I didn't know about it until I came back from school and she was gone already.

RANDAL: All right, I want you to bring her spirit here. She has just had this heart attack and passed away. What would you like to say to her?

SOPHIE: Why did you leave me? Why?

RANDAL: When I touch your shoulder switch and be your grandmother's spirit and respond. What is your name when you're thirteen?

SOPHIE: Sophie.

RANDAL: Okay, respond to thirteen year old Sophie. (Randal touches Sophie on the shoulder) "Why did you leave me?" What do you have to say to her?

SOPHIE: She's tired.

RANDAL: So be her. Say, "I'm tired."

SOPHIE: (in a tired voice) I'm tired. (sigh) I love you but I'm tired. I've given you...(breaks into sobs) I've given you all my love and I'm just tired.

RANDAL: Okay, switch and be Sophie and respond to your grandmother. (Randal touches Sophie on the shoulder)

SOPHIE: How can we stay together? Because I want you to go wherever you need to go, but I want us to stay together at the same time. I know that's possible.

RANDAL: Switch and be Grandmother. (Randal touches Sophie on the shoulder) Grandmother or Grandma, what do you call her?

SOPHIE: Mammy.

RANDAL: All right, be Mammy. What does she say?

SOPHIE: She says that she is there in my memories.

RANDAL: Become her and say "I'm there in your memory."

SOPHIE: I'm there in your memories of us together and those beautiful emotions that are shared...that were shared and still are shared. That's how I'm still with you.

RANDAL: Good. Switch and be Sophie. (Randal touches Sophie's shoulder)

SOPHIE: I feel okay with that, I really do. I don't feel the pain anymore inside of me.

RANDAL: Okay, you can accept that. You understand that just as she said, it's her time to go. She's tired. It's time to move on but she can be there with you in those ways. Both with what you've had and what you still have together.

SOPHIE: (crying) But I miss her.

RANDAL: Say that to her.

SOPHIE: I miss you so. It would be so wonderful to have you around. But maybe it wouldn't be so wonderful to have you around. I don't know. I just miss you. I love you.

RANDAL: Good. Switch and be Mammy. (Randal touches Sophie on the shoulder) What would you like to say in response?

SOPHIE: (with a little laugh) I'm taking care of you from up here.

RANDAL: Uh huh. I thought so.

SOPHIE: Just be open to it. Ask me for stuff if you need to. Think of me when you need strength and love and courage and comfort. I'm still here for you.

RANDAL: Good. (Randal touches Sophie on the shoulder) Be Sophie.

SOPHIE: Well, I will ask you to help me to have the strength of letting you go. I find that difficult.

RANDAL: Be Mammy. (Randal touches Sophie on the shoulder)

SOPHIE: Everything is perfect the way it is. You have to let me go. I'm with you of my own free will. (switching to herself) What I'm getting is, I don't have to worry about keeping her from going where she wants to go.

RANDAL: Are you Sophie talking about Mammy?

SOPHIE: Yes, back to Sophie again. She's telling me that there is no need to worry that I'm keeping her from going elsewhere in the universe. She's with me because she wants to be with me, she loves me, and that has nothing to do with me keeping her here. That's what I get.

RANDAL: How does that feel?

SOPHIE: It's a relief.

RANDAL: She's been with you all along and you were naturally out of touch with that, although perhaps feeling it on some level.

SOPHIE: I think I was pretty much not in touch with it.

RANDAL: Consciously you were not at all in touch with it, but I don't know about subconsciously. Tell her how you feel about knowing that she's there for you.

SOPHIE: It gives me a lot of comfort. It makes me feel safe in the world. Protected. Very much protected. Thank you for being there.

RANDAL: Now switch and be Mammy. (Randal touches Sophie on the shoulder) Is there anything further you would like to tell Sophie at this time?

SOPHIE: She's laughing. She used to laugh a lot. (pause) She's just hugging me now.

RANDAL: Good, take it in because right now you can really feel her hug.

SOPHIE: I can hear her laughter, too.

RANDAL: Good, feel that warmth and hear that lovely laughter once again. And you can come back and feel her hugs and hear her laughter whenever you want from now on, because she is there for you. (pause) Is there anything further you'd like to say or ask her? Is there any appreciation you'd like to give her?

SOPHIE: Well, I want to thank her for...

RANDAL: "Thank you."

SOPHIE: Thank you for the incredible amount of love you had and still have for me. And how generous and beautiful you are. You're a strong woman. Thank you for your laughter and your joy. Most of all thank you for your deep, deep care for me.

RANDAL: Be Mammy. (Randal touches Sophie on the shoulder) Do you have any appreciation you'd like to give Sophie?

SOPHIE: (pause and then laughter) I don't want to say that out loud.

RANDAL: Okay, say it silently to her. That's fine. (pause) Be Sophie and take it in. What are you feeling right now?

SOPHIE: So lucky.

RANDAL: This is Sophie talking, right?

SOPHIE: Yes, this is Sophie talking. I'm so fortunate to have her as part of my life.

RANDAL: Say "to have you as part of my life."

SOPHIE: To have you as part of my life. Because I don't think I would have made it if not for you. I'm sure I wouldn't have made it to where I am today. I owe it all to you. I really feel that. (crying softly)

RANDAL: Great.

SOPHIE: I love you more than I've ever loved anybody in my life.

RANDAL: All right, be Mammy. (Randal touches Sophie on the shoulder) What would you like to say in response?

SOPHIE: Is it okay if I don't say it out loud? Because it's so big.

RANDAL: Say it silently. Just take it in. Be Sophie and hear her telling you that now. (pause) And if she's done you can signal with your "yes" finger. (Sophie signals) Okay. You know that you can contact her any time you want. Do you want to say goodbye to Mammy now? And hear Mammy say goodbye to you. A silent goodbye is fine.

SOPHIE: Okay.

RANDAL: You know you deserve this, Sophie. You deserve to have this wonderful woman who loves you so completely and unconditionally. It's no accident that she's been there for you both in life and after life. You and she have a very special connection. And just as you gained so much from her, she gained so much from you. You're a joy to her. You can use that tremendous strength and joy and love she's sending you. Feel it expanding within you, moving throughout your body and into your heart. Expanding you with every breath that you take. You know that you can feel her love with you and you know deep down that she's been there with you all along. That helps you over and over again in situations in which you find yourself. It gives you courage and strength. You can just feel that energy emanating from her. That love really has a profound effect in helping you feel all the more peace and tranquillity and satisfaction.

It's such a relief to know that it was just her time. So often, you know, children blame themselves or feel directly rejected when someone leaves or passes on, but that's just the reality of life and death. It was time for her to go on and she knew that she would be there with you and now you can feel it too. It might be true that she lived much longer because of you, because she had you to live for all that time. That was one very special part of her life.

Is there anything further you would like to say or to ask before you come out of the hypnosis? (Sophie shakes her head) As you were doing the last parts of the dialogue there, were you experiencing yourself as the child Sophie or the adult Sophie?

SOPHIE: As the adult.

RANDAL: So you're back here as adult Sophie. Breathe down into your stomach. Feel your body and describe what it feels like. Are there any parts you're especially aware of?

SOPHIE: I'm aware of my forehead. There's a little bit of energy stuck there.

RANDAL: Does that feel like a process that's working itself out?

SOPHIE: (laughing) Actually, it's going away now. That's interesting.

RANDAL: Put all of your attention on your forehead and allow that feeling to just be and do what it wants to do. Just embrace that feeling.

SOPHIE: It's like a big vacuum cleaner that sucks out whatever needs to get out.

RANDAL: Let that vacuum cleaner suck out whatever doesn't belong there. (pause) Is that complete now? Does your forehead feel fine?

SOPHIE: It feels good.

RANDAL: Does your body feel good?

SOPHIE: Yes.

RANDAL: All right. I'm going to count from one to five. With every number that I count you become more and more alert, awake and aware. At the count of five you open your eyes and you are then fully alert, wide awake, refreshed and invigorated. Number one, slowly, gently and easily begin to return to your full conscious awareness, continuing to have a sense of peace and wisdom and joy. Number two, as I bring you up out of hypnosis I'll make a few more points here. In the days ahead you are continuing to realize how your grandmother has been with you and you are all the more aware of her presence from now on. On number three, more and more alert, awake and aware. You're finding that energy and feelings are moving more freely and smoothly. You're feeling more grounded and more at peace. On number four, getting ready to open your eyes. On the next number you are fully alert, awake, aware, invigorated, and feeling good. Coming back, number five. Take your time. (as Sophie opens her eyes) Good job. (Sophie sits up and hugs Randal)

SOPHIE: It is such a big relief to know that she's okay. That was bigger than the loss of her. I really wasn't aware of that when we started. I thought I was in grief and yes, I do miss her. But the bigger thing was that I didn't know if she was okay.

RANDAL: Another big thing was discovering and letting go of your hidden guilt. As for your grief, you don't have to be in grief for her or yourself anymore because she's fine and you haven't fully lost her. She isn't here physically but most importantly she is here spiritually.

SOPHIE: Right, and I couldn't get that straight in my head.

RANDAL: It's beautiful that in hypnosis you can get it so much more deeply. Not just intellectually, but you can really experience it.

SOPHIE: Yes, because I never was able to really get it. Something didn't make sense. I couldn't really believe it and now I believe it. I just know it. It's great. I have my Mammy again! (class applauds loudly)

CLASS MEMBER: She has you, too.

SOPHIE: Gee, that's true. She has me, too.

RANDAL: She has you all the more now because now you know she's here. Loss is such a universal experience. (Sophie lies back down) Great! Just relax. Enjoy yourself. (to the class) I felt this was the place to go with Sophie. I could have done an affect bridge and tapped her into her feeling of sadness and then gone back to any earlier time, whether that meant going back to her grandmother or not. But the issue with her grandmother was clearly important and Sophie was obviously in touch with her emotions so I felt it was appropriate to just go there. When someone has lost a loved one it can sometimes be helpful to take them to the death bed. In this case the grandmother died so quickly and unexpectedly in the night that it felt right to take her to just after that.

(to Sophie) When you wondered whether there was some part of you that was to blame for her death you were already in the process of being receptive to whatever she had to say. So often people need to deal with feelings of guilt in having lost someone and it was so important that you let go of that. (to the class) Doing a Gestalt dialogue with the person can often take care of that fairly quickly. Are there any questions?

BOB: (to Sophie): Did you ever use your grandmother as a guide?

SOPHIE: When Randal gave me the suggestion to recall times when she was there for me, I remembered being in a lot of trouble when I was a teenager. Deep trouble! But I would talk to her and she was always there. I had forgotten about that. Something would happen and I would be all right.

RANDAL: Now Sophie can use her as a guide knowing she is there. Some people may have a hard time with such a concept, but I've seen it work over and over again when people feel a deep connection with someone who's passed on. (to Sophie) You've got it! (applause)

Interview two weeks later

RANDAL: How have you been doing since our session?

SOPHIE: Interestingly, the last two weeks have been very challenging emotionally. There is a lot going on with finding emotional support within myself. I'm experiencing losses, which is pretty interesting since I experienced the loss of my grandmother for so many years.

RANDAL: Having just dealt with the loss of your grandmother and in a way finding her as a result of that session, I'm wondering if that's been helpful in what you're dealing with?

SOPHIE: I'm sure it fits in because it all started after that. It's easier to deal with some of this stuff now because she is there.

RANDAL: That's what I would think. You have such a tremendous connection with your grandmother. When people lose a loved one it's such a big issue to say goodbye and this was an experience of saying hello as well as goodbye. Of course your grandmother has been with you all along. Now that you feel her there I would certainly think you could use her as a guide to help you through what you're dealing with in your life now. Have you been doing any specific hypnosis work with her in the last couple of weeks or with her and your inner child?

SOPHIE: I've done work on myself with the inner child and also with other people. I didn't think about integrating her into the hypnosis, although I do talk to her pretty often.

RANDAL: I would suggest that you do some self hypnosis sessions in which you tap in and make an even stronger connection with your grandmother. Does it sound good to do a few sessions like that over the next few weeks and a few with yourself and your inner child as well?

SOPHIE: Yes! I'm going to be busy.

RANDAL: Busy doing good things. When you go to bed and realize you haven't done that in a few days, you can do it right there in bed. Is there anything else you'd like to say about your feelings regarding your grandmother or anything about the session?

SOPHIE: I want to say thank you so much for helping me make that connection.

CHAPTER 9

Ericka's Difficulty with Boundaries

The Little Girl Who Had to be Grown-Up

ERICKA: This morning I woke up with pain throughout my body and I related it to a lot of emotional stuff. We're processing so much in these classes and I tend to take on other people's traumas. Then it becomes overwhelming for me and instead of just being able to let it run through me, I take it in. It's something I've had a problem with all of my life.

RANDAL: How would you summarize the core of what this issue is about?

ERICKA: I don't want to be separate from people but I don't want to be a sponge, absorbing their fears. I sense it and think "I can handle this" and then I wake up in the morning or I come home at night and I'm drained.

RANDAL: So there is an issue of boundaries and of saying no to people in certain ways.

ERICKA: Absolutely.

RANDAL: We may go back to earlier times in your life when these issues came up, and I'll ask for signals from your subconscious early on to determine the appropriateness of that.

ERICKA: Okay.

RANDAL: Can you give any more detail about this issue?

ERICKA: Actually, I'm realizing that a dream is part of it, too. I keep having a recurring dream that I'm having to go back to my last job and work there. One of the issues or patterns in my life is that I go in and rescue businesses that are failing. I run them as if they were my own and make them very successful while the people that own the businesses abuse me the whole time. The more they abuse me the better I have to be at it until I reach the end of my tolerance and leave screaming. That's the boundary thing again, being able to say no and keeping balance.

RANDAL: Do you feel you have to do it better because then they will stop abusing you?

ERICKA: Exactly.

RANDAL: These details give me an even better sense of where we may go with the regression.

ERICKA: (laughing) It's definitely a pattern that I'd like to give up.

RANDAL: That's reasonable. Okay, you can sit here in the recliner. (Ericka sits in the recliner) Are you ready for the hypnosis?

ERICKA: I'm ready.

RANDAL: Roll your eyes up and look at that light.

ERICKA: First I have to say that I feel scared. (taking a deep breath) All of a sudden I just got this fear.

RANDAL: Where do you feel your fear?

ERICKA: A little bit in my chest.

RANDAL: What do you feel in your chest?

ERICKA: Vulnerability.

RANDAL: Can you feel it as a kind of sensation?

ERICKA: Yes, it's a whole lot of energy in my chest and it's lightening up as I just express it, which is something I've trained myself to do. I express my fear and it tends to move, whereas if I don't acknowledge it, it will stay blocked. It's moving right now.

RANDAL: That's great. Are you ready now? (Ericka nods) Look back up at that spot and take a deep breath. (pause) Relax now. Take a second deep breath and switch to looking at my two fingers as they move toward your face. Now follow my fingers until your eyelids close down. (Randal's hand moves down in front of Ericka's eyes and they close down) That's right. I'm going to count from three down to one. At the count of one your eyelids lock tightly closed. You try to open them but the harder you try the tighter they lock together and the deeper into hypnosis you go. Three, stuck together. Two, sealing together. One, go ahead and try to open them but the harder you try the tighter they lock. (the muscles in Ericka's face tense) When I touch your left shoulder relax, stop trying, and go deeper. (Randal touches Ericka's shoulder and the muscles in her face relax)

Now I'm going to lift up your left foot and you can let it hang loosely and limply in my hand. (Randal picks up her foot) Take a nice, deep breath and fill up your lungs. As I drop your foot on the exhale, send a wave of relaxation down your body and go much deeper. (Randal drops her foot as she exhales) Now we'll do the same thing with your right foot. (Randal picks up her foot) When I drop your right foot send another wave of relaxation down your body and go much deeper, way down. (Randal drops it as she exhales) That's good.

This time I'm going to push down on your shoulders and as I do, let that be a signal to you to move down much deeper in hypnotic relaxation. Take a nice, deep breath and fill up your lungs. On the exhale, Ericka, feel yourself go way down (Randal is pushing down on Ericka's shoulders), deeper, deeper, deeper. That's good. Your whole body is becoming loose and limp and relaxed. Let every sound around you bring you deeper into relaxation. As I rock your shoulders you feel yourself going deeper. That's excellent.

I'm going to touch your left hand. When I do I'd like you to feel as though your hand from that time forward is getting heavier and heavier. Okay, I'm touching your hand now. Feel your hand getting heavier and heavier. I'm going to count from five down to one. At the count of one you try to lift up your left hand and the harder you try the heavier it becomes and the deeper into hypnosis you go. Number five, your left hand is growing heavier and heavier. Number four, just sinking down like it's made of cement. Number three, heavier and heavier. Number two, your arm is so relaxed that if you tried to use those muscles it just wouldn't work. On the next number I count you make an effort. The harder you try to lift up that hand the heavier it becomes and the deeper into hypnosis you go. Number one, go ahead and try. (Ericka tries to lift her hand) It's heavier, heavier, heavier. That's good. Very heavy. When I touch your left shoulder relax, stop trying and go deeper. (Randal touches her shoulder) When I touch your left hand again any sensation of heaviness is taken away. (Randal touches her hand) You feel a very comfortable feeling in your left hand and left arm just as you do in your right hand and right arm.

I would like you to visualize the word "yes" in your mind. There is a certain finger that is your "yes" finger. You keep thinking, feeling and seeing the word "yes" until a certain finger begins to move. (Ericka's index finger rises) Okay, the index finger of your left hand is your "yes" finger.

Now there is a certain finger that is your "no" finger. Feel, see and hear the word "no" until a certain finger begins to move. Keep thinking the word "no." I've seen it move already but I want to get a stronger response from it. Keep hearing, feeling and seeing the word "no." (Ericka's thumb rises) Okay, your thumb. Your thumb was twitching before but I wanted to get a clearer signal from you.

If I were to ask your subconscious a question and for some reason your subconscious mind did not know the answer, then a certain finger will give that response. Keep thinking the words "I don't know" until a certain finger begins to move. (Ericka's ring finger moves) It's the ring finger. And if for some reason your subconscious mind does not know how to answer a question or chooses not to, then let a certain finger become that finger signal. (Ericka's little finger moves) Okay, your little finger.

Ericka, you were just talking to me about a recurring dream you have that has to do with rescuing a failing business. While you are rescuing that business people treat you badly and you work harder hoping that they will stop abusing you. What I want to do now, in whatever way is appropriate for you, is to take you back to an earlier time when you felt as if your life were going that way. My question now is for your subconscious response. Is it safe and appropriate for you to consciously recall any and all memories or experiences in your past that were in some way like this dream? (Ericka's index finger rises) The answer is yes. I have another question for you. As you recall the memories, is it safe and appropriate for you to be open to your emotions? (Ericka signals with her thumb) The answer is no. All right, I will respect that.

I would also like to encourage you to use methods like the following ones with yourself on a regular basis to help you in your process of grounding and centering yourself. You are a very powerful, aware, and intuitive person, as you know. These techniques can help you take in the positive energy you want from others but reflect away any energy that is not appropriate to take on.

I want you to feel a grounding cord going from the base of your spine all the way down to the center of the earth. Be aware of the effects of that cord. Feel a beam of light, like a healing laser, going through the side of your head just above and in front of your ears. Feel another beam of light from your forehead, your third eye, to the back of your head, the lights intersecting in the center. Go to the center of your head right now and feel that intersection within you. Meanwhile, be aware of breathing down into your belly.

Also feel grounding energy from the earth coming up through your feet, continuing up through your legs, your torso, your head, and out through the top of your head. And feel some of that earth energy go all the way up from your feet to your shoulders and then down your arms and out through the palms of your hands. And some of this energy goes up to your hips and then circles back down and out your feet, allowing this energy to further ground you.

Feel a beautiful star of light over you. You can visualize and experience this as any color. I'd like to get a finger signal from you. Would white be the color of the star that is best for you? Yes or no. (Ericka signals with her thumb) The answer is no. Would blue be the best color for you? (Ericka signals with her thumb) The answer is no. Would green be the best color? (Ericka signals with her thumb) The answer is no. Would gold be the best color? (Ericka signals with her index finger) The answer is yes. Okay, a golden star above, showering your whole being with golden light. Any tension or negativity is draining out of your body through the palms of your hands and the soles of your feet, and transmuting into positive energy in the atmosphere. Feel yourself being showered with this golden healing light, like an aura of protection around you.

Now you're going to go on a journey but you'll go on the journey in such a way that you remain detached. You will observe from the point of view that we call the hidden observer. You'll go back and take a look at a girl who had certain experiences that are like that dream you recounted. You're going to look at it from this very grounded and centered place. You can observe the scene from a distance, as if you were observing a movie. In fact right now imagine you're walking down into the basement of a theater where there are rows of thousands of old reel to reel films. These are films within your subconscious mind from your many past experiences. You're going to pick one or more reels of film of past experiences that have to do with that recurring dream.

As you get ready to pick that film, I'll ask you to begin to recall that dream. Remember to stay centered as you do this. Recall it now from a distance, calmly and coolly, seeing that woman attempting to rescue a failing business, working hard at it and yet people are treating her badly. If you are recalling that dream now, signal with your "yes" finger. (Ericka signals with her index finger) Good. As you watch that dream from a distance something from this woman's childhood relates to that, and we're going to take a look at it on that film.

(after a pause) You've got the reel to reel films now and you're going back up the steps, through the lobby area, and continuing up to the projection room. There is a projectionist getting ready to roll the film and there is a seat next to the projectionist. You can sit in that seat while the projectionist sets up this film and as you sit there you can see in the dim light that the theater is empty except for a woman, Ericka, who is walking down the isle and finding a place to sit. You are about to watch her watch this film. You're actually going to watch her seeing it, so you have that further detachment.

Now you may feel no feelings at all, or you may have some identification with the character as you might do in a movie, although you are further back from that. You have compassion that is grounded in your centeredness, so you are coming from a therapist's viewpoint. You are there in the projectionist's room to support this woman in what she is going to see.

The film is beginning to run and I'm going to count from ten down to one. At the count of one there will be an incident or an

Ericka's Difficulty with Boundaries 113

experience or a memory showing up on the screen from this woman's childhood. An incident that has to do with her helping people out and people abusing her. In response she may try harder to please, harder to make things work out. I'm going to count from ten down to one and at the count of one you'll begin to see the film from that detached place.

Ten, nine, eight, seven, six, theater lights are dimming. Five, four, the film is coming on. Three, the film is beginning to run. Two, the film is running. One, you're beginning now to sense the memories. When you get a memory signal with your "yes" finger. (after a pause Ericka's index finger rises) All right, study that memory. When you feel like you've gotten a good look at it then signal again with your "yes" finger. (after a pause Ericka's index finger rises slightly) Okay, I got a small signal.

Now I'd like you to study this scene you've been watching from the projection booth. You were studying what was happening with this girl. I'm going to ask you some questions and you'll be able to give me verbal answers when I tap you on the shoulder. In the memory that you've just seen, was this girl under twelve years old? Yes or no. (Randal taps her shoulder)

ERICKA: Yes.

RANDAL: Is this when she was under seven years old?

ERICKA: I don't know.

RANDAL: Is this memory from around the age of seven or eight?

ERICKA: Yes.

RANDAL: Is this memory in her home or outside of her home?

ERICKA: Both.

RANDAL: Is this one memory that evolves or more than one memory?

ERICKA: Two memories.

RANDAL: Okay, one memory inside the home and one memory outside of the home. Is this memory with her family or with others?

ERICKA: Both. One is with my family and the other is at school.

RANDAL: You're doing very well. So you observed from this film two different memories that are similar to this recurring dream. Let's look at the memory with the family. Which room is she in?

ERICKA: The living room and the kitchen.

RANDAL: Besides the girl, are other people involved in this memory?

ERICKA: Her mother, her brother, and her father.

RANDAL: What is the memory that you see on this film?

ERICKA: (sighs deeply) I see a fight between my mother and my stepfather.

RANDAL: When you say a fight do you mean an argument or a physical fight?

ERICKA: An argument. My heart is really pounding.

RANDAL: Is that what you're seeing there or you're experiencing here?

ERICKA: Here.

RANDAL: Do you want to get some further detachment with that?

ERICKA: I'm okay.

RANDAL: You're doing fine. It's okay that your heart is pounding. It's natural as you see what's occurring to identify with the characters but you also have a certain compassionate detachment as a good therapist. Keep your ground now. How is this girl reacting to the argument between her mother and stepfather?

ERICKA: It's very upsetting. It's like I see the answer they can't see.

RANDAL: Her mother and stepfather don't see it, but the girl sees how to work out this argument. Does she attempt to help out in some way at that time?

ERICKA: No.

RANDAL: Does she feel she's not going to be taken seriously as a young girl?

ERICKA: No, she's told to stay away.

RANDAL: How does that affect her?

ERICKA: She's frustrated.

RANDAL: Watching that girl's reaction and noticing that she feels frustrated, does she do anything at that time with her frustration?

ERICKA: She cries.

RANDAL: That's good because it helps to get some of her feelings out. Does she do anything else with it?

ERICKA: Not yet.

RANDAL: Does she do something as a result after that experience?

ERICKA: She just starts acting older.
RANDAL: She forces herself to mature more quickly?
ERICKA: Yes.
RANDAL: What is the purpose or benefit of her maturing more quickly?
ERICKA: Understanding.
RANDAL: Is it her feeling that understanding will help her to deal more effectively in some way with such a painful experience if it were to occur again?
ERICKA: Compassion helps her to understand. Wise compassion.
RANDAL: So very early on she develops a kind of wisdom and compassion beyond her years, to help her to deal with such painful experiences.
ERICKA: Yes.
RANDAL: Does she begin to actually use that wisdom in her life then?
ERICKA: Yes.
RANDAL: Give an example, whether it's a general example or an incident, of how she goes about doing this.
ERICKA: She becomes a diplomat.
RANDAL: Would you consider her becoming a diplomat to be her primary response to this or one of the primary responses?
ERICKA: One of the responses. Caretaker, too.
RANDAL: Does she begin even when she's still a young girl to act as a diplomat and a caretaker? To attempt to smooth over some rough edges, so to speak?
ERICKA: She does.
RANDAL: Does she begin to act this out in part within her own family then?
ERICKA: Yes.
RANDAL: All right, let's take a look and see what happens at school. Is she around the same age or a different age?
ERICKA: I think she's a little bit older. Maybe ten.
RANDAL: What is the incident that you observe at school?
ERICKA: Violence.
RANDAL: Did something violent happen?
ERICKA: (voice quivering) My right arm.

RANDAL: All right, keep your ground now. Was this violence to your right arm?

ERICKA: Yes.

RANDAL: You're observing it now from a distance. If necessary you can back away from that.

ERICKA: I'm okay.

RANDAL: All right, you're doing fine. Stay with it. Did some child or a group of kids hurt her right arm?

ERICKA: A group of kids. Look at my right arm. There's a scar.

RANDAL: (Randal looks at her arm) Yes, I can see it. How was this right arm hurt?

ERICKA: It was cut.

RANDAL: With an instrument of some kind?

ERICKA: (Ericka's voice is very small and shaky) A knife.

RANDAL: Okay, back away from that. You don't need to feel that anymore. Come back to the projection booth. You're going to turn that film off now. You have the memory of it if we need it but you've seen what you need to see and you can respond accordingly. The film is off and you're calming down. You're doing very well. Are you ready to continue to look at that from a distance?

ERICKA: Yes.

RANDAL: I'd like you to get a sense of what the girl did. Why was that film shown just now? Did she play the diplomat or caretaker or was it about something else?

ERICKA: Martin Luther King was assassinated. I was attacked because I was white. (Ericka begins to cry)

RANDAL: It's all right to cry. (after repeated communication from Ericka that she was okay with the feelings coming up in spite of the detachment suggestions, Randal encourages her to release the grief that she had developed the habit of repressing)

ERICKA: I really loved my teacher and she was black...(Ericka cries softly) and she took me to the hospital. She was really upset about Martin Luther King and she was sobbing. And it was also her son's thirteenth birthday. My parents weren't around so I had to go to the birthday party after I got sewn up.

RANDAL: How was that for you?

ERICKA: It was really a hard time. I knew her pain and I was in pain. It's like I was pretending.

RANDAL: You were pretending not to be as hurt emotionally and physically as you were to help her out?

ERICKA: Yes.

RANDAL: That had to be very difficult for you. (Ericka sobs quietly) For a little girl like that, only ten years old, to have such a terrifying experience and have to be an adult about it. To actually take care of those around her when she herself needed to be taken care of. (pause)

Let's back away from that experience now. Go back to the projection booth. That memory is still available but you're relaxing and calming down. Bringing examples of these very difficult experiences to your subconscious mind is helping you to see how she developed certain ways of coping in the world that she is continuing to use now as an adult.

I'd like you to analyze the experiences of this girl now in such a way that you discover a misconception that was developed and that she has been carrying inside up to the present. A misconception that developed in a normal and understandable way under the circumstances. When you get a realization you can signal with your "yes" finger. (after a pause Ericka signals) All right, when I touch your shoulder you'll be able to talk about it. Three, two, and one. (Randal touches Ericka on the shoulder)

ERICKA: That I don't have to not be heard any more.

RANDAL: In other words, as a young girl you learned to cope with the great difficulties around you by not expressing yourself. You needed to do that for your physical and emotional and mental health. (Ericka is nodding) At the time that was a reasonable response. You learned that it worked well for the very difficult circumstances then, but that became a conception about the world and about yourself, that you better not make yourself heard or you will get hurt. Is that correct?

ERICKA: Yes.

RANDAL: So that became an ingrained habit of mental expectancy. And yet by virtue of the way you answered the question, you are also communicating that some part of your subconscious mind, as you review this experience, understands that this is a misconception. You no longer need to keep from being heard. Do you recognize that you no longer need to hold back from being heard?

ERICKA: (sigh) I don't know.

RANDAL: You have mixed feelings about that. Let me put it this way. There are many circumstances in the world. There are times when it is appropriate to keep our feelings to ourselves. I think that's part of the response I'm getting from you. It's an intelligent and appropriate response, that we need to have control over our communication. Do you recognize that this habit of avoiding being heard has gone too far and has kept you from the appropriate expression sometimes of your feelings?

ERICKA: Yes.

RANDAL: Good. So you are clearly seeing that this girl learned something that can still be appropriate to this day. She learned a lesson that under certain circumstances is important to remember. However, it's time for this girl to recognize that there are many situations in which it is appropriate for her to be heard. I'd like you to talk to this little girl who is seven. Is her name Ericka or is she called by some other name?

ERICKA: Ericka.

RANDAL: Adult Ericka, I want you to talk to seven year old Ericka. You can put your arms around her and tell her whatever you would like to say to her. (Randal has handed Ericka a large pillow which she is holding awkwardly)

ERICKA: (crying) I'm really sorry. I'm sorry for leaving you behind. (Ericka motions for Randal to come close and whispers to him as she continues sobbing)

RANDAL: (whispering back) Do you love this girl?

ERICKA: I don't know.

RANDAL: Become this seven year old girl. (Randal puts his arms around Ericka and the pillow, gently stroking her arms and hands; she cries periodically as they continue whispering quietly and then Randal moves away, speaking in a normal voice) Let me help you. (to the class) She's given permission to say this. She said that her mother didn't love her and she doesn't know if she loves little Ericka. (to Ericka) I want you to tell her that you love her. Try it out and see how it feels. "Ericka, I love you."

ERICKA: (Ericka sighs and sobs) I'm trying to do it.

RANDAL: Does it fit? Do you love this girl?

ERICKA: I don't know. Her mother hated her so much. (sobbing) She must be bad.

RANDAL: Let's bring in Ericka's higher self here. Ericka's higher self is a powerful therapist and radiant being. See her up there? She's a beautiful, powerful soul. What does she say right now?

ERICKA: She says to take care of her.

RANDAL: For you to take care of this girl?

ERICKA: Yes.

RANDAL: What does higher self Ericka say to the little girl about the fact that she says, "My own mommy didn't love me."

ERICKA: Your mommy wasn't well.

RANDAL: That's true. Her mom wasn't well. Her mom couldn't be well if she didn't properly show love to this little girl. (after a pause Randal whispers to Ericka, and then emotionally says) Tell her you love her.

ERICKA: (whispering) I love you.

RANDAL: How did that feel?

ERICKA: She feels good. (Ericka has her arms around the pillow now and looks much more comfortable holding it)

RANDAL: It feels good to hold her or the little girl feels better?

ERICKA: The little girl is feeling better.

RANDAL: (to the class) This is a classic situation. You see it over and over again in therapy when a child has had a withholding parent. The child tends to blame herself or himself because the parent does not express love. The child feels, "I must not be lovable. My own mommy doesn't love me." But Ericka's higher self can feel it. She knows this is a beautiful, lovable girl. (to Ericka) She's a beautiful little girl. (still holding Ericka and whispering softly) She's a wonderful little girl. Become that seven year old girl, that ten year old girl, and take it in. Are you starting to open up? Do you feel it? (Randal continues to hold and rock Ericka) Now be adult Ericka, loving this girl. I want you to tell her what you love about her and what you like about her.

ERICKA: I love that you care. And I love that you're so responsible. I love your magic. And you're so pretty. And you're so silly.

RANDAL: Good! Those are wonderful qualities for a little girl to have.

ERICKA: I love your brightness. And I love your understanding. I love your strength (sobbing) and I love that you didn't give up.

RANDAL: She's a very courageous girl. Those were very difficult circumstances. She needs and deserves a good mommy that really appreciates her because she's a wonderful little girl. Now be the little girl and take it in. The little girl within you can feel the love from adult Ericka, the mommy that is within you. So much is becoming clear now. It was her mommy back then that was messed up. This is a beautiful girl, who had all of these special qualities and still does. It's way past time for her to have a good, loving mommy and that's what you, adult Ericka, are to her from now on. Is that right?

ERICKA: Yes.

RANDAL: And you want to be that?

ERICKA: Yes, I do.

RANDAL: So little Ericka, what do you want to tell your new mommy who really appreciates you for who you are?

ERICKA: (sigh) Thank you for coming back to get me. (sobbing)

RANDAL: Feel how good it is to be rescued. Everything is going to be fine. It's a whole new world. You've got this very powerful, loving, beautiful, intelligent, talented mother here to take care of you and to protect you. You're also very powerful at protecting yourself. You'll find that there are a lot of beautiful things out there in the world. It's a different place now. You've got so many more resources to help you. Is there anything else as mommy Ericka that you want to say to young Ericka?

ERICKA: I just want to hold you for a long time.

RANDAL: You don't have to say anything. Just hold her and love her. Now switch and be young Ericka. Feel your mommy holding you and hold her back. Feel how good that feels. You've got a beautiful new mommy and she's wonderful. She has so many qualities that that other one didn't have. This is the mommy you deserve. Just feel it. Take it in. (pause) If there is anyone who would like to say something to seven year old Ericka, please say your name and then say something from where you're sitting.

KAREN: Ericka, this is Karen. I love you as a mommy and I love you as a child.

JANICE: Ericka, this is Janice. You're beautiful and wonderful both as a child and as a mother and I embrace you with love.

KATHY: Ericka, this is Kathy and I'd love to invite you to come out and play with me because I really love you a lot.

VIRGINIA: Ericka, this is Virginia. I want you to know that you are lovable and that you've always been loved.

JUDITH: Ericka, this is Judith. I'm going to blow you a big kiss. (smack!)

MONA: Ericka, this is Mona. I want you to know that you are good and you always have been and you always will be.

RANDAL: You've got a tremendous team here, Ericka. You've got a loving mommy that is yourself and you've got a beautiful, amazing little girl inside. You've got a very wise and powerful higher self. If you ever get stuck at any time you can ask her for assistance. You've got an adult Ericka who can get things done and be successful and express your talents and be powerful in the world. But that adult Ericka gets a lot of her juice and excitement and fun from that little girl of various ages within her. Not just seven year old but ten year old and three year old and thirteen year old Ericka. All these different ages of Ericka that are learning to play. She grew up too fast and it's time to have that childhood back. You will find more and more ways to let that child of yours come out and play. There are a lot of safe places to do that. (pause)

I'm going to bring you out of hypnosis in a little while and I want you to know that you can spend plenty of time loving the little girl within you and being that little girl feeling loved. You can have many more moments like this. Before I bring you out I'd like you to imagine, if you had an ideal father, what he would look like. It might be the father you had but he would be different in various ways. He would be very loving. Or maybe he could be a famous person or someone you've never seen. I'd like you to get a sense now of what that ideal father is like. He's very proud of his little girl. Do you have an image in your mind, a sense of what he looks like and what he feels toward his beautiful daughter?

ERICKA: He's Cary Grant. (laughter)

RANDAL: Good for her! This little girl is starting to get what she deserves. (to the class) She's getting it, folks. Thank you all for helping. (to Ericka) Especially thank you, Ericka, for taking it in and getting it from yourself. You've got all this opportunity now to catch up on everything that was missing all that time and that's going to feel so good. There is a lot of love coming your way. You've got beautiful adult Ericka loving you and you've got Cary Grant, who is your perfect father. He loves you just the way you are. You don't have to perform or do anything but just be yourself.

Now I'm going to count slowly from one to five and with each number that I count you become more and more alert, awake and aware. At the count of five you open your eyes and you are then fully alert, rested, refreshed, and feeling good. Number one, slowly, calmly, and easily returning to your full conscious mind. Number two, more and more alert, awake and aware. Number three, coming back gradually, taking your time. Feel yourself being receptive to the love around you. Number four, feeling grounded as you come back, with a powerful aura of protection around you. On the next number I count you open your eyes and are then fully alert, rested, and refreshed. Taking your time coming back. Number five, all the way back. (Ericka is still holding the large pillow and peeks out at the group in a shy, playful way)

RANDAL: Isn't she cute? (laughter) Look at all these people. Aren't they beautiful? (Ericka giggles) What a beautiful world it is out there! Maybe in a little while when you feel like it, you can come out and play. Take care of yourself and do whatever you want to do. (Ericka is still peeking out from the pillow and looking around) I love this work. See how smart you all are for getting into hypnotherapy? What in the world could be more satisfying?

ERICKA: (putting the pillow down) It's amazing how numb my body got when I was recalling things, especially my right side here. It was like it wasn't even there. That's why I was asking you to check my right arm because I thought it had completely disappeared.

RANDAL: Well, it was still there. Are you feeling your right side back now?

ERICKA: Yes. There was all this white light and it was numb.

RANDAL: Take your time and just hang out in this chair for awhile. (Randal and Ericka are giggling and looking out at the group) I can see quite a few playmates out there for you.

ERICKA: (Ericka shakes her feet into the air, laughing) I've got my tennies on!

RANDAL: I know, I love those bright red tennies! (Randal helps Ericka up and they hug before she goes back to her seat in the audience)

I'd like to say something about this session. Occasionally someone will signal, as Ericka did, not to be open to her emotions during the regression. Most often, the person will stay detached throughout when various methods are employed encouraging detachment. In this case emotions eventually began to surface and she communicated she was able to handle them. This became a compromise for the subconscious, which eventually trusted that she could open up to the emotions.

SANDY: You offered to make her more detached and she said, "No, it's okay." What would you have done if she had needed to be more detached?

RANDAL: There are a number of things I could have done. I could have taken her away from the memory to her inner sanctuary, or to a pleasant scene. I could have encouraged her higher self to talk to her. I could reiterate or further develop previous detachment suggestions and remind her about the filming. I could have her turn the lights on in the theater and suggest, "Let's walk out of the theater now and go to the beautiful park across the street." There are many symbolic ways in which you can lighten it up or just take the person away from the scene completely and put them in a pleasant, nurturing place. I had suggested detachment in many ways, and when emotions still come, more often than not the person wants them to come at that point. Sometimes the initial desire for detachment is a cry for "I don't know what I'm getting into and I want to be cautious about this."

MARK: I'd like to ask why you brought the father into this?

RANDAL: Of course this was not her father, but an ideal father. What we were creating is something I often find very helpful in therapy, and that is an internal ideal mother and ideal father who can be there for the inner child. In this case she was the obvious ideal mother, especially in her need to learn to appreciate and nurture herself. Whether any problems with her father were relatively minor or as great as they were with the mother, this inner child, who really deserved so much love and had not been getting it, could benefit from bringing in an ideal father figure.

ERICKA: I'd like to say that a part of me was conscious that Randal was telling me all of those positive things and I was also imagining that it was my father. And I was thinking, "Wow, I don't have a complete family here," so I was glad that he said that.

RANDAL: Thank you. It's good to hear that.

ANN: In regard to the actual parents, is there a point where people come to the realization that their parents were themselves treated badly or equally damaged and are passing this on because they don't know how to act?

RANDAL: That can be a classic recognition that comes near the conclusion of a Gestalt dialogue between the parent and child. Often the client already knew that intellectually but needed to get it on a deeper subconscious level. Also, it's often good to do a little hypno-analysis late in a regression session. I especially like to have clients analyze for themselves regarding any mistaken subconscious attitudes and expectations still continuing as a result of traumatic experiences. That's another time the client may experience and communicate this wiser or deeper realization about the parent.

I want to acknowledge Ericka for dealing with these very personal things and being willing to be vulnerable in the class. (to Ericka) I know from a previous discussion with you that there's a lot more you could say about what happened in your childhood. You had some tough times. I really admire you for how far you've come. Is there anything else you want to say to the group?

ERICKA: I want to share how it felt for me to do this. When I first sat down I said that I was fearful and I wanted to take this opportunity to get past my dream and the pattern in my life. I was really committed to that, but I was afraid to experience it here because I might be too vulnerable or I'd be ripped off or I'd go someplace I didn't want to be or whatever. What was amazing to me is that the only time I was even aware that the group was here was when I couldn't love my seven year old and I asked you (Randal) to come closer because I didn't want the class to hear that I couldn't love myself. I had felt that if I came across anything heavy I wouldn't be able to open up and share that, but it turned out to be easy. The whole thing was a good experience and it wasn't as frightening as I thought it would be.

RANDAL: Ericka did a great job. I generally tend to be as loving as I can but I'm not so much in the person's physical space. The fact that this was in a class setting made it feel comfortable and appropriate to be supportive in that way. When Ericka was whispering that her mother didn't love her and she didn't know if she loved her seven year old self, I was just melting. Here was this beautiful child who had been so blocked off from love. I'm sure many of you were feeling that empathy.

ERICKA: Thank you.

Note: Ericka has been in touch at various times and enthusiastically refers to the results of her session as "life transforming."

CHAPTER 10

Kenn's Terror of Further Neck Surgery

The Former Gambler Stooped with Shame

RANDAL: (to class) Kenn is here today regarding an injury. (to Kenn) What would you like to say about the injury?

KENN: I got hurt on the job a year ago in June and had to go on Workman's Compensation. The following January a cervical laminectomy was done on my neck. They went in on the sides to make the holes bigger for the nerves to come down into my arms because the injury had caused numbness in my arms. After I started recovering everything seemed to reverse itself and I lost more and more strength in my hands. Just before surgery my strength was measured at 42 percent of normal on the right and 21 percent on the left. Four months later it was something like 15 on the right and 7 on the left.

I went back to the surgeon six weeks ago and we decided that he was going to have to go back in because when they opened up the back of my neck it created a weakness on the front part. Now my spine is curving in the opposite direction and getting worse so that it's pinching my central nervous system and affecting the use of my hands. The doctor told me that with the surgery I could expect to either have some overall improvement in my condition, possibly twenty–five percent improvement, or I could look forward to becoming a quadriplegic.

I didn't like the odds and it happened that I got a phone call from Randal about the same time telling me about a recent graduate of his that lived in Modesto, where I live. His name is Charlie Simon and Randal recommended him highly but I thought, well, I don't trust anybody but myself and Randal, so I neglected to call Charlie. Then Charlie called me. This was about five weeks ago and he agreed to come over and do a couple sessions with me.

Prior to seeing Charlie I couldn't tie my shoes or even button my shirt. My hand was like this (holding his left hand with the fingers curled into a fist) and the only way I could straighten the fingers would be to lay them flat with the other hand. I couldn't depress the top of a shaving cream can, that's how weak I was.

So Charlie came over and we hit it off right away. I was impressed by him, and we've had six sessions since then. Now I'm off of all pain medication, I'm able to tie my shoes, and I can button all but the top button of my shirt. (applause) I'm really impressed with Charlie's work and I know he gained a lot from these classes. Then I called Randal to ask if he would possibly do a session with me because by the sixth of December I have to make a decision. Either I'm going through with the surgery or I'm going to avoid it. I thought if I could get a booster from Randal, then it would be easier to make this decision. That's why I'm here today.

RANDAL: Initially you had weakness in your arm after an injury, which led you to delicate surgical work on your neck. Then you got even weaker afterwards in spite of your strong desire to recover and in spite of working hard to do whatever rehabilitation exercises you could. What happened when you talked to the physician about that?

KENN: Well, the physician kept telling me that it takes a long time to recover from the surgery. He said he's even had patients that took up to a year for the feelings to return to their fingers. He wasn't too concerned about it. He just felt like I was going through some difficult times, which I was, and I didn't get across to him that instead of recovering I was getting much worse. Then four weeks ago he decided to do an MRI and get more x–rays. The MRI showed that my neck is so severely bent that it's depressing my nerves. If we don't reverse that I'm going to be in a wheelchair.

RANDAL: It was at that point that he felt you needed to have further surgery?

KENN: He said I need another surgery and I need to have it right away.

RANDAL: Did he feel that things hadn't gone right with the first surgery?

KENN: Oh, no. He never admitted a mistake and I'm not saying he made a mistake. I thought that the surgery he did was adequate and well done. But because part of the vertebrae on my upper neck was patched up on one side and made stronger, it had a tendency to make this weakness on the other side more prevalent. And it's the weakness now that's giving me trouble, right in front of where he went in for the laminectomy.

RANDAL: So something else happened in this other area after the first surgery that needs to be corrected.

KENN: Right. Now it's the front of my neck that's giving me the problem. My head bends the wrong way. And the surgery in back left part of my vertebrae open so there's no strength back there to keep it from bending further, which it did. Now it's bent to the point where the nerve going down into my legs is cut off.

RANDAL: Can you briefly describe further what kind of surgery the doctor is now proposing to do?

KENN: He wants to cut out the front of my third, fourth and fifth cervical vertebrae, open them up so the spinal cord has room to operate in there without being pinched, and then put a brace from my seventh cervical vertebrae up to my first cervical vertebrae. So basically I'll be able to look at you like this. (Kenn stiffens the upper part of his body and holds his head back, facing slightly upwards)

RANDAL: In other words your neck would be stuck in position.

KENN: And I won't ever be able to nod my head yes (demonstrates with neck), so I'll just have to say no. (laughter)

RANDAL: Have you gotten medical opinions from any other physicians?

KENN: I'm getting a second opinion on the sixth of December.

RANDAL: I'm not a physician and I have no idea what needs to be done with this. All I can say is that I would recommend a second, third and fourth opinion as quickly as possible. I got opinions from several doctors before I received surgery and it wasn't nearly as major as this. I want to encourage you to go to other doctors in the Modesto area where you live. Do it immediately. This is an incredibly important decision. In many cases people get different opinions from different doctors. I'm also wondering if the second opinion you've scheduled is with an associate of the first doctor or is it somebody you found on your own?

KENN: I asked for a second opinion through my family doctor because I didn't want a close association with the original surgeon.

RANDAL: Good. Depending on whether you decide to go through with this procedure after getting more opinions, how soon might you need to go in for surgery?

KENN: The first surgeon said surgery post haste. Now if the second doctor says, "Yes, we should go to surgery and we should go tomorrow," then I'll have to really give it careful consideration.

RANDAL: Is there any possibility of getting an earlier second opinion from this other doctor?

KENN: No. They told me I was fortunate to get one within a month's time even though the first surgeon was saying we don't have any time to waste.

RANDAL: Okay. I do feel that the time is urgent even though you've gotten some significant recovery. I also feel that this decision is so extremely important that I urge you to check around. Can you try to get at least one more opinion before you meet with the next doctor?

KENN: Sure. I'd like to interject here that while Charlie was working on me we made the most progress when we used visualization to replace my spine with the little wheels on tinker toys that I used to play with as a kid. We stacked them up with the same number of vertebras that were in my spine and we found out that the tinker toys are more flexible. What we're trying to do is reverse this curvature so it begins to straighten out. We also use visualization to replace the spinal fluid with a golden healing liquid that we get from God. Something is working because I was wearing a brace every day up to the time that I saw Charlie. And no strength in my voice at all. I really didn't care whether one day followed another. It was all one pain.

RANDAL: Kenn, you have one of the strongest spirits of anybody I know. I've seen your tremendous will. May I quote from the letter you sent to me? (Kenn nods) "My need to see you is mounting. I'm scheduled for a second opinion on December sixth. They want to go back into my neck and I have a foreboding reluctance to re-experience such a traumatic and debilitating piece of hatchery." That was your feeling when you heard about the possibility of a second surgery.

KENN: When I was through with surgery the first time and in recovery I found myself in front of two doors. I could open one door and go through and not have to worry about all the pain and debilitation and frustration I was going through with this condition. Or else I could go through the other door and come back to this life. I didn't feel as though I had really accomplished what I had set out to do and if I didn't come back I would be leaving my wife in a very precarious position. I had the choice. It was very tempting to go to the right and take the easy way and start again in another lifetime. But I took the left hand door and I'm pleased with the way things are going because I feel like I had a certain amount of humility to learn from this. Now I feel like I'm very humilitized (laughter) and when they say another surgery red flags pop up in my mind. If I get to the same two doorways I feel like I'll have a tendency to go to the right hand door this time because now my wife is very well taken care of. I have accomplished a few of the things that I wanted to accomplish, but not all of them. I have bad feelings about another surgery. My intuition tells me not to do it.

RANDAL: Also, it may not be a black and white issue. I'm not the one to tell you what decision to make and whatever we do today is not going to take away from the importance of getting that second and third medical opinion and then giving serious consideration to what the other doctors have to say. If you get more opinions you may get entirely different kinds of responses. I don't know what those could be but to speculate, for example, perhaps another doctor might say, "Yes, do surgery, but do it in a different way. We can do something not as dramatic as going through these six vertebrae here." Or maybe one doctor would say not to do surgery yet but to try something else, such as working with an osteopath. There might be various kinds of possible medical opinions.

I know you've gotten a great response from the six sessions you've had. You were really going down hill and now you're improving. I'd like to introduce Charlie Simon, who I have invited to join us for this session today. (to Charlie) Welcome, Charlie. (to the class) Charlie is a very talented hypnotherapist. His insight and creativity stood out right from the beginning. I knew how particular

Kenn was when I said, "This is a great person to see you and he's right there in Modesto." Like Kenn, he has a lot of heart and enthusiasm and I felt they were kindred spirits. (to Charlie) Is there anything you would like to say or any details you want to add about your work with Kenn?

CHARLIE: Working with Kenn, who was already a hypnotist, really gave us a leg up because I didn't have to explain hypnosis or any of those things. Kenn was in agony when I went to see him. He was taking I don't know how many drugs, just to ameliorate the agony somewhat. He hasn't mentioned the pain that was in his belly all the time. I believe he said he was never without it.

KENN: My stomach hadn't been right since the first surgery. I was constipated five out of seven days a week. When I wasn't constipated, boy, I was on top of the world. Since I started seeing Charlie five weeks ago, I think I've taken a laxative twice. I don't have the constant pain.

CHARLIE: We used visualization techniques and my little tinker toy metaphor. He latched right onto that as a visualization. Then with the post–hypnotic suggestions I gave him he found that he could indeed recover these things when he needed to.

KENN: I was able to reach back inside of myself and come up with answers I had been struggling with for years.

RANDAL: That's great. Thank you. Tell me some of those answers, Kenn, so we can use them in our session. I want to get your ideas.

KENN: I think I've started recovery and I feel like what might be stumbling blocks on the road to recovery are my feelings of guilt and shame that go way back. Before I met Randal five years ago I was a drunk. I was a three pack a day cigarette man, a compulsive gambler running my own casino, and a womanizer. Fortunately I wasn't into hard drugs. I remember my childhood being excellent, a very happy childhood, and well done by my parents. Even so I came up with every compulsive, addictive behavior. I've even experienced eating disorders. I don't know why but because of all these disorders I have a tendency to place a lot of shame on myself.

RANDAL: That's what I want to work on in this session. I certainly will be able to give you some positive suggestions at the end of our session but I could give more in the way of visualizations to help your neck further if we knew whether you are going to be having surgery or not. It would be good to hear from you just after you get your second and third opinions to find out what the doctors have said and what you decide to do. Then if you do need to have surgery we can have a hypnosis session after the surgery for further healing, or if you don't have surgery I definitely feel that a hypnosis session right after the second and third opinions will be important. Does that make sense to you?

KENN: Yes.

RANDAL: Good. As far as the surgery goes, you may get several different opinions and then you can make your decision based on an informed choice and what your gut feeling tells you to go with. I just want to be really clear about all of that.

KENN: I understand.

RANDAL: Now you mentioned your feeling that there is some shame deep down that might possibly be affecting you and that's something we can work with. I'd like to ask if you have more strength in your right hand than your left hand?

KENN: About double.

RANDAL: Have you been able to use ideomotor responses at all?

KENN: Yes.

RANDAL: Now you mentioned to me during the break that your hands and arms were very cold and clammy before you started the hypnosis work and now you're getting some warmth and circulation.

KENN: I didn't have good circulation at all. Now I do.

RANDAL: (feeling Kenn's hands) Yes, they're very warm. That's good.

KENN: At the time Charlie started I would not be able to squeeze your hand like that.

RANDAL: So you've really made some very dramatic improvement at this point.

KENN: Yes.

RANDAL: And when you do ideomotor responses do you usually do them with your right hand or with your left hand?

KENN: I've been using my left hand. All we've been using is yes or no.

RANDAL: Okay, show me your "yes" finger and your "no" finger.

KENN: This is yes. (lifting the index finger of his left hand) This is no. (lifting the thumb of his left hand)

RANDAL: Now that is your weaker hand but you still have had no problem getting ideomotor responses from that hand?

KENN: No, and the reason we use that hand is because when I go into a trance state my right index finger will come up. I designed that so that I would definitely know without a doubt when I'm in a trance state. Now my right index finger just automatically lifts and I don't have any control over it.

RANDAL: So we will use the left hand.

KENN: As long as we confine it to yes and no. Before I couldn't raise these two fingers at all. (Kenn barely lifts his ring finger and little finger) Now I do have movement in them but it's difficult.

RANDAL: What I may do in that case is have you use the thumb or middle finger of your right hand for alternative answers in this special circumstance.

KENN: Okay, but we'll keep yes and no here. (wiggling the thumb and index fingers of his left hand)

RANDAL: Can you move the middle finger on your right hand?

KENN: Yes, a little bit. (moves middle finger slightly)

RANDAL: And your thumb?

KENN: Yes. (moves thumb easily)

RANDAL: For the length of the process I would like to have you lie down if that's comfortable for you.

KENN: Yes, but I'll need a pillow.

RANDAL: We do have pillows here and we have a mat. (Kenn gets comfortable on the mat and Randal kneels beside him) Do your hands feel comfortable where they are? (Kenn's hands are on his chest)

KENN: Yes.

RANDAL: Okay, that's great. Your hands will be close together. In terms of touching or manipulating your body, Kenn, how would it be if I were to gently push down on your shoulders or drop your hands?

KENN: No problem.

RANDAL: I probably won't drop your hands but it's good just to know. Are you feeling comfortable?

KENN: Yes.

RANDAL: I'd like you to look into my left eye. (bringing his face in front of Kenn's) Stare at my left eye. Feel your eyelids beginning to get heavy. Getting heavier and heavier. The next time they blink they get harder to open. Your heavy eyelids are closing, closing, closing. Feel your eyelids getting heavier as your eyelids close down. (Kenn's eyes close) Good. Now your eyelids are tightly closed and continuing to get heavier still. Your heavy eyelids are now locking more and more tightly together. Your eyelids lock tightly closed. Get ready to try to open them but the more you try the tighter they lock and seal. Go ahead and try but they're stuck together. When I touch your left shoulder stop trying, relax and go deeper. (the index finger on Kenn's right hand lifts) That's good. You've already got a good, pleasant feeling of hypnotic relaxation moving throughout your body. Going deeper with every easy breath that you take.

I'm going to lift up your left foot just a little ways. Let it hang loosely and limply in my hand. When I drop it send a wave of relaxation down your body and feel yourself going much deeper. Take a nice deep breath and on the exhale feel yourself go twice as deep. (Randal drops his foot) That's good. I'm going to do the same thing with your right foot. Take a nice deep breath and fill up your lungs. When I drop it feel yourself go three times as deep. Going down (Randal drops his foot), going down. That's good.

Now I'm going to count from three down to one. At the count of one only your eyelids open and you stay in hypnotic relaxation. When your eyelids open I'll snap my fingers and say the words, "sleep now." At the finger snap you close your eyes and go deeper, even deeper than you are at this very moment. Getting ready now. Three, two, one, open. (fingers snap) Sleep now, close your eyes and go deeper. And again. Three, two, one, open. (fingers snap) Sleep now, close your eyes and go deeper. And again. Three, two, one, open. (fingers snap) Sleep now, close your eyes and go deeper. That's your signal. Whenever I snap my fingers and say the words "sleep now" you instantly go into a very deep, pleasant state of hypnotic relaxation.

You continue to go deeper now with every easy breath. I'm going to count from ten down to one and as I do you feel yourself going deeper with each number. Deeper in very pleasant relaxation. Number ten, nine, feel yourself going deeper. Eight, deeper with each number I count. Seven, deeper with every sound that you hear. Six, with every easy breath. Five, with every easy beat of your heart. Four, turning loose each muscle. Three, just letting go. Two, deeper and deeper relaxed. And one. That's good.

All right, Kenn, I'm going to do a couple of practice ideomotor questions here. Is the month that we're in now the month of November? Yes or no. (Kenn's left index finger rises) The answer is yes, as you have correctly signaled with the index finger of your left hand. Next question. Is the year that's coming after this year going to be the year 1993? Yes or no. (Kenn's left thumb rises) Of course the answer is no, since next year will be 1992. Kenn, I'll be asking you some more questions now. Your answers may be as immediate as they were just now or they may take more time. You have plenty of time to allow the subconscious mind to come up with the correct answer.

Now in terms of the physical difficulties you have been experiencing in your neck area, does at least part of that difficulty have to do with feelings of guilt or shame? (Kenn's left index finger rises) The answer is yes. Would it be valuable for you then, as part of your healing process, to deal with this guilt or shame? (Kenn's left index finger rises) The answer is yes. I want to use one word now, so let's use the word shame. In dealing with the shame that you feel in your life, is it appropriate and safe for you to recall any or all memories from your past? (Kenn's left index finger rises) The answer is yes. As you go back into memories from your past, is it safe and appropriate for you to be open to any emotions that may arise? (Kenn's left index finger rises) The answer to the question is yes.

All right, Kenn, continue to go deeper with every easy breath. I want you to feel the energy in the room. There are a lot of loving people here. I want you to feel my loving energy for you. I want you to feel the good energy of the universe here to help you to stay with the process and to work through it as I know you're going to do very well.

I'm going to count from one up to ten. With each number that I count you become more and more aware of a feeling that you sometimes have. It's an unpleasant feeling. You're going to become aware of that feeling for now as a way to deal with it. It's a feeling of shame. With each number that I count you become more and more aware of that feeling. Number one, two, three, becoming more and more aware of that familiar feeling of shame. Four, five, six, you know it's a deep feeling. Sometimes you feel very ashamed of yourself. Seven, feeling that feeling more strongly now. Feeling it more and more intensely in your mind and in your body. Number eight, like the flood gates of a dam, feeling that feeling gushing forth within you. That feeling of shame, of being ashamed of yourself. Number nine, on the next number I count you're right there with that feeling. Number ten.

Now I'll count from ten down to one and you'll go back to an earlier time in your life when you felt that shame. Number ten, nine, eight, going quickly back in time now. Seven, six, going back to an earlier time in your life. Five, four, three, going back to an earlier time in your life. Two, on the next number I count you're right there feeling that feeling of being ashamed at an earlier time in your life. I'm going to tap your forehead. One. (Randal taps Kenn's forehead with his finger and Kenn's body jumps) Okay, where are you now? Are you inside or outside? You can speak.

KENN: Inside.

RANDAL: Nighttime or daytime?

KENN: Daytime.

RANDAL: It's daytime and you're inside. Are you under twenty years old? Yes or no.

KENN: Yes.

RANDAL: Are you under ten years old? Yes or no.

KENN: Yes.

RANDAL: Are you under seven years old? Yes or no.

KENN: Yes.

RANDAL: Are you under four years old? Yes or no.

KENN: Yes.

RANDAL: Are you under two years old? Yes or no.

KENN: No.

RANDAL: How old are you?

KENN: Three.

RANDAL: All right. You're three years old. You're inside. Is there anybody else around?

KENN: Yes.

RANDAL: Okay, who else is there?

KENN: Mother.

RANDAL: Are you in your house or some other building?

KENN: House.

RANDAL: Which room in the house are you in?

KENN: The bedroom.

RANDAL: Your bedroom? The room that you sleep in? (Kenn nods) So that's the scene. You're with your mother, you're in the bedroom, you're three years old. And how are you feeling?

KENN: Ashamed.

RANDAL: What is happening? Give me more details of this scene.

KENN: Being scolded.

RANDAL: Did your mother feel that you did something wrong?

KENN: Yes.

RANDAL: Now go back. Experience that scene and get a sense of what is was that you did wrong.

KENN: I wet the bed.

RANDAL: Have you wet the bed before?

KENN: Yes.

RANDAL: Has she scolded you before for it?

KENN: Yes.

RANDAL: So this is something she has repeatedly done with you. She has scolded you for wetting the bed. I'd like you to hear her scolding you now. What is she saying to you?

KENN: Can't you control your bladder?

RANDAL: And what do you say back to her? How are you responding as a three year old?

KENN: I didn't know it was happening.

RANDAL: Did you say that to her then?

KENN: Yes.

RANDAL: What does she say in response?

KENN: She said, "You're a naughty boy."

RANDAL: I'm going to count again and as I count downward from five to one you go back to another time when you felt ashamed. Five, four, going back to another time when you were a young child or an infant and you felt ashamed. Going back into another early time in your life. Three, two, going back. On the next number I count you're right there. (Randal taps Kenn's forehead with his finger) Number one. All right, this time are you inside or outside?

KENN: Inside.

RANDAL: Nighttime or daytime?

KENN: Daytime.

RANDAL: Daytime and inside again. Are you under four years old? Yes or no.

KENN: No.

RANDAL: How old are you?

KENN: Six.

RANDAL: You're six years old. Are you inside your house or somewhere else?

KENN: School.

RANDAL: Okay, you're six years old and you're in school. What's happening?

KENN: Program for circumcision.

RANDAL: A program for circumcision?

KENN: Yes. Anybody could get circumcised at the school.

RANDAL: I see. And what are you doing or thinking about?

KENN: My mother is taking me and I'm very scared.

RANDAL: Can you see yourself in the room now where you are going to be circumcised?

KENN: Yes. I threw a fit and it was never done.

RANDAL: What was said by either your mother or someone else at that time or immediately afterwards?

KENN: That I was irresponsible. That I was a naughty boy because I didn't want this done.

RANDAL: A naughty boy again. Irresponsible. Who is it that's telling you this?

KENN: Mother.

RANDAL: I see. I want you to go back to that scene when you were three years old, Kenn. Three, two, one, back to that scene of being scolded for wetting your bed at the age of three and being called a naughty boy. How do you feel as your mother is saying these things to you?

KENN: Terrible.

RANDAL: Do you feel ashamed?

KENN: Yes.

RANDAL: I would like you to imagine that you could talk to your mother as a three year old and that you could have me here with you. We're recreating the scene in such a way that you can now speak up to her. You can stick up for yourself in whatever way you feel is appropriate. What would you like to say to your mother as she is scolding you for being a naughty boy at the age of three for wetting your bed?

KENN: I'm not doing it on purpose and it's over before I realize what's happened.

RANDAL: Now I'd like you to switch and be your mother. What does your mother say in response to that?

KENN: She's saying, "Well, you're just being lazy and I want you to get up at night and go to the bathroom."

RANDAL: What do you say in response to that?

KENN: I'm not even aware of what's going on.

RANDAL: And what does your mother say?

KENN: Try to get up.

RANDAL: And what do you say?

KENN: I will. I'll be good.

RANDAL: I'd like you to bring in adult Kenn now. Adult Kenn, what would you like to say to your mother as she's there in that room with three year old Kenn?

KENN: Mrs. McGee, it's a fairly common thing among young children and it's been found to be linked to genetics.

RANDAL: Uh huh. That's all true.

KENN: It's something that your young son has no control over and he'll probably grow out of it.

RANDAL: That's right. What does she say in response to that?

KENN: Well, we'll see.

RANDAL: As you said that to her three year old Kenn has been listening to you. Now be three year old Kenn and talk back to big Kenn. Having heard what big Kenn said what do you want to say to him?

KENN: Wow. I wish I could have stood up and talked to her like that.

RANDAL: And big Kenn, what do you want to say to the three year old?

KENN: Well, as you grow up you'll understand and you'll become wiser. You won't have to feel the shame.

RANDAL: I want you to talk some more to little Kenn about the shame he's been feeling about wetting the bed. He's really impressed with what you had to say and that's good news to him. Now he knows that it's something normal that other kids go through, too. You can check out how he's feeling. What do you want to say about his experience at this point?

KENN: You no longer have to feel that shame. It's something that happened in the past. Something you're entirely not responsible for so you no longer need to carry this shame.

RANDAL: In fact would you tell him that even when it happened there was nothing to be ashamed of?

KENN: Yes.

RANDAL: Now be little Kenn. What do you want to say in response to that?

KENN: I'll try.

RANDAL: You'll try what?

KENN: I'll try not to feel the shame.

RANDAL: All right. You've heard what big Kenn has said to you and it's different than what your mother used to say, that you should be ashamed for this or that you're a naughty boy. What I want you to do is have three year old Kenn speak up for himself about that. Make a stronger statement than "I'll try." Say something to your mother about how she's been talking to you.

KENN: You know that I wet the bed and I'm just human. I'm your little boy and I really don't feel as though I deserve all this brow beating.

RANDAL: Good for you. Remember you have big Kenn to help you, to encourage you to say whatever you feel. Now be mother and respond.

KENN: You're right. I have been too harsh on you and insensitive to something you have no control over. I'll try to be more understanding.

RANDAL: Very good. Now be little Kenn and respond to your mother.

KENN: Thank you, mommy.

RANDAL: And mother, do you have anything more you'd like to say to little Kenn?

KENN: You're a good boy.

RANDAL: Good. Do you have any further appreciation to give little Kenn?

KENN: No, other than the fact that you're so helpful.

RANDAL: All right. And little Kenn you take that in. What does your mother call you? Kenn or Kenny or what?

KENN: To my mother and only to my mother, I'm Kenny.

RANDAL: Okay, only to your mother when you were a young boy, then you were Kenny. Being Kenny and talking to your mother do you have any further thing you'd like to say to her? She's just acknowledged that you're a very good boy and you're very helpful.

KENN: Only that I'm growing up.

RANDAL: What is it about your growing up that you want your mother to know about?

KENN: What a good person I am.

RANDAL: That's good. And she's already called you a good boy. All right, be mother. Do you recognize that your little son is growing up and do you feel that he is a good person as he said?

KENN: Yes, I do.

RANDAL: Be little Kenn and say goodbye to your mother for now.

KENN: 'Bye mommy.

RANDAL: And be mother and say goodbye to Kenny for now.

KENN: Goodbye Kenny.

RANDAL: Very good. We've just cut a cord from certain associations in your subconscious mind that can have amazingly positive ramifications. You've just come a long way. You may be amazed, Kenn, even in spite of the dramatic work you've seen done with hypnosis, at how quickly changes can come and how easy it can be. It's a process that works itself out.

Now I'd like to check things out with your finger signals. Having done this process regarding the shame you felt at various times with your mother, do you feel like you are now able to let go of that shame and of the effect those experiences had on you? (Kenn's left index finger rises) The answer is yes. Are you now letting go of the effects of that shame you felt in terms of your relationship with your mother? (Kenn's right thumb rises) Okay, the thumb on your right hand indicates an answer other than yes or no. When I count from three down to one you'll be able to speak. Three, two, one. What would your subconscious mind like to say?

(Note: These kinds of ideomotor questions can be very valuable in helping to uncover resistance or misconceptions or information that the conscious mind is not aware of.)

KENN: I don't know.

RANDAL: Okay. There's some other information your subconscious mind is wanting to say. I'm noticing that your hand is now raising upward. (Kenn's entire right hand is lifting up) I can imagine various possibilities here about what your subconscious mind may be communicating. For example, perhaps there is something further you want to verbalize. Or perhaps the subconscious is not clear on an answer right now. Another possibility is a very strong "yes" signal that is lifting the entire hand up. Another possibility is that the way I asked the question makes it too complex to answer in a simple "yes" or "no" manner. These are just samples of possibilities.

Right now I'm only referring to the initial sensitizing events of your relationship with your mother. I will be checking in about issues regarding any other possible shame in your life also. I'm going to ask a question now for an ideomotor response. Does the signal of your entire right hand lifting up primarily have to do with the feeling of a very strong "yes" signal? (Kenn's left index finger rises) The answer is yes. Very good.

As you let go of these feelings of shame that your mother mistakenly gave you as a child, this is having a very positive effect on you and the rest of your life. You are experiencing things differently on a lot of different levels. A great deal of healing is taking place. I'd like you to analyze in your mind now what effect your mother's mistaken attitudes had on you at the time and later in your life. Analyze how those attitudes that you used to have are changing and in the process of healing. When you are ready to talk about that I'd like you to signal with your "yes" finger. (After a short pause Kenn's left index finger rises) All right. When I touch your shoulder say what you'd like to say about that. (Randal touches Kenn's shoulder)

KENN: We went back to when I was three when the problem started but the problem continued up to the time I was about thirteen. It was very embarrassing. If I spent the night with a friend or something I would wet the bed. Consequently I was very shy and reserved and self–conscious all through school. Even though I was a good student I would never volunteer answers to the questions or do anything that would force me in front of the class. And I didn't learn about this genetic part until maybe two or three months ago. I've been carrying this shame a long time.

RANDAL: All that time. Have you also learned, Kenn, that this is actually a very common problem among boys? Much more common than with girls. Most boys eventually grow out of it, as you did. A significant percentage of boys wet their beds frequently for a period of time. Of course ten or twelve year old boys are not going around saying, "Hey, I wet my bed last night." It's something that feels very embarrassing, especially if you don't know that it's a common problem. You mentioned that all this time you've been carrying that shame around, even all the way through your adult years until just two or three months ago. How did that affect you two or three months ago when you learned that there was a common genetic link to wetting the bed?

KENN: I felt like I wasn't such a bad little boy after all.

RANDAL: No, you weren't. In fact you were a fine boy. You hadn't done anything wrong. Having explored this now directly with your subconscious, working it out with your mother and clearing this experience that started by the age of three and went on for all those years, how do you feel? Are you getting additional insights or a deeper understanding?

KENN: I think it's important to recognize shame for what it is and know the difference between shame and guilt. Guilt reminds us that hey, we probably shouldn't have done this. But there is no reason to carry shame. It's something that happened and as long as we're living our life today as we would want to live, there's no reason for the shame.

RANDAL: Yes. And you recognize that there is no reason to feel guilt, either, for the issue you've been working on here? There's nothing to feel guilty about.

KENN: Yes.

RANDAL: Good. It is very important that your recognitions are going beyond the conscious and having a very profound affect on the subconscious. Now I'd like you to focus on the mistaken attitude of your mother, recognizing that she was naive and made some mistakes. Do you feel a sense of acceptance, understanding and completion with her, or is there any resentment? Look at your mother and get a sense of how you feel for the mistaken ways she treated you when you were a child.

KENN: I realize that she was doing the best job she could. I love her deeply. There's no problem between my mother and I.

RANDAL: It felt like you had probably completed that but I wanted to be sure. Very good, Kenn. I'd like you to look over your life and get a sense of knowing that this habit of shame that was so deep is now being transformed into a deep acceptance of yourself. It was a mistake to feel shame and guilt over something you didn't have any control over, and there are all kinds of changes and new habit patterns that are being formed. Feel a sense of relief, a sense of peace, a sense of self–acceptance, a sense of self–love. It's not only having a beautiful affect on you, but it's going to have a beautiful affect on all the people you'll be helping in your work as a hypnotherapist as you continue to become more and more healthy.

And already, beginning in the near future, you'll be able to work again as a hypnotherapist. It's something that you're very good at and you'll be using your tremendous abilities to do a lot of healing work in this world. I'd like you to look over your life now from this new perspective and get a sense, Kenn, of how you feel. Is there anything that you feel some kind of deep shame about at this time?

KENN: No.

RANDAL: Very good. I'd like you to analyze the experiences you were describing before this hypnosis that you did feel ashamed about at that time. Analyze those experiences and get a sense of how you feel now, coming from a whole new perspective of what you've just experienced. Recognizing what a beautiful, exemplary life you're living now. When you get a good understanding from your deep subconscious you can talk about those experiences from your new perspective. When you're ready you can signal with your "yes" finger. (Kenn's left index finger rises) All right, when I touch your shoulder you can speak. (Randal touches Kenn's shoulder)

KENN: I realize the amount of time and energy that I expended on my shame was really a waste and I could have been using it better in a different direction. And now that I'm aware that I even carried that shame I'll be able to use this energy in a more constructive way.

RANDAL: Looking over your life now is there anybody that you feel you need to say anything to or do you feel clear at this time?

KENN: I feel clear.

RANDAL: Okay. This was a process that you were going through internally with yourself, this feeling of shame that you were carrying with you for years. This habit pattern went deep down. You've made some mistakes in the past but you've worked through that. You've transcended certain difficulties and come to be a good, loving husband and family man, a good, responsible person and a good hypnotherapist. Would it be correct to say that?

KENN: I feel that I've had a problem with forgiveness, but I think I've been able to work through this by asking for forgiveness from various people. And I think that's all I can do. As long as I ask for forgiveness and extend forgiveness.

RANDAL: Do you accept their forgiveness? Can you take in that forgiveness from others?

KENN: Oh, yes.

RANDAL: Most importantly of all, do you feel a total forgiveness of yourself for any mistakes you may have made in the past?

KENN: Yes.

RANDAL: I'd like to double check that. Talking to Kenn's subconscious mind now, do you release and forgive any mistake that you may have ever made in the past? (Kenn's left index finger rises) Good. The answer is yes and that is wonderful. You, Kenn, are a miracle worker. You have done so much good work with yourself and other people. And you've just done some very good work in quickly breaking through with yourself. This is beginning to have incredible benefits for you.

Now I'd like you to turn your attention to your neck. I'd like your subconscious mind to signal whether the experiences you've just gone through, the realizations that you've made and the transformation you're making in your life, are going to have some powerful healing influences on your neck. (Kenn's left index finger rises) The answer is yes. All right.

Now I'd like your subconscious mind to come up with a powerful healing image to accelerate the healing progress of your neck. It may be one that you used with Charlie or an entirely different one. Even if you've already used it on yourself it will now have a much more powerful effect. When your subconscious mind comes up with a very powerful image to help to heal your neck I'd like you to signal with your "yes" finger. (Kenn's left index finger rises) Okay. When I touch your shoulder you can tell me. (Randal touches Kenn's shoulder)

KENN: All I can see are tinker toys.

RANDAL: That's great. I'd like you to describe these tinker toys and what you are doing with them.

KENN: I'm stacking them one on top of another. I started with twenty four and then I found out that I needed thirty three. I added some more tinker toys and I'm piling them one on another and they reach way up into the sky and it's flexible and I can easily change the contour to suit my best health. I'm concentrating in the cervical area and bending the tinker toys to the rear so that I'll be able to function in the future.

RANDAL: Great. And you're functioning in a more and more flexible and healthy way every day.

KENN: Yes.

RANDAL: Besides working with this image what will you be doing in the days ahead to help the spinal cord in your neck to heal?

KENN: I'll be doing a lot of visualization and I've started an exercise program. I'm doing some walking and working out with Richard Simmons on the TV. I think he calls it something about exercising with the oldies. Well, I fit the category so I'm working with him.

RANDAL: You also have your young side and you're going to feel younger every day.

KENN: I've been doing a lot of strengthening exercises with my hands.

RANDAL: Are these exercises that you learned from a physical therapist or your doctor?

KENN: It's something I picked up in physical therapy.

RANDAL: Are you continuing to see a physical therapist?

KENN: Not any more. And I'm also working with some neck exercises that Charlie showed me, trying to get more flexibility there. I'm concentrating on the flexors and the tensors.

RANDAL: You're aware as you do these exercises that it does take time to heal although it can be miraculous how fast that can sometimes happen. You can use the intuition of your subconscious mind to keep working with these healing exercises in a way that feels right, not going too fast, not straining yourself, and at the same time you're able to continue progressing. Does that feel appropriate for you? (Kenn's left index finger rises) The answer is yes. And you can be clear too, if you're ever in doubt about something, that you can go back to an appropriate, responsible expert, such as a physical therapist or a doctor, to find out more information if necessary. Are you committed to doing that? (Kenn's left index finger rises) Very good, Kenn.

I'd like you to look within your subconscious mind to sense now whether we've gotten this major issue out of the way so you can feel clear and love yourself fully. Using your finger signals, are there any other blocks in your subconscious mind that we need to remove to help you to go through this healing process? (Kenn's left thumb rises) The answer is no. Hallelujah! (Randal puts his hand over Kenn's)

Kenn, you're going to do great. I want to tell you that I really admire you. I'm so glad that you've let go of the shame and the guilt because you never deserved it. You're a good person. For years you've been living a beautiful life. When I think of everything you've been through in your life, all the changes that you've made, I want you to know that you're an inspiration to me. You're an inspiration to everybody in this room. And you've got a lot more to do in your life. You've got great kids and a wonderful wife and they want to see you live for a long time. You want to live a long healthy life and you deserve it. You've got a lot of healing work to do in the world.

I have been impressed by you in so many ways. When I gave you special homework to do as a way to get additional advanced training in hypnosis, you were so thorough. You combed through all those books I had given you and so many more, and wrote thoughtful critiques. And you were so excited about the hypnosis work you were doing with people. Now you're moving into this whole new career. It's just beginning. That old career is over and you can move into the new one in full force in the days, the weeks, the months ahead. You have transformed yourself so much and now you can use everything you've gone through in your life as a way to help other people to heal. The most powerful healers in the world, I feel, are people that have faced adversity and succeeded with flying colors, and that's what you're done.

Every day you continue to heal physically, mentally, emotionally and spiritually. And this joy that you feel you can express to your loved ones, to the people around you, and to your clients. That joy is infectious. It blesses everyone that you contact. Every day you are becoming stronger and healthier. You are a radiant, enthusiastic and loving person who is so excited about life and so excited about helping other people to transform their lives, just as you continue to transform yours. You have so many powerful ways to use your life and your subconscious mind to heal people and to heal yourself.

You're getting into the habit now of focusing on loving feelings about yourself and doing visualizations as well as doing the actual physical exercises. And you are healing every day. You have heard about people who weren't supposed to recover from severe physical problems and had spontaneous remissions. Working through subconscious blocks is one way that can often produce miracles.

Is there anything you would like to say or to ask, Kenn, before I bring you up out of the hypnosis? (Kenn's left thumb rises) The answer is no. All right, is there anybody in the room that would like to say something to Kenn before I bring him out of the hypnosis?

GLENDA: I would just like to say that my heart is so open to you and all of my energy and my loving thoughts and all of the divine connections we have with God. Your guides travel with you today and for all the days of your future so that your healing may be thorough and complete and filled with joy and love. May your work grow and be an inspiration to all who come in touch with you. Our love is with you.

ANASTASIA: As I've been watching this process I feel a tingling energy in my body that is a beautiful energy. It's real and it's healing me and it's for you, too. I feel it's working in every dimension, physically and spiritually and emotionally. You have a lot to live for.

JOANNE: You have so much to give to us. Thank you, Kenn.

SALLY: Have lots of fun, Kenn. Tomorrow begins today.

RANDAL: (to Kenn) Take it in. Feeling pretty good, huh?

KENN: Great.

RANDAL: Good job, Kenn. You deserve all the love and affection and support and approval from yourself and the many beautiful people around you. People in this class, clients that you are reaching out to and who are reaching out to you, and your family and friends. Just feel the new day dawning. The sun is shining and you're in the process of beginning a whole new life. It's better than anything you've ever experienced before and you deserve it all. (Kenn's hand has been rising and is now several inches up) Feel the energy, the truth in your subconscious mind as your right hand is lifting upwards. Your fingers are proclaiming "yes!", lifting so high they're carrying the hand with them.

Now I'm going to count from one to five and with each number that I count you become more and more alert, awake, aware and invigorated. When I reach the number five you open your eyes and you are then fully alert, rested and refreshed. Number one, slowly and calmly begin returning to your full awareness once again. Number two, more and more alert, awake and aware. Coming back to a very special kind of awareness where you continue to have more insights and healing and healing dreams. Good feelings are coming up and love is welling from within you, blessing people around you, and first and foremost, yourself. On number three, more and more alert, awake and aware with each number. On number four, getting ready to open your eyes. On the next number you open your eyes and are fully alert, awake and aware. Coming back now. Wide awake and refreshed and feeling great. Number five. You can open your eyes and stretch if you'd like to. Take your time. (Kenn opens his eyes and sits up and the class applauds)

KENN: (stands up) I would like to say that there's something very special I gained from taking this class and I want to pass it on to you. We should all learn to love ourselves. It's very important. Thank you for all of your support. Each one of you I'll remember always. (more applause)

Interview Seven Months Later

RANDAL: We had a session a few months ago, at a time that you had a big decision to make on whether or not to have more surgery. You were going to get a second opinion as to whether you needed further surgery on your neck. You felt that an underlying sense of shame was affecting your ability to heal and we worked on that. Then I recently got this letter from you which shows spectacular improvement in the quality of your handwriting. I'd like to read from the letter if that's all right? (Kenn nods)

Dear Randal, if you can compare the strength of this penmanship to that of our prior correspondence you will have some indication of the vast improvement of my physical condition... It goes beyond saying that I am deeply indebted to you for permitting me to be a part of a class demonstration. Thanks to your masterful therapeutic skills I was able to face and turn loose a shameful notion that has clouded my evaluation of myself since the age of three. Letting go of the shame association with chronic bed wetting was paramount to one of the greatest moments of my life and has already opened new doorways to an exciting and fulfilling future.

Then your letter continues about leading your first self–hypnosis class. You've started small but you have high hopes and aspirations of using your experiences to help others. (reading from the letter) *It will be my desire to help those less fortunate than myself. I love you and thank you.* (to Kenn) So bring us up to date. What's been happening since I saw you in November?

KENN: After I saw you I renewed my efforts to exercise more and to have a better feeling about myself. Though my progress was slow and gradual, each day I could see a little improvement in my condition. I had an appointment with the doctor in January to see about further surgery. By the time I got to my appointment he examined me and said, "Well, because of your vast improvement I can't justify surgery at this time."

RANDAL: This was the same doctor who prior to that had said that you needed to go in for surgery as soon as possible?

KENN: Yes, he had wanted me to go in the following week but I begged off by getting a second opinion. The second opinion also said surgery was indicated. Then when the first surgeon told me he didn't feel I needed surgery I actually kind of felt let down. I was totally exhausted by the whole program. I languished around and sat on my behind for a couple of weeks and I felt a little bit sorry for myself. Then I had a couple more sessions with Charlie and got back on the program and today I feel that even though I have a ways to go I'm past the hurdle.

I wanted to let you know what's going on so I wrote the letter to you. I learned a lot of humility with this program but I also learned that if you have the desire and a direction or someone who can put you in the right direction, you can do just about anything you want. The body is capable of so much more than we're aware of. I had a condition that they told me was irreversible. I was either going to be a quadriplegic or I was going to have surgery in which they wanted to put a strip in my throat so I'd go around the rest of my life looking up. I know that's not going to happen now.

This last week I learned I could squeeze a toothpaste tube again. That's something I haven't been able to do. My hand was like this. (Kenn makes a fist with his left hand) My wife would say, "Open your hand," and I would force it open (demonstrates forcing the fingers of his left hand open with his right hand), then I'd put it on my leg to hold it open. Now it's almost back to normal. (Kenn wiggles the fingers of his left hand easily) I still have a little bit of weakness in this arm.

This past week my wife and I joined the "Y". We're going to start with the Nautilus program. I'm pretty happy with the way things are going. (to the class) The thing I want to impress upon you is, if you want to do something badly enough you can find a way. Anything is possible. I've beat the surgery, thanks to you.

RANDAL: Thanks to you. Let's give him a hand. (applause)

Note from Kenn Nine Years Later

Congratulations on progress with the new book on a subject I feel is often overlooked and underused. Anyway, no botched surgery, no downhill convalescence, no furtive plea to *Randal the Magician*, no regression, nothing left but a deeply buried caldron boiling, bubbling, spewing rivulets of shame into an all too susceptible vehicle. Having found the source of the shame and exposing it to be nothing more than a fairly common childhood event, Randal and regression therapy were able to relieve me of a very heavy load.

I feel this is one of the defining moments on the road to full recovery and it certainly enhanced my belief in the amazing curative powers of the human body and the truly therapeutic value of regression therapy.

CHAPTER 11

Questions & Answers

The following are actual questions and answers taken from the transcripts of this book.

Q: Do you ever get stuck when you're working with someone? How do you know what to do next?

A: I stay in the here and now. One of the beauties of Gestalt is that there are so many options. Negatives reframe easily into positives. Suppose a client is "resistant" in some way. Honor it. Encourage it to manifest. Have him or her become the resistance. Everything is awareness.

One little trick if you're not sure what to do next with somebody is that you can always encourage the person to go inward. That's a common Gestalt process. "Go inside to your internal experience. What are you feeling right now?" I'm not saying that when I normally do that I don't know what to do next, but it's something that can be done when you don't know what to do next. It often leads somewhere important. I generally do that when I feel that there is some feeling developing or being blocked in some way, or I'm noticing some tension or physical movement or the sound of the voice is telling me that something is going on. I want to check out the internal process at that point.

Q: When you're doing a process with the inner child would you call the inner child by the name the individual was called as a child?

A: I usually use the name the person was called as a child to help him or her identify with being that young child, like Joey instead of Joe. An exception would be when there was great difficulty in childhood and the person is used to associating that name with those difficulties or with a highly dysfunctional family. I may have the child pick a different version of his own name or a different name.

Q: Is having a person respond with finger signals in hypnosis preferable to having the person verbalize?

A: It depends on the situation and the stage of the therapy session. Let's say that your client had an auto accident several months earlier and is dealing with some aspect of that fully remembered and understood trauma. After basic ideomotor questions to determine the appropriateness of recalling the memory and feeling the emotions, you could probably have the person verbalize from the beginning of the regression because it would be easier, faster and more direct. But if your client doesn't understand a particular emotional response or if there is something that the person has no conscious memory about, then he or she may not be able to give an accurate verbal answer. Ideomotor questioning may work best in that situation. As a realization begins to occur with the use of ideomotor questions, then the work may naturally switch to verbal responses.

Q: Is it possible not to have any ideomotor or verbal responses in a session?

A: In many cases it's valuable to just give direct or indirect suggestions in hypnosis with perhaps some metaphors, without necessarily any need for communication from the individual in hypnosis. But during uncovering work to get to issues that happened in the past to clear them away, in most cases ideomotor and/or verbal responses will be important. Obviously some work can be done without checking responses but some interactive process will usually facilitate speedy progress.

Sometimes asking for a verbal response can be distracting because the person has to use the part of the mind that involves speech and that could lighten the state or be somewhat interruptive, so there is a positive and a negative side to that. In some cases, a few ideomotor finger responses may be elicited to confirm the client's engagement or focus, for example.

Q: What do you think of the NLP idea of tapping into minimal cues?

A: I remember seeing a video tape from an Ericksonian conference in which the therapist was working with a husband and wife to demonstrate couple's therapy. He induced hypnosis without first having an interview or asking any questions of them at all. He had both of them recall an experience in which they felt they were doing something together. He had them pay attention to that experience and then go to another experience, all the while giving indirect suggestions. I would have felt it was a good demonstration if he had done this with a group because you can't usually do many specifics in a group, although even then he could have first encouraged information in a group interview. But here he had all of these opportunities to check things out with simple ideomotor responses to make sure they were aligned, rather than assuming alignment or acceptance, perhaps because he saw a shift in the breathing or a slight change in the color of the face. He even avoided feedback with them after bringing them out of hypnosis, immediately encouraging them to not say anything, explaining they could discuss their experiences with each other in private later.

I think tapping into minimal cues is good. You can notice various subtle clues in the body. But to focus on that exclusively and not to ask for verbal or non-verbal responses, whether with finger signals or a nod or shake of the head, is usually too limiting. You may still get a good session out of that but you are all the more likely to get better results if you elicit specific feedback.

Q: I've worked with post traumatic stress, for example, with clients who are survivors of sexual abuse, and sometimes that appears through a dream. I'm wondering where you would go with that.

A: I'll answer first in terms of regression and then talk about dreamwork. Let's say I'm working with a man who was frequently beaten as a child and I'm going to be using regression to deal with the effects of that trauma and how he is repressing himself as a result of that. Sometimes I do a classic Gestalt process, figuring that in one way or another, most people internalize what happened. That doesn't mean that the man is necessarily going to beat his children, but he might habitually beat himself up mentally, for example.

At other times I avoid a traditional Gestalt dialogue of becoming the other part by adding some detachment: "Now what does the other person say?" And if necessary I can have the person do some grounding and centering techniques or visualize healing light for protection to create some distance from that other part, even if ideomotor signals have given approval for working with the emotions. It isn't possible to formulate some scientific point at which to create some limited detachment during a dialogue. I often use my intuition with that. However, I can request ideomotor responses to tell me whether there is some significant or positive aspect in that person that needs to be integrated, or if there is some negative aspect of that person that has been internalized that is hurting him or her. If that's the case then I would usually go with a regular Gestalt dialogue.

When I'm doing Hypnotic Dreamwork™ I never assume I know what the dream is about. The Gestalt modalities are powerful in helping people work on current issues left over from past traumas, and I let the dreamwork evolve in whatever direction it goes. If there is a section of the dream that is a memory of an abuse experience, or the dreamwork triggers a traumatic memory, then there is the possibility of moving into a regression. But it usually works just right to stay within the framework of the dream therapy, treating the dream as reality and working through it. In a dream session I can have a person play the parts and let them be transformed and integrated positively.

Q: Do you find that you rarely or usually work directly in Gestalt in traumatic cases?

A: I can usually work directly in Gestalt because generally there is some related internal unfinished business, which is part of the reason why this person is still having struggles with that. The energy that has been imploded is having a negative affect on the person and it may be having a negative affect on others as well. Let's say that one of the parents had drunken rages and had beaten this child severely at times. Sometimes I will do ideomotor questions to check with the subconscious mind to find out whether a significant part of this abusive figure has been imploded. If it has, then I think the classic Gestalt dialogue is appropriate to begin to work with integrating these sides, except that I may have the person stay in one position. If the person is lying down in hypnosis I'm not going to have the person get up and alternate sitting in opposite chairs as is done in traditional Gestalt. That usually works great in dreamwork, but after a relaxing induction it would be too distracting.

Q: If you were working with a client who was having a cathartic experience or release from all these issues emerging, how would you bridge that over a period of weeks? How do you close a session and start the next one so that the person doesn't go out of your office feeling raw?

A: I would generally start with a first fifty minute session in which I ask a lot of questions and get to know the person better. I move more quickly when I do work in my classes, partly from experience and partly because I know each of my students to some degree. But if I haven't met someone before I want to get a greater history, take time to discuss hypnosis, and give an overview about potential directions and procedures over a brief series of sessions. In the next session we'll be able to get into a regression just a few minutes into the session if that's where I'm going to go, and allow up to two hours for it. That gives us time for a thorough session. There will be more insights to come and more to work on in life and usually in subsequent sessions, but my clients almost always feel a sense a completion at the conclusion of a session. If a lot has been uncovered or a lot of feelings have come up, a suggestion can be given at the end such as, "Some uncomfortable feelings may arise at times but this is a great growth opportunity as you find creative, healthy solutions to begin to work through them."

During the initial hypnosis an individual may not necessarily reach a completion of forgiveness, for example, but motivated clients can get to the point where they have released a lot. They've communicated their anger or felt their grief. You've given their feelings a chance to get expressed so the individual feels finished with that. Organize your schedule so you have plenty of time for regression sessions. You don't want to leave the person unfinished in terms of being in the middle of expressing a feeling. I've heard of some therapists doing that, saying, "Well, your time is up."

Maybe something more comes up in the next session regarding associated issues, but your clients have begun their explorations and expressions and said what they need to say, at least significant aspects, during the processes of the previous session. As therapists we can take a person whatever number of steps, but the objective is not to feel obligated to try to make your client go all the way from A to Z in one session. Don't try to accomplish too much. You could keep looking for every little thing in a perfectionistic way but the idea is that there is a lot a person can accomplish and get a sense of completion from and move on.

Q: So if a person has been feeling a certain emotion, anger or grief for example, you encourage the expression of that so they can get it out of their system?

A: Sometimes people need to go through a period in their lives where for the first time they are getting in touch with an appropriate expression of some feeling such as anger or grief. They are sometimes going to feel it and that's life and that's okay. The point isn't to get it out so the person never has to feel it any more. The point is that the person may have been holding back on all kinds of feelings and by releasing the feeling this time, something that they may not have done at all before, they're able to begin to unleash all kinds of self-expression and communication that can lead to becoming more at peace, confident, alive and self-actualized.

Q: Is there some point in a session when you might decide that the client needs to go into a past life regression?

A: I would never decide that a person needs to go into a past life regression. I just go where that person goes. The vast majority of my sessions with regression are in this life and that's what I generally assume. But if I count a person back in a regression and then ask, "What age are you? Under ten?" And if a person keeps going back past a birth experience and begins to describe some incident with other people that happened before birth, I might ask, "Okay, where are you?" and "How old are you?" I never want to suggest that a person go to a past life unless that person has come to me initially requesting a past life regression.

In another example, suppose the regressed client keeps saying or signaling an earlier age as we go back in time to an initial sensitizing event. Eventually we'll get to a question like, "Was this before the age of one month?" If affirmative, I'll ask, "Have you been born?" If not, I don't assume it will become a past life regression at that point because we first need to check the possibility of birth trauma. If that doesn't apply, the next step would be the womb. Many of my clients have gotten a sense of some significant experience or realization in the womb, such as a sense of not being wanted by the mother. When all the other possibilities are signaled to be irrelevant, I can ask, "Did it happen before the womb?" In that way a session may develop into an apparent past life regression.

Q: Are there other possible explanations for past life memories?

A: During an age regression if a client reports something that seems to be of a very different time and culture, I would usually first check out various possibilities, including being influenced by a movie, book, fantasy or dream. Eventually the questioning might lead to a question such as, "Is this an experience you had in this lifetime?"

Whether you believe in the possibility of reincarnation or not, whatever comes up can be a symbol for this life. The symbolism in dreams, for example, is a reality during the occurrence of the dream, and when I work with dreams I treat them as a reality. I can treat any image that comes up during hypnosis as a valid subconscious connection. Experiencing reality in various metaphorical ways is common within subconscious states and a lot of valuable work can be done with imagery that develops in hypnosis, including with imagery that is metaphorical or combining various experiences and expectations.

(Note: The subject of past life regression will be explored in much more detail in this book's companion volume, *Catharsis in Regression Therapy*.)

Q: To what extent is it safe to use regression with someone who has extremely negative memories?

A: You can work with any sane person who wants to do regression work, as long as you're thoroughly trained and use appropriate modalities. I'll carefully ask a person's subconscious in hypnosis whether it's safe to recall any and all memories having to do with a particular issue and if it's safe to be open to the emotions, then direct the regression accordingly. People can do amazing healing whether it's through their life's experience over time or in dramatic work in hypnotherapy or some other good therapy.

CHAPTER 12

Beneath Janine's Sabotage of Her Success
The Real Issue Explored

RANDAL: Janine has volunteered to work on an issue having to do with sabotaging success. What would you like to say about that, Janine?

JANINE: I've been thinking about it a lot this week because I knew we were going to have this session and a lot of people right now would think that what I have is pretty successful.

RANDAL: And on a lot of levels it is.

JANINE: Yes, on a lot of levels it is. For a long time though, for over twenty years, I've done things that have kept me from achieving everything I could achieve. I've made choices that kept me from realizing my full potential. I'll give you some examples because I think you need to know how this has worked. When I was at school I always got top grades. I even talked a teacher into giving me extra work so I could get from an A to an A plus because I wanted to have straight A plusses. No problem there until I got to be a senior in high school. Then I was taking calculus and I could have understood it, no problem, but somehow I decided I was going to get a D in that class so I got a D. It just wasn't as important to me after all those years of doing really well.

RANDAL: Obviously some part of you has some perfectionism in terms of wanting A plusses instead of A's.

JANINE: Yes, exactly.

RANDAL: How did you get a D in that class? You say you decided to.

JANINE: I don't think I consciously decided to, I just sloughed it off.

RANDAL: So maybe you didn't do your homework or you just didn't pay as much attention as you could have in class, that kind of thing?

JANINE: Probably. But I can tell you a better example possibly. The first year I went away to college I did fine. But then I went back in my second year and, after all those years of doing really well and knowing I could do really well, I made an A, a B, a C, a D, and an F. That was really stupid. The thing I got the F in, and I had it changed to a D ultimately, was in French and I had lived in France and spoken French for years. My French teacher said my work was so bad that nobody could have cheated or copied and done that bad. Well, I hated that guy and he hated me.

RANDAL: You're obviously very intelligent and you have a lot of skill and learning capability. With these two examples you've given, like the D in calculus, I'm thinking, so what? Maybe calculus wasn't that interesting. In your second year in college you got those different grades and maybe it wasn't that important to you. There are other things that are important besides getting good grades. Did you deliberately try to get bad grades or what happened?

JANINE: I didn't try. I just didn't go to class and I slept in until eleven o'clock.

RANDAL: You said that your sophomore year stood out for you. Other than your sophomore year did you get good grades in college?

JANINE: I did the first year but then I never finished and that has plagued me until today.

RANDAL: (exaggerating the words, in mock shock) You didn't finish college?

JANINE: (gasping and laughing) You see! I told you.

RANDAL: I wish you had told me that before we started the session. (laughter) Okay, I'll work with you. (more laughter)

JANINE: You see, it's stuff like that. Not having completed college. Now I wish I had. And I let that drag me down and keep me from achieving because I have this feeling like, "Oh God, I didn't finish it." Basically, I would like to stop sabotaging myself. I would like to be able to drop this if necessary or complete it and get on with my life feeling whole.

RANDAL: Does the issue with sabotaging success tend to be that you can start out fine and then you find a way to stop being successful or to not finish the project or whatever it is?

JANINE: I finish a lot of things just fine, so I don't know if that's the case. (big sigh) This is a really big statement, but things that I like I finish.

RANDAL: Maybe you didn't like college. It's okay that you didn't finish it. Some people have gone on to incredible accomplishments without ever going to college.

JANINE: I know. That's another part of my belief system. I see people who haven't had some of the benefits I've had in my life, who have taken off and done wonderful things because they've believed in themselves. And I really admire people who have lifted themselves up and flown by the seat of their pants and just done it. So you see I have these conflicting feelings about not having finished college on the one hand, but seeing all kinds of people who have done incredibly well without it on the other.

RANDAL: Does this issue of not finishing college stand out when you think of how you've sabotaged success?

JANINE: That is a real big one, and another thing I consider a symptom of the same issue is being overweight, because the weight keeps me from interacting with people on a level that I think would be more successful. I love people and I have friends and all of that, but I guess there is a part of me that is using weight as a buffer. I feel the weight is another symptom of the same underlying issue.

RANDAL: Let's be specific about college and about your weight. When you've tried to go back to college or when you've tried to stick to a diet, does some fear come up, "Oh, if I were successful," with a catastrophic expectation?

JANINE: I don't feel like it's a catastrophic expectation, but I do feel that if I were successful in some of these areas then there would be a whole lot more expected of me in some way.

RANDAL: So there could be a fear to that. "If I'm successful much more will be expected of me." It really struck me when you talked about getting *almost* all A plusses and no, you wanted *all* A plusses. There is a part of you that has very high expectations. And there is another part of you, I'm just throwing this out so correct me if it doesn't fit, that is afraid that if you really achieve then the other part of you will demand more and more and you don't want to have all that pressure. Is something like that going on?

JANINE: That's true. And my ideas of what I consider to be success have gone through big changes. I don't want to be the driven executive making barrels of money. I want to be a happy person making barrels of money. (laughing)

RANDAL: So let's talk about what you want to accomplish. Is making a lot of money important to you?

JANINE: Meeting my needs is important to me and meeting some desires is important.

RANDAL: You're not meeting all your needs?

JANINE: Things are nip and tuck sometimes. I'm making it. And I'm making it on a level that some people only hope for. All in all I'm very aware of how lucky I am.

RANDAL: Tell us about some of the ways you're lucky or successful or getting your needs met.

JANINE: Okay. This is one of the ones that is teetering on the brink as we speak. I have this condo that I lease out in Puerto Vallarta. I go there at Thanksgiving and Christmas, but during the summer when I can't sublet it out it's killing me financially. In the winter time lots of people want to go so there's no problem keeping the financial end up. And when friends want to go to Puerto Vallarta they stay there instead of a hotel.

RANDAL: It sounds wonderful to have that but you have to determine whether it's financially feasible.

JANINE: Yes, but I'd like to be able to keep it. That would be one of my desires, but not to have to worry about the short times during the summer. Even with the loss in the summer I'm still making it in every other way, but it's very tight.

RANDAL: Are you just allowing your friends to stay there or are you charging them?

JANINE: They always pay for their time.

RANDAL: So that's an example of success. Do you want to give another example?

JANINE: It's hard to come up with some of these things. I guess I can talk about how lucky I am to have my apartment and to be able to share it with a compatible person so I can enjoy this beautiful place.

RANDAL: So you have a beautiful apartment. How do you feel about your work?

JANINE: I hate it. It sucks. That's why I'm at this class. I love being with people.

RANDAL: So you like to have gobs of money but you hate your work. That's an interesting combination.

JANINE: Pretty bad. (laughing)

RANDAL: What kind of work do you do?

JANINE: I underwrite loans on apartment buildings so I get to travel all over.

RANDAL: So you don't hate everything about it. You like some things. Does it pay well?

JANINE: Yes.

RANDAL: It's interesting that your comment came so quickly about hating your work. I'm wondering if that's too strong.

JANINE: Maybe I just hate aspects of it. It gets down to, and this is going to sound so disgusting. What's been bothering me all week about coming up here and being honest is that it's not all pretty.

RANDAL: I know. I'm shocked about all of this. (laughter)

JANINE: I just don't give a rat's ass about whether the borrowers who come to us get their money or not. They apply for millions of dollars. They always do get it because I wouldn't do anything to hurt them, but I don't care.

RANDAL: Do you feel a little critical of yourself or guilty about not caring?

JANINE: No, I don't feel the least bit guilty about that.

RANDAL: Good. So it sounds like you do your work well?

JANINE: Yes, I do my job.

RANDAL: You give them a good run for their money and they usually get it, so that's fine. There's no problem with that as long as you're being responsible and doing a good job. Life seems to be going just fine. (*Note: This statement is made in part to reframe, and in part to coax or challenge her to elaborate on what she wants.*)

JANINE: (laughing) And that's why I feel so weird about being up here complaining about not having a decent life. But I know it could be better. There are ways it can be better. And I'm standing between me and getting those better ways.

RANDAL: How can it be better?

JANINE: One of the things I'm doing to make it better is that I'm here and I'm learning that I can do things I like doing. I would much rather be interacting with people on a one to one basis and being helpful in some way that I feel is real. Helping people to get millions of dollars doesn't do anything for me because yes, they get it, but that's where it stops. With something like doing hypnotherapy you can get such fantastic return because you get to see the success and the happiness in the people. This is why I'm here and it's one of the steps I'm taking to change the way things are.

RANDAL: I always recommend that people go gradually into hypnotherapy to test the waters and to have a stable income until you get more solid and established.

JANINE: Exactly.

RANDAL: Is your work full time? Do you have enough energy left over to do some part time work on Saturdays or a couple of evenings a week or something like that?

JANINE: (laughing) I will when we don't have classes anymore.

RANDAL: Go ahead, blame it on me. (laughter)

JANINE: I take classes now in the middle of the week and on the weekends and I'm perfectly okay with it. In fact I've been pleasantly surprised at the energy I've had to get it all accomplished.

RANDAL: That's quite a lot when you're working full time already. It sounds, Janine, like you have a lot. You have a successful job, a beautiful apartment and a lot of good friends. You've got the everyday problems of, "How do I work this out? How do I make ends meet?" Things like that that we all have. But you also have high standards for yourself and I'm inspired by the fact that you feel excited by the prospect of work that can make a difference in people's lives. I think that developing work you love and hopefully making at least as much money as you were will come a long way toward helping you to feel more peace of mind and happiness. I can certainly appreciate that.

JANINE: Yes, but there's something in me that keeps me from achieving what I think I really want. There is some stumbling block. I see things that I'd like to have and maybe I don't even make an effort.

RANDAL: So we're really focusing in on what it is that keeps you from your achievement. You said that if you really like something you finished it, so I was wondering if it's kind of an attitude or if your standards are too high. It sounds as though there really is something here that sabotages you from doing something that you really want to do. Do you associate this more with work or with other kinds of things?

JANINE: I think I associate it more with career type things. I know that in the next six months or so there might be a job opportunity with substantially more money. It's doing the same kind of thing with much better benefits in a better place. And I don't even feel like I want to get my resume together. It's really crazy.

RANDAL: So this is a good example. You need to be realistic and not expect that within six months you'll have a full time hypnotherapy practice. Therefore to switch and do the same kind of work in a better place and get much better pay and benefits would be a perfect example of something to go forward with, and yet there is a part of you that feels resistance to that.

JANINE: That doesn't even want to try. Well, actually, I'll probably get the job because I have a friend there who knows me and knows what I can do. So when the time comes for that job to open I can pretty much have it if I want it. But the thought of sending my resume for a professional position and it saying no college on there. That's the most sabotaging thing I've ever done to myself by not completing something I could have done and could have been good at.

RANDAL: After your grades fell in your sophomore year did you just quit?

JANINE: When I had opportunities I would go back and take a couple of classes and of course I'd make A's in those classes. I guess because things were different or maybe it was because I was paying for it

RANDAL: But you didn't finish. Was there something that came up for you at the time? Were you aware of a fear of success that seemed to sabotage you or it just wasn't important?

JANINE: One of the things that happened is that the first year I went to college I went to Michigan State. I liked it there. Then at some point in that year, eighteen year olds can be such idiots, I wrote this letter to my mom and dad about why things could have been different than they were. Not that I didn't have decent, loving parents. I did. But I was telling them in this eighteen page letter all of the ways I wished they had been different.

RANDAL: Whew!

JANINE: They were thinking, guess what, I could have been a better kid once or twice. Three times maybe. (laughter) They were just really crushed. They yanked me out of Michigan State and stuck me in UT in Texas, and that was the beginning of the bad grades. I guess it had a lot to do with punishing them but it ended up punishing me, too.

RANDAL: It's interesting because this fear of criticism is something significant. Here you have a job almost being handed to you on a silver platter and the real issue is that not having completed college is probably not going to keep you from getting that job, it's just an embarrassment for you.

JANINE: Yes, it's an embarrassment.

RANDAL: It feels like the big part of what you're dealing with is more a fear of criticism.

JANINE: That could be.

RANDAL: Of having a critical parent inside yourself that is not okay with you, that is beating you up for not having accomplished this.

JANINE: That sounds true, Randal.

RANDAL: Aha, we're getting down to it now.

JANINE: Could you just say, "Boo!" and make it go away? (laughter)

RANDAL: Certainly in this case we could do that. But I'm wondering if that's the bigger underlying issue here, the core issue. I mean, hey, someone might raise an eyebrow when they read your resume. That's passing. You'll get your job and everything will be fine. Maybe someday you can go back and finish college if it's really important, although it doesn't seem to be. I'm more concerned by the way you're so hard on yourself.

JANINE: Yes, I think that might be a big part of it.

RANDAL: Okay. Are you ready for some hypnosis?

JANINE: Yes, please. I can't wait. (laughter)

RANDAL: (Randal helps Janine into a reclining chair) If we do ideomotor do you use your right or left hand?

JANINE: My right hand is fine.

RANDAL: Here we go. I'd like you to look at my two fingers here. Watch them as they rotate and move toward your face. (Randal induces hypnosis with a combination of rapid induction techniques) Now I'd like you to focus your attention on your right hand. See and hear the word "yes" until a certain finger begins to lift and to rise. (Janine's index finger signals for "yes," then her middle finger signals for "no," and her little finger signals for "I don't know") If your subconscious mind doesn't know how to accurately answer a question with yes or no, then you can signal with your thumb for that.

I have a couple of practice questions for you now. Is the hand that you're currently doing the ideomotor questions with your left hand? Yes or no. (Janine's middle finger moves) The answer to the question is no, as you've correctly established. Is the hand that you're doing the ideomotor responses with currently the right hand? (Janine's index finger moves) Of course the answer is yes.

Janine, I would like to focus on the fear of criticism that came up. Being concerned about how someone is going to feel about you because you haven't completed college is a sample of that. Being concerned that people might criticize you. I'd like you to signal with your "yes" or "no" finger to the next question. Is it safe and appropriate for you to be open to any or all memories having to do with criticism or issues of being criticized? (Janine's index finger moves) The answer to the question is yes. Is it safe and appropriate for you to be open to your emotions as you recall any memories of being criticized or being in a critical environment? (Janine's index finger moves) The answer to the question is yes. Do I have permission from your subconscious mind to go in this direction to work with your issues of being hard on yourself and feeling sensitive to other people's criticism and so on? (Janine's index finger moves) The answer to the question is yes.

I'd like your subconscious mind to understand, Janine, that this issue is directly relevant to your feelings of success or sabotaging success. Dealing with this issue of your relationship to criticism will have a direct effect on feeling at peace with yourself and moving forward with freedom and comfort in your life in many ways.

I'm going to count from one up to ten and with each number that I count you become more and more aware of a feeling that you sometimes have. A feeling of being criticized. A feeling that someone is going to criticize you. You become more and more aware of that feeling. As I count upward you stay in hypnosis but you tap more and more into that feeling that you know so well and that goes back so far. Number one, two, three, becoming more aware of such a feeling. Number four, becoming afraid of being criticized. Number five and six, being afraid that someone is going to criticize you. Number seven, feeling that more and more strongly. Number eight, perhaps feeling that somewhere in your body as well. Number nine, more and more intensely afraid of being criticized. Afraid of being put down. On the next number you're right there with that feeling, number ten.

Stay with that feeling. I'll count from ten down to one and you're going to go back to an earlier time when you had that feeling. Stay with that feeling. Ten, nine, eight, going quickly back in time. Seven, six, five, going back to an earlier time when you felt this feeling of being criticized, maybe being criticized unfairly. Four, three, two, on the next number I count you're right there with that feeling. One. You can speak now and stay in hypnosis. Are you inside or outside? Pick one.

JANINE: (crying softly) I think I'm inside.

RANDAL: Is it nighttime or daytime?

JANINE: It's daytime.

RANDAL: Are you alone or with others?

JANINE: With others.

RANDAL: Are you under ten years old? Yes or no.

JANINE: (whispering) I don't know.

RANDAL: Are you a child or a teenager? Do you have a sense of that?

JANINE: No.

RANDAL: You say you're inside. Do you know whether you're inside your house or somewhere else?

JANINE: I can't picture it.

RANDAL: What's going on with you right now? What are you feeling?

JANINE: It's like I want to cry. It hurts. (patting her chest)

RANDAL: You're pointing to your chest area.

JANINE: It's my heart.

RANDAL: It hurts in your heart. What is that feeling like?

JANINE: (crying) It's so sad.

RANDAL: What do you feel sad about?

JANINE: It feels like maybe I'm not what I should be.

RANDAL: What makes you feel that maybe you're not what you should be?

JANINE: I guess I'm not what whoever is saying this wants.

RANDAL: Is that something that happens sometimes? Go back to childhood. Are you sometimes not living up to what people's expectations are, whether that be your mother or father or teacher or someone else?

JANINE: I think I was a teenager.

RANDAL: This feeling is coming up from a time when you were a teenager?

JANINE: Yes.

RANDAL: Are you feeling like you've failed in some way?

JANINE: It's my mom.

RANDAL: Are you afraid that she's upset with you or disappointed in you?

JANINE: (crying) She wants all these things for me. I just don't know if I want to do them. She has this thought of me doing all the things she didn't have a chance to do.

RANDAL: So she wants to have you do or get or achieve the things that she didn't do herself?

JANINE: Right.

RANDAL: Give me an example.

JANINE: I think that even though she got married when she was twenty six so she had time to be herself, I think she feels like she gave up a lot. Some of her dreams. She sees me as having the opportunity to achieve all the dreams she had. She wants me to live her dreams.

RANDAL: But they're not necessarily your dreams, are they?

JANINE: Some of them are but some of them aren't.

RANDAL: Let's talk to your mom about that. Imagine your mom is right here now and you're a teenager. Your mom really wants you to be able to have all the things she dreamed of having and wasn't able to get. What is it that you'd like to say to her?

JANINE: I'd like to say that some of them are okay, mom, but some of them just aren't me.

RANDAL: All right. When I touch your shoulder switch and become your mom. (Randal touches her shoulder) What does your mom say in response to that?

JANINE: I can't understand why you don't want to do that. You've got the capability. How could you not want it when you can?

RANDAL: Is Janine the name you go by when you're that age? (Janine nods) Okay, switch and be Janine.

JANINE: (sobbing) You know sometimes I just don't even know what I don't want, just the way I sometimes don't always know what I do want. And you are expecting me to do things or want things but I don't even know what I want for myself. It's too much.

RANDAL: Switch and be mom.

JANINE: I worked hard to achieve the things I've achieved and I managed. I got married and I had to finish college late but I not only finished, I got a master's degree. And it wasn't everything I always wanted to do but I achieved it, even if I had to give up so many things. And now you have this opportunity to achieve anything and you have the capability. I want you to do that.

RANDAL: Now switch and be Janine.

JANINE: (still sobbing) I guess I feel your wanting every day.

RANDAL: Tell her how you feel about that.

JANINE: There are some things I want to do well but I can't live your life. I'm not the same as you.

RANDAL: Say, "I won't live your life."

JANINE: I won't live your life. I can't. I'm not the same as you.

RANDAL: Now switch and be your mom.

JANINE: I just can't give up what I want for you.

RANDAL: Change that to take responsibility, Mom. Say, "I won't give up what I want for you."

JANINE: I won't give up what I want for you. I only want the best for you. Can't you realize what's best for you?

RANDAL: Switch and be Janine.

JANINE: What's best for you and what's best for me could be two different things. We're so alike but we're so different. It's the generation thing, Mom.

RANDAL: So say, "I won't do everything you want me to do."

JANINE: I won't do everything that you want me to.

RANDAL: Good. Now switch and be Mom.

JANINE: Well, that's obvious.

RANDAL: So tell Janine how you feel about that. It's obvious that Janine isn't doing everything you want her to do.

JANINE: It hurts me.

RANDAL: Say, "I hurt." Once again, take responsibility.

JANINE: I hurt because I see you not taking advantage of opportunities you could have to do anything. It hurts me that you won't move forward and take those chances.

RANDAL: Switch and be Janine.

JANINE: Mom, there are some things that I will take chances on. I'll take chances on people. I'll take chances on love. I'll take chances on some of the things that are out there in front of me, but you can't make me be perfect by how you understand perfect.

RANDAL: Now switch and be Mom.

JANINE: I just feel so bad. How did I fail you? How did I not instill in you these feelings of wanting to be... How did I miss?

RANDAL: Be Janine.

JANINE: I think you just need to understand that things that are important to you just aren't as important to me and things that are important to me you don't care about. You just don't see. I'd say that you're just going to have to get over it.

RANDAL: Switch and be Mom.

JANINE: I don't think I'm going to get over this.

RANDAL: How about taking responsibility and saying, "I choose not to get over it." Say it and find out if that feels right.

JANINE: I choose not to get over it. That works. I choose not to.

RANDAL: What do you say to Janine now? Anything in addition to that?

JANINE: I find it unbelievable that you let these things happen. I find it unbelievable that you have made these disgusting grades.

RANDAL: Be Janine. How do you feel in response to what she just said?

JANINE: Mom, I know I did this. I know I got that D from that shithead of a professor because I didn't like him. And I got those other bad grades because I was fighting you.

RANDAL: Tell her how fighting her caused you to get those bad grades.

JANINE: (sobbing) It was almost as though if I got the bad grades it would break some connection or some control that you had on me. And I hurt myself in the process.

RANDAL: You can tell her that you chose to rebel against her by getting bad grades.

JANINE: I chose to rebel against you by getting these grades.

RANDAL: Now be Mom and respond to that.

JANINE: Well, I don't know what to do with you. I just don't know.

RANDAL: Tell Janine what you want from her.

JANINE: I'm glad you understand why you did it. Now I understand. I still feel that you had all this potential and that you're refusing it, and I guess you're refusing to realize it because you're rebelling against me. I still don't like it. I'm so unhappy with you.

RANDAL: Okay, switch and be Janine.

JANINE: (sobbing and big sigh) Oh, Mom. I probably love you more than anyone else in the world, but you can't do this to me.

RANDAL: I want you to tell her what's wrong with her now. She's been saying what's wrong with you and now you tell her what's wrong with her.

JANINE: What's wrong with you, Mom, is that you must feel like a failure yourself for giving up your dreams and you must have felt miserable lots of years of your life when you weren't doing what you thought you could do. (sobbing) And all those things you dreamed of doing. I really feel that you thought you would feel better if I did those things for you. And I know that some of your unhappiness was so attached to this issue. And I think that you should leave your unhappiness behind and not force me to be you.

RANDAL: Good. Switch and be Mom.

JANINE: Yes, you're right. I've had my unhappy times. My thoughts of how disappointed I am that I didn't do certain things. But I have achieved a lot in my life and I receive some satisfaction from that and if you can't have my dreams maybe you can have some of yours. But I guess one of the things I'd like for you to have is the satisfaction of having done something you think is important.

RANDAL: All right, let's switch.

JANINE: I've done some things, Mom, that I'm happy with.

RANDAL: So when she says she wants you to feel that kind of satisfaction from some accomplishment, you feel you have that satisfaction?

JANINE: Not many things, but in some.

RANDAL: She just said she wanted you to have a kind of satisfaction, and you can sense having had it. How did you feel about your mom saying that if you can't have her dreams you can have your own?

JANINE: Mom, we've fought about this for so long. It's nice when you relinquish even a little bit of hold.

RANDAL: Now tell her what you want.

JANINE: Mom, I want to be successful. (sobbing) I want it. And I want to feel good about the things I do. That's what I want.

RANDAL: Okay. You want to feel successful and you want to feel good about the things you do. What do you want from her?

JANINE: I want her support.

RANDAL: "I want your support."

JANINE: I want your support.

RANDAL: All right. Switch and be Mom.

JANINE: When you were twenty eight, I came to grips with you and I decided that maybe you were finally doing something I could feel good about. Things got better then, didn't they? It's not so much that I gave up on my dreams for you, it's just that I somehow managed to accept you. In some ways you didn't do all the wonderful things you could have done but you were doing something that was okay. Somehow I could deal with it better. And if you'll remember, we got along so much better. It took me ten years but I could finally find something you were doing that I liked.

RANDAL: Does Janine know what that is?

JANINE: Yes.

RANDAL: Thank you. Now switch and be Janine. How do you feel about the various things your mom just said?

JANINE: I feel like it was a long time coming and I'm not happy with you for being so rigid.

RANDAL: Good. Now get into it. Your mom has so often wanted you to do things differently and wanted you to do things better. It's time for you to tell her what's wrong with her.

JANINE: I think you are so brilliant but for a brilliant woman you are so stupid. You know you pushed me away when I didn't do things your way. I would never, never do that to a child of mine. (shouting) I can't believe you did it! I can't believe you treated me that way.

RANDAL: That's good. Speak out and tell your mom how you feel.

JANINE: Mom, you piss me off. It was all I could do for those ten years to not keep your grandson away from you and to not do the spiteful things that you did. It was all I could do to be bigger than that. I guess that was one of the great lessons of my life. How to be nice in the face of your carping and disapproval. And to not be to you the way you were being to me.

RANDAL: It's so good to speak your truth. It's so good to tell your mom how you feel and to get that out. Go ahead.

JANINE: I didn't like that about you. I was full of disbelief that a mom could do that to her own kid. We were so close for so long. Then for ten years I couldn't do anything right. And you know, some of those years I was just searching. I was trying to find who I really was because I didn't know and because I didn't take a direction you wanted I was wrong. Well guess what? I wasn't as wrong as you were.

RANDAL: Say that again.

JANINE: I wasn't as wrong as you were.

RANDAL: You've said a lot. You've gotten a lot off your chest. Now switch and be Mom.

JANINE: I was so wrapped up in myself that I guess I just couldn't let you be who you were. All I could be was unhappy. It wasn't just you. I was unhappy with me, too. And dissatisfied on so many fronts. But you were my focal point because I had invested all of my dreams in you. What a disservice.

RANDAL: Thank you. Now switch and be Janine.

JANINE: It's a good thing those ten years past. It's a good thing because things got better. There were times after that before you passed on that we had some really wonderful moments and I was grateful for those. But what a waste those ten years were.

RANDAL: There is still some more so get into those feelings. Go inside your body. What do you feel in your body right now?

JANINE: I want to say empty but I don't know if that's really it. I guess a sense of loss. I feel there's a loss inside.

RANDAL: Do you want to tell her any more about that?

JANINE: Yes. Those years were just as bad for me as they were for you because I didn't like being at odds with you. I didn't like being so angry and you being so angry. It's just not my nature. I don't like it but I can do it. I can be angry even though I don't like being that way.

RANDAL: Is there anything more that you're upset about? Anything that you want from her or to tell her?

JANINE: No, I think I'm over a lot of the upset part but I know what I want.

RANDAL: Tell her what you want.

JANINE: I want you to be with me. Stop dragging me in a different direction. I want you to be with me in my direction.

RANDAL: Now switch and be Mom.

JANINE: Don't you know I do that? Don't you know that I'm with you now? I've learned so much and that's why you notice the time when it's on 11:11, my birthday. That's why you know to see that. I'm just showing you that I'm there with you.

RANDAL: Thank you. Switch and be Janine.

JANINE: Yes, I notice the time, Mom, when it's 11:11. I think of you when I see it. And I feel better, I guess.

RANDAL: Is there anything more that you want to say to your mom?

JANINE: Yes. If you put your mind with mine there's nothing we couldn't do. (laughing) God, I wish you would do that because I can use some help getting some places I want to go.

RANDAL: Make that a clear statement. "I'd like you to do that. I could use that help."

JANINE: Yes, mom, I would like you to do that. I could use that help. If only we could put the energy into good things, like good thoughts and good plans and hopes. Just help me get there.

RANDAL: Switch and be Mom.

JANINE: I try. I'm better at it. You'll be better.

RANDAL: When you say you try, and you do say you're better, can you make a stronger statement? You know what she's asking you to do. Will you do it?

JANINE: Yes, I can do it and I will do it. I've learned a lot and I've realized a lot about what I did. Unfortunately it came too late to do much about it in this lifetime. But I know the help she needs.

RANDAL: Say that to her. "I know the help you need."

JANINE: Oh, I know the help you need, Janine.

RANDAL: Okay, be Janine.

JANINE: I'll try to be open to it, Mom.

RANDAL: There's that word try again.

JANINE: I'll be open.

RANDAL: Would you like to be?

JANINE: Yes. I would like to be open. I love my mom.

RANDAL: There is something called a Gestalt prayer and I'd like you to say this to your mom now as we close the conversation. Please repeat after me, and you're talking to your mom now, "I am I and you are you."

JANINE: I am I and you are you.

RANDAL: "I am not in this world to live up to your expectations."

JANINE: I am not in this world to live up to your expectations.
RANDAL: "And you are not in this world to live up to mine."
JANINE: And you are not in this world to live up to mine.
RANDAL: "I do my thing and you do your thing."
JANINE: I do my thing and you do your thing.
RANDAL: "If by chance we find each other it's beautiful."
JANINE: If by chance we find each other it's beautiful.
RANDAL: "If not it can't be helped."
JANINE: If not it can't be helped.
RANDAL: Now switch and be your mom. How did that sound? Do you have any response to what Janine just said?
JANINE: It sounds like a pretty sane thing to me.
RANDAL: Good. I'd like you to say it to Janine now. "I am I and you are you."
JANINE: I am I and you are you.
RANDAL: "I am not in this world to live up to your expectations."
JANINE: I am not in this world to live up to your expectations.
RANDAL: "And you are not in this world to live up to mine."
JANINE: And you are not in this world to live up to mine.
RANDAL: "I do my thing and you do your thing."
JANINE: I do my thing and you do your thing.
RANDAL: "If by chance we find each other it's beautiful."
JANINE: If by chance we find each other it's beautiful.
RANDAL: "If not it can't be helped."
JANINE: If not it can't be helped.
RANDAL: How does it feel to say that to Janine?
JANINE: It's kind of a new idea but you know, I think it's true.
RANDAL: That's good. Now switch and be Janine. What do you want to say to your mom in response?
JANINE: I'm happy that you think it's true. It's such a relief.
RANDAL: Do you have any closing statement for your mom?
JANINE: I just want to say that I miss you.
RANDAL: Switch and be Mom. Do you have a response for Janine?
JANINE: I'm with you more often than you know.
RANDAL: Is there anything else you'd like to say to Janine?
JANINE: (sobbing and whispering) I love you.
RANDAL: Janine, do you have any response to what your mom just said?
JANINE: No, not really.

RANDAL: Okay, take it in. Can you say goodbye to your mom for now?

JANINE: 'Bye Mom.

RANDAL: Be Mom. Can you say goodbye to Janine?

JANINE: Goodbye.

RANDAL: Now switch and be Janine. See your mom going now. Feel that sense of completion. Feel the good feeling of you and your mom both growing a lot through this and deep down understanding that Gestalt prayer. For you to take it in and accept it is so freeing for both of you. If your mom can be accepting of you and interested in supporting you in your dreams, then that's great. If she's not interested in doing that then that's the way it goes. You can do great on your own and you can do great with your mom. You'll be yourself and in being yourself, Janine, who you are is an incredibly powerful person. You are not in this world to live up to anyone else's expectations. You're in this world to actualize yourself, to be yourself. Who you are is a magnificent person. It's a matter of you doing what you want to do. Give yourself that freedom. You are someone who has already accomplished many things in your life.

You're going to find that the more comfortable and accepting you are of yourself, the more positive you feel and the more energy you have to make whatever improvements you want to make. Whether it's in your work situation or your relationship with food or in any situation in your life. You can do whatever you set your mind to do. One of the things you can do is to accept who you are right here and now. You are not only okay, you are great just the way you are. I know you'll go on and do other things as well because you want to do them. That's happening. Enjoy the journey. Enjoy smelling the flowers along the way.

What you've got, Janine, is the world at your fingertips. If you want to do this other job for now you find that it's easy for you to fill out that application. You can feel great and you're proud of yourself. The fact that you're involved with helping people get large amounts of money is an example of your success. You did that without a college education. That's who you are, that you were able to propel yourself forward in ways that other people wouldn't be able to do. You have a tremendous amount of awareness, alertness, intelligence and people skills. People are inspired by you. You are very good at what you do.

All of those skills that you have, along with your heart and your compassion, help make you an outstanding hypnotherapist, so you are also moving in that direction. As these classes are completing and more time is freeing up you move into the kinds of opportunities in which you can serve people in ways that satisfy you to your core. You're not out there to make changes for other people, they have to make the changes for themselves, but you can come from a centered space and from detached compassion. The Buddhist concept of detached compassion is such a powerful way to help people become more powerful.

Using these skills of tapping people into their subconscious minds can help them to move mountains and that's a wonderful feeling. As the best comes out from you, the best is returned. And the loving energy that goes out to people's subconscious minds is so rewarding. You know that when you're doing that work, you're doing something that can be profound for them and also profoundly rewarding for you.

You are finding yourself physically to be more healthy and more attractive, and that's just because of who you are. You deserve to live your dreams. You become your dream, whatever that dream is. That's what you're on this earth for and you deserve all of that. Maturation, in the Gestalt sense, is going from environmental support to self support. You are feeling your own support because deep within you, you love and appreciate yourself as you are.

I'd like you to do some self-hypnosis over the next several weeks. When you're going to bed at night or during some other time, take a few minutes to embrace the child within. Also embrace that teenager within and let her know that she is perfect just the way she is. I'd like you to imagine doing that right now. Please signal with your "yes" finger when you have that image. (Janine's index finger moves) Good. I'd like you to keep doing that. Really love that girl, whatever age you're feeling her to be right now. You can imagine different ages at different times. She can be a young teenager, she can be a child, or whatever age needs that at the moment. Give her all of that love and support and acceptance for who she is.

Now I'd like you to be that teenager or that young girl. Feel that love from this inner mother who is you, this inner mother who is completely accepting and loves you for who you are. Take in that love and acceptance and approval that you deserve. You've deserved that all along. You're beautiful and wonderful just as you are. We all love you for who you are. You don't have to do anything or to achieve things. You do things and you achieve things anyway, that's just part of being who you are in the world. Not to satisfy others but to satisfy yourself. You're naturally a giving, loving person in many situations, and especially with yourself. (pause) Is there anything else you would like to say or to ask before I bring you up out of the hypnosis?

JANINE: No.

RANDAL: Getting ready now. (Randal gives suggestions as he counts her up out of hypnosis)

JANINE: (opening her eyes slowly) Thanks.

RANDAL: We're going to take a break in just a minute and before we do I'd like you to look around at all these beautiful faces.

JANINE: (looking around) Oh, God.

RANDAL: You'll see the way the world really is.

JANINE: Not without my glasses. (laughter)

RANDAL: You can do anything! But I'll make it easier for you. (Randal hands Janine her glasses)

JANINE: (putting them on) I can see!

RANDAL: (reaching for his own glasses) Okay, I'll use my glasses, too. Look around at all these beautiful people. See the complete and total acceptance. See the love that's there. There are people here that you haven't met until today and others that you know.

JANINE: (with a big sigh, voice teary) Thank you for being here and giving me this opportunity. It's really important. Thank you.

RANDAL: Is there anyone who would like to say something to Janine from your heart before we take a break?

NANCY: We love you and thank you.

BOBBY: Thank you for being my friend.

JANINE: You are so welcome.

JAN: This room is so full of love for you. You just did a beautiful job.

JANINE: Thank you.

JOE: (mimes sending a hug)

JANINE: (laughing) Thank you.

RANDAL: You're going to get more than the visualization of a hug in a few minutes. I kind of sense these things with my psychic awareness.

JANINE: Hugs are one of my favorite things.

MIKAYLA: You're magnificent and I see so much of myself in you. Thank you for doing that work for me, too.

DOUG: I'm so glad to be in on this session. I'm taking away as much as you are, Janine. I'm glad you shared in this because it's really helped to heal all of us.

JANINE: It was a little scary. I've been waiting for this, to find out what it was.

CAROL: How do you feel now, Janine?

JANINE: (Janine's voice continues to be soft and teary) It's kind of different. I don't feel joyful or anything but what I do feel is a little bit of sadness because of the way the situation was. A little bit like I came to grips with parts of the relationship with my mom who really...when she died, the thought that went through my mind was that I love her more than anyone else in the world. That's how close we were and that's why that ten year gap was such a big thing. But I feel that she loves me. She didn't always know how to be that loving parent and I didn't always, believe me, know how to be a loving daughter. (laughs) But I feel like we've come to grips with each other.

CAROL: What's your sense of her now?

JANINE: My sense of her is, well, about three years after she died, which was about fifteen years ago, I had this really vivid dream of her. In this dream she was back to being her healthy self and she said to me that she was fine now. She knew I was worried about how she was because of the way she died and all, and she said, "I just want you to know that I'm fine and I want you to take care of Randy," who is my son. That was a good thing and I remember saying in the session that I notice times when I know she's around. It's like she makes me see her birthday when the time is 11:11 on the clock radio, or whatever. So now I do feel that she's more supportive and I do feel that she understands some things that she was too involved in during her own life to understand then.

RANDAL: I feel like you really were in touch with your mom. You were working on two levels. It was beautiful to see how far both of you came. I would trust your instincts in that but at the same time I want to say that whatever or how much of this she really does get, I know that what you get within you is the most important. You can't change her. The Gestalt prayer goes both ways. You need to accept where she is and you may have an inkling if she has had some further growth from this experience. You may get more of a sense of that in the days ahead.

The residual sadness that you feel is part of being an authentic person and being in touch with the reality of the loss you experienced. That's very fresh in your experience now. It's part of what you're going to be in touch with, for the moment anyway, and it may pass fairly quickly. You're still dealing with the completion of that. Okay, we'll take a break.

RANDAL: (after the break) The pre-induction interview was somewhat longer than I usually do in class because I wanted to get a handle on what I felt was the essence of the direction to go. I kept coming back to the perfectionism Janine had mentioned early on. That was the key that helped me to figure out where I wanted to go with this. Then it really clicked when Janine was so embarrassed about turning in an application for that job, which was pretty much a slam dunk, because her lack of college wasn't likely to have any significant effect.

During the session we got into quite an involved Gestalt dialogue. When I'm doing emotional clearing work, I'm not going to try and rush it or cut corners. I say that partly in context with preparing for a session. If I know in advance that I may be doing a regression with someone, I like to reserve a couple of hours. There is so much that can be accomplished with this and it's so valuable. Things can go more quickly, but this was a lifetime of stuff between Janine and her mom.

You'll notice that I didn't push Janine or her mom to try to get to a compromise or resolution. In fact, when anything came up for either her or her mother, I encouraged both of them to really get into it and not to try to be nice about it. If the mom was upset about the grades or whatever, just get it out. Let's get everything on the table. Say it as strongly as you can and get it out of your system. Even though she was quite possibly working on two levels, the most important part from the standpoint of the therapy was working out the internalized critical parent for herself. There was also loss and just by feeling it and saying all she could possibly say about it, it has started to dissipate so she can move on with her life and put it behind her.

It doesn't always come all the way to a completion as this did. When there is nothing more left to be said often the final statement will be "I love you" and she came to that. Sometimes, especially if you're working with a client who has done very little therapy before that, it may not get that far. Don't feel like you have to keep working for hours and hours. The object is that I was going to be very patient with Janine in going back and forth as long as she needed to. Sometimes people reach a point where they have been holding their anger in all their lives and they need to be in touch with the fact that this is important. "It's okay for me to be angry. I have a right to be angry about this," which may mean expressing the anger or it may be a matter of standing up for themselves or taking charge. It's fine when it gets to that, too. I think it's so healing to actually be able to feel a sense of completion and letting go, and it's great when you can get that far.

EVELYN: If you didn't have the Gestalt method to use for this, what else might you have done?

RANDAL: There are always various ways to deal with things. I could have done some ideomotor work, asking her a series of questions to get down to it. I could have her observe the experience in a detached way and then go straight to getting a sense of underlying issues. Once I got clear on the pervasiveness of Janine's fear of criticism, I felt it was obviously something from the past that had been entrenched for many years. After confirmation of ideomotor signals, it felt like Gestalt would become part of the therapy of choice. There are so many good forms of therapy, but Gestalt is often so very effective in regression. Janine, do you want to come up here and say anything?

JANINE: Yes, there is something I want to say. Intellectually I've known for a long time that people don't generally criticize me, but I do their work and mine, too. I might get a little criticism here and there, but I'm pretty hard on myself.

RANDAL: One of the reasons you don't get a lot of criticism is that you've tried to live your life so well and in such a way that you're not going to.

JANINE: Exactly. So I pretty much do most of it. And I don't want to do that anymore, so thank you. (laughing) I'll keep you all posted.

RANDAL: Great. I'll check in with you later in class.

JANINE: When I came up here today I thought there was something else that was the problem. I knew that I beat myself up with criticism but I didn't think that was it. But that is it. I was talking all around it.

ANASTACIA: I have a question for Janine. I've been in a process with Randal and I remember almost feeling removed. When I was answering questions it was like someone else was answering. And I was struck by the distinct personality differences between you and your mom. I was curious how you felt that difference within yourself.

JANINE: The sense I got was that I felt the disapproval when I spoke as my mother and when I spoke as myself I felt the wanting of that approval.

RANDAL: It's so good to turn the tables when you're doing Gestalt. You were so used to trying to protect yourself from other people's criticism, so to internalize that and become it right at the source was a way to get the two sides to come together.

JANINE: There is something else I want to say. The desire to get help takes you beyond the feelings of whatever it is, like in my case, thinking, "Oh God. The class is going to think I'm just a whiny bitch." Or whatever. Then at the end when the group gave their feelings, it was such a wonderful thing. I really appreciate it. I know that the other people who have done this always appreciate the love that comes from the group and from Randal.

RANDAL: Thank you all very much and thank you, Janine. (applause)

Interview the Following Day

RANDAL: In our session yesterday what started out as an issue of sabotaging success became an issue of dealing with a fear of criticism. Is there anything else you'd like to say to the group about your experience or insights since?

JANINE: I do have something I'd like to say. After I left here yesterday and went home all these memories were bubbling up and continuing to bubble up today. Some of them were the same battle stuff and one was the worst memory I could possibly have of something my mother did to me. Because she didn't agree with my choices she actually talked my dad into disinheriting me for awhile. I had totally forgotten that. And then my dad was trying to be a peace maker. When I found out about it and was storming out of the house he came out and said, "You know, Janine, if you just do what your mother wants everything will be okay." And I said, "Daddy, you can take the money and stick it." And I just walked out. But then I was also telling some people this morning of this beautiful memory I have of my mother, and this was probably after ten years passed and we were back to feeling good about each other.

RANDAL: I'm glad that happened before she died.

JANINE: I am, too. I'm so incredibly grateful that we had some years of love before her passing. I realize now that when she decided she could love me again was when I got into being a real estate appraiser. I was making the amount of money that both she and my dad combined were making and she couldn't criticize me any more. All of a sudden maybe I had achieved some of the dream that she'd had in store for me. I think that underneath all this confusion on her part and on my part there never was a disconnection of love. It was just everybody being so messed up in different parts of their lives that the combination was incendiary.

RANDAL: You know, the opposite of love is not hate. The opposite of love is indifference, and one thing you never had was indifference.

JANINE: There was never indifference. (laughing) But this wonderful memory popped in when I was on my way home last night and inching my way up one of the hills in San Francisco, of one time when I'd had some surgery done. I was coming out of the anesthesia and she was there. She didn't know I was conscious yet and I wasn't really. I was teetering on the brink of awareness and she said to the nurse, "You know...(crying softly) Just a second. (pause) That's my daughter. Isn't she beautiful?"

RANDAL: A perfect time, too, when you were as vulnerable and suggestible as you were. That's great. Was that a time when you were or weren't getting along so well?

JANINE: We had started back on the right track.

RANDAL: So that was part of what helped you to get better fast.

JANINE: And then later when she got sick I felt so good that I could be there for her. (crying)

RANDAL: That felt like a real healing for you to be nurturing toward her.

JANINE: It was.

RANDAL: And to give back in spite of all of her stuff. She was your mom and you loved her a lot. Our parents give us so much and if a parent is not really abusive we can't possibly give back all of the positive things that a parent will give. In most ways your mother was a good mother to you.

JANINE: Yes, she was. The most satisfying thing that I gave back to her was toward the end, when she had stopped looking at people's cards and flowers because she just didn't want to see them. I think she had already come to the understanding that she was going. She just wanted to be in her little world and not know. I couldn't stand to see the aloneness in her and the fear. At that time I didn't know a lot of the spiritual things I know now that I could have maybe helped her with. She couldn't hear at that time either, but I made her this big sign with great big letters that said, "I LOVE YOU MOM." And I held it in front of her face until she read it. That was awesome because she knew that even though she felt alone, she wasn't. (crying softly) These are just some of the things that have been sifting to the top.

RANDAL: It's great that you're turning all of this into diamonds in the rough. The positives and negatives. You're having a chance to really be with your relationship with your mom. Just let those memories come. There will be painful ones and blissful ones. This is a way of acknowledging and owning these very important aspects of your life. And a way of saying goodbye to your mother, as well as a way of saying hello to her again. If you intuitively feel that she's still there it's good for you to really pay attention to this aspect of your life and have a kind of closure with it. Before we finish that closure sometimes we need to be present with these very important things.

JANINE: Yes, and you know, I've had little glimpses of feeling that alignment with her that I could have used all these years, of her understanding my need to go in a different direction. During the day I was wondering, who do I take after, anyway? Everybody used to think I was kind of like my mom and in many ways I was. And I thought, am I like my dad? Then I figured maybe I was like my grandmother. You know, all of a sudden I can't really see who I'm like anymore.

RANDAL: Maybe you're like yourself.

JANINE: Maybe I am.

RANDAL: Does anyone have a question for Janine?

SHARON: Between last night and tonight what I have observed is that where you're showing emotion now is on where you love her. When you talked about that disinheritance due to her input, it didn't seem to hit you inside anymore.

JANINE: No, it doesn't hit me like it once did. It was a pretty big issue when it happened.

SHARON: And now feeling that reconnection and the reunion. I just wanted to comment on that.

JANINE: The fact is that she and I had three or four really close years. There are some very funny and some very good stories from those years that are also coming back and it's amazing. (to Randal) So thank you. And I want to say something about the feeling I had with the ideomotor responses yesterday. I was blown away by the fact that even though I was thinking "yes" that there didn't appear to be any connection between what I was thinking and my finger movement. It was such a strange sensation and it made ideomotor responses very real for me.

RANDAL: Good. So that's an example of that. Thank you. I've appreciated all your sharing and openness with the group. (applause)

Interview Two Weeks Later

RANDAL: Hello, Janine. Do you want to tell us something about how you're doing?

JANINE: I'm doing very well, thank you. A couple of things that have happened this week are that I've come to understand so much more of my mom and to feel quite empathetic with her. I still can't understand some of the things she did but I got to the root cause of her behavior, and I've certainly gotten to the root cause of my behavior. It was me becoming me, basically. But I'm also coming to feel quite a bit of empathy for my dad because he was in the middle of these two raging lunatics, trying to make everybody happy and not succeeding. (laughing) My heart really goes out to him now. But he and I made our peace when he was dying.

RANDAL: He's passed away, too?

JANINE: Yes. He was in a coma for about four months and I'd come into town to be with him when he was in that state. I said so many things to him that I was really happy about so I feel at peace. And actually I have to say that I feel at peace with my mom, even though I don't know where some of her ideas came from.

RANDAL: When you say some of her ideas, do you mean why she would disinherit you, that kind of thing?

JANINE: Exactly. What in the world was in her mind to do that?

RANDAL: There are certain things many of us do that there simply isn't any excuse for. For example, we've all experienced saying something stupid and thinking, "Why in the world did I say that?" or "How could that have happened?" Of course the situation with your mother was very different. It wasn't something spontaneous that was blurted out. I'm sure you could find reasons for it in your mother's background and upbringing and so forth, which isn't an excuse. I would see it in part as a feeling of powerlessness on her part, that she felt obsessed with wanting to give you the things that she needed when she was a kid and didn't get. That's a classic kind of a thing. People can get so obsessed with giving their children what they didn't have and yet that's not necessarily what their children need. You are not your mother and you don't need what she missed. I think she may have been offended when you weren't responding to all the things she was doing for you, that when it comes down to it, she wanted for herself.

JANINE: A couple of other things that have surfaced this week is that I have other issues connected to this. Like I think my attitude toward money has been jarred and it's still not back in place. And I can think of some specifics where my attitude toward relationships has been impacted.

RANDAL: When you say your attitude toward money and relationships, do you mean jarred by the issue you had with your mother and you're still working through that?

JANINE: Yes, I think there's still some work to be done in those two areas and that they're connected to the issues with my mom.

RANDAL: In spite of that you and she had and have a very strong connection. Even when she was taking away your inheritance, still deep down she really loved you a lot.

JANINE: Of course she did.

RANDAL: And you can see that.

JANINE: Yes, I can. It was an extremely valuable process for me because I had buried these things so deeply that I hadn't thought of them in years. I probably thought about them for a year after they happened and then they slipped under the surface and caused all this mayhem. Now that it's out so many things are falling into a better perspective. I still have those two areas to work on but now I can see a way to do it.

RANDAL: And you're working on them just by seeing that you have them to work on. You've come a long way in your life regarding money and relationships and this is taking the next step.

JANINE: I'm clearing out the rubbish and leaving the good stuff, which is the whole point.

RANDAL: Earlier today you mentioned something else that is happening, too.

JANINE: (laughing) Yes. I'm very thrilled about this. Apparently I don't need to be feeding that hurt teenager anymore and since our session I've lost seven and a half pounds. It's like the weight is going away now. (applause)

RANDAL: Seven and a half pounds in two weeks. You're not eating the same way you were before?

JANINE: No, I've shifted that a little bit.

RANDAL: So you're not eating for the teenager inside.

JANINE: Yes, the weight is just going away and my clothes are starting to fit better.

RANDAL: Now you're eating for the physical sustenance your body needs rather than for the emotionally starved girl that was missing the love of her mother or her appreciation.

JANINE: Exactly. It's a wonderful feeling to not even have to try. Since the beginning of this class I've been on a regimen to lose weight and I was really good on it. I did everything the program said to do and I didn't lose an ounce. All of a sudden now it's just going and I'm not even having to try. (laughing) Awesome.

RANDAL: That's great. So there is a lot that's going on. Have you been doing some self-hypnosis?

JANINE: Yes, I do self-hypnosis. Well, I use a tape but I find a place in there to put in loving the teenager.

RANDAL: Continue doing that. There are shifts that are obviously happening on a number of different levels and you may not even need any more sessions, other than giving yourself nurturing support in self-hypnosis. You may find that with your own process this will continue to evolve.

CAROLINE: (to Janine) How are you doing in writing out your application for that job?

JANINE: I haven't done it. It's not coming up for six months, but I have to tell you that my attitude has undergone a transformation.

CAROLINE: Do you feel you've released the shame about that?

JANINE: Yes, I feel that I have. Now instead of focusing on the lack I find myself realizing the strength I have in that regard. I know I can do a damn good job. I'll get it if I want it. I just might not want to move to Texas.

RANDAL: This sounds like a woman with a lot of abundance who is in charge of her life.

JANINE: I'm working on it.

NANCY: Do you really think losing those pounds was a result of working with that inner part of yourself?

JANINE: Oh, yes!

NANCY: Did you think about it or not think about it the next day? What went on for you?

JANINE: After that session I went home and I was pretty shaken. I made myself four pieces of toast with butter and I ate them. (laughter) But then I didn't eat anything else. The next day, I'm always fine during the day but then in the evening I had something that was less fat, but it was still closer to something I do that isn't so great. The day after that things just shifted and all of a sudden I didn't have to do that.

NANCY: You didn't have to consciously think about it?

JANINE: No, I didn't have to consciously think about it. It just showed up in my behavior and it felt right. I think that I'm feeding the real me now, not someone else. It's a good feeling.

RANDAL: Thank you, Janine. (applause)

Janine Writes Three Years Later

I loved reviewing my session. It really brought it all back to me - tears and love and all.

Things have been pretty amazing since the time of the session. Not only did I get the new job I went to when I was leaving California, but I have also gone on to another one with even better pay. Luckily my career path has made me quite a valuable commodity on the job market, because I may be getting an even better position than I have now. I have been very happy with the results of my interviews. I walk in feeling confident, and it must really show. It is good to feel powerful.

I've taken charge of my life in other ways too. My husband (I'm married now) and I bought a home in Mexico - not in Puerta Vallarta, but in Merida, a really charming city on the Yucatan peninsula. We're planning to retire there in a few years. Our house is located right across from the English Library, which is a perfect location for my future hypnosis practice. All the English-speaking people in Merida will go past my hypnosis shingle when I hang it above the door.

I've also taken control of my weight issues.... I've lost 24 pounds already, and firmly expect to lose all the rest within a year. By Christmas I'll be thinner than you and all my hypnosis class friends have ever seen me. And I will feel wonderful too. As a matter of fact, I already do.

So things have changed very much for the better. While on occasion I am still concerned about how others see me, their opinions mean a lot less than they once did. I think I've now gotten to the point that I know myself well enough to understand when someone else's opinion is a function of their own biases and not a true reflection of who I am.

So you see, the session must have really gone deep. I've grown so much since then. I have one thing to say: thank you from the bottom of my heart and from the recesses of my psyche. With your help, many of my life issues were brought to light.

CHAPTER 13

Jacque's Attraction of Unhealthy Relationships

Nary a Sensitive, Successful Man to be Found

RANDAL: This is an opportunity for someone to work on an issue that has been a significant problem, perhaps for a very long time. Do I have a volunteer? (Jacquie raises her hand) All right, Jacquie, come on up here. (Jacquie sits next to Randal and whispers something) Can I say that to the group?

JACQUIE: Yes.

RANDAL: Jacquie is feeling scared right now. That's normal. I think most people would feel that in this circumstance. (to Jacquie) Both to work on this and to do it in front of the group?

JACQUIE: Yes, because it's a big issue for me.

RANDAL: (to the group) I want to remind you that everything that is done in a therapeutic context in class is totally confidential outside of the class, except for any specific agreement to the contrary. (to Jacquie) I think you're wise to break through your fear and be here. I feel this is a very compassionate group. You can look around and see a lot of friends here. So tell us about this important issue.

JACQUIE: I have a pattern with men that I just can't break. It's a pattern that gets me into unhealthy relationships. I seem to attract people that end up...I feel like I'm getting engulfed. It feels like they take my energy from me but I know that it isn't them taking it from me.

RANDAL: That's your experience, as if they are taking it from you.

JACQUIE: It's like they're attracted to something in me but I'm not clear what it is. It becomes intense real fast normally, and I get protective and pull back. The more I pull back the more they come on. It seems to be men who are really needing some sort of mother energy and when I get hooked by that, which I usually do, it's almost like then I move into needing to heal them. I need to be with them. Somehow I get attracted into that, too. Being needed is an attraction for me. I always get left short changed, I think, because I'm the giver. I realize I must be receiving something or I wouldn't be in it but I do a lot of giving myself and that's the big pattern. I give up a lot of my energy to make them okay and in order to make the relationship work.

The reason I'm so vulnerable around that is this has really caused a lot of pain in my life. For more than half of my life I was in a relationship with my ex-husband, and the pain that I lived with, I didn't realize it but I woke up to it seven years ago, has been really devastating. I was terribly careful about the last two men that I got in a relationship with after him. I made sure they were distant relationships because I was so scared of getting into anything too close, but I still repeated the pattern. They were men that were drawn to something in me that I...the whole pattern repeated. Just recently I decided to try it again, the third time around since my marriage.

RANDAL: You're beginning a new relationship?

JACQUIE: Well, I'm not beginning a relationship, but since my marriage I've never dated anyone close by. They have always had to be about two thousand miles away. I would always go there or he would come here. It was like a honeymoon kind of thing.

RANDAL: That certainly keeps a certain amount of intimacy at bay and keeps some distance, figuratively as well as literally, doesn't it?

JACQUIE: Yes. So now I decided those two relationships didn't work. The other pattern in my relationships is that the guy is never truly available. It's like I've got this place in me that says I can only be loved by people who are not really available. And I have the intention of breaking that cycle and that pattern. I've done a lot of work within myself and with therapy in the last six months. I'm very aware of the pattern. I've worked on the father stuff and all of that and decided to try to date again. Now I've been out four times with this man, which was a big step for me. It's the first time I've gone out with someone who lives in this area in five years. I kept it real clear with a lot of boundaries and said I just want to be friends and then last night it started again. All of a sudden he got hooked into some energy coming from me and there was this intensity of his wanting to be with me all the time.

I see that pattern happening again. I get scared and pull away and the more I pull away the more he wants me and yet there's a part of me that gets attracted to that. It's like, oh God, he needs me that much, he's that attracted to me. It makes me attracted to him even though I wasn't attracted that much in the beginning. It's a little confusing.

RANDAL: Many relationships and developing relationships go through similar patterns. It's so ironic. There is part of you that really doesn't like it, in fact it has kept you from dating because you don't like being in a position where you feel like you're giving more than you're receiving. Yet there is some part of you that enjoys being the giver and needs to find a balance between the giving and the receiving so you don't feel like your energy is getting sucked out, so to speak. This is an aspect of life, an aspect of relationships. Being the giver is an easy role for you to fall into and you need to be on guard about that. You said you worked on father stuff, so is that part of what this goes back to?

JACQUIE: This is totally connected with my father. He never saw me and never knew who I was. I had to achieve all the time and be perfect. I think that what I've done with guys is try to win and get daddy to see me and love me for who I am. You know how you recreate that.

RANDAL: Right. So your father didn't really appreciate you for who you were so if you just kept working hard enough he could at least appreciate you for what you did. It goes down that deep. And you feel that this pattern tended to happen in a similar way with both your ex–husband and men in general.

JACQUIE: I need that connection with a man, which I needed from my father and didn't get. I think somehow that winning his attention is something I'm putting out that men get hooked into. It makes me wonder if I need to connect with a guy because I'm still trying to do the daddy thing even though I think I've worked through that. I put out that energy which I know will hook them but I'm doing it unconsciously. I really don't think I'm doing it consciously, at least not this time around. I'm so careful because I've seen what I've done in the past. And it still seems to happen, like last night. Here we go again.

RANDAL: Part of my sense is that you have a lot of nurturing energy, which is a positive part of you. But having had the father you had, that energy makes for a tricky combination of circumstances. You said you have worked on this. Have you done any hypnosis work?

JACQUIE: No.

RANDAL: We may end up going into some areas you've worked on in other kinds of counseling but we'll work with hypnosis. Many people have been amazed at how much more clarity they were able to get in hypnosis, or how they were able to move beyond some place that felt stuck even after substantial therapy. With hypnosis we can get down to the basic issue within the subconscious mind, which is the seat of emotions, imagination, memories and habit patterns. Even when working on something you've worked on before, connecting directly with the established attitudes, emotions and expectations of the subconscious mind can be much more powerful and have far greater effect. And we have many ways we can work in hypnosis.

JACQUIE: I'm glad. I feel like this is on a subconscious level. I've done very focused work on myself and on relationships for seven years. One thing I want to add is that I have a sexual abuse incident. Not just one incident but a period of time when I was six years old. I've done a lot of work on that. The man it was with was sixty five years old. He was truly a very gentle man. It's hard for me to accept but there actually were some positive things in that situation because it was not at all aggressive, although obviously sick. I know it stemmed from getting nothing from my father and getting a lot of attention from the man next door who put me on this pedestal and made me a little goddess thing.

I'm wondering this morning if in some way, even as a child, I did this healing number with my energy on this man and that's where this pattern started. Now when I get with a man, if I'm needing attention or if I'm needing to feel special or to have some kind of connection, I feel like I have to give my whole self, all of my energy. It's weird. I don't know if it's connected.

RANDAL: Certainly this is very important, whether or not there is a strong connection to an initiation of this pattern. Is there anything else you can think of that would be helpful as far as your adult or childhood history?

JACQUIE: Well, I just know that another pattern I have with men is this power struggle, this dance that is a subordinate/dominant thing. Sometimes I'm in the dominant position and I'm real clear how I do that. I do it with spiritual energy, goddess energy, sexual energy and image. And heart energy, I think I use that. I don't know that I do it consciously but I think it all ties in to the mother nurturing energy. And then on the other side of that dance I give myself away and let the guy have all the power. I'm aware that I've done that all my life.

I really believe in the power of thinking and intention, and about five months ago I realized that I want to be an equal partner. I want to be able to just be with a man. I think I've done this dance because it's a way to avoid intimacy, because you never truly just are. You're always making something happen and avoiding intimacy. And I never could just be with my father. He was a nervous wreck and we didn't have that opportunity. My intention a few months ago was that I'm really willing to let go of this old pattern, to let go of the power struggle and the daddy issue and recreating that. I really desire a true equal partnership and I'm willing to wait even if it takes the next five years.

RANDAL: Are you willing to have it happen a lot more quickly?

JACQUIE: What?

RANDAL: Well, after seven years of therapy you're willing to wait, and it's fine to take some time to wait for that to happen. Are you willing to allow a miracle to happen?

JACQUIE: The reason I said that is because I want to start a career and I'm so scared that if I get hooked up with a guy all my energy will go to him and I won't be able to do my thing.

RANDAL: Close your eyes and imagine how you could hook up with a guy, whether it's six months from now or tomorrow (Jacquie shakes her head and throws her hands over her eyes, laughing), and have it be amazingly easy. I mean there are always dances and so forth and that's life. But can you imagine hooking up with a guy and not giving away all your power to that? What would that look like?

JACQUIE: That would mean that he would be so powerful that he wouldn't need my energy and he would overpower me.

RANDAL: Now keep your eyes closed and see if you can visualize or think of a couple that doesn't seem to have that power struggle in their relationship. One that's different from you giving all your power away or you having all the power.

JACQUIE: Okay, I can think of about one couple that I know of.

RANDAL: Are these friends of yours?

JACQUIE: Actually they're mentors of mine, Hal and Sidra Stone.

RANDAL: Describe what the relationship is like within this context of being equal partners.

JACQUIE: I've looked all around and there is hardly any couple I've looked at and thought I'd like to have that kind of relationship. But I've really looked at them and they're equal. He has different gifts than she has. They teach together and that's why I get to see them working together. They have this real nice rhythm where she gives him his space to do his thing when he's teaching and then he steps back and allows her to have her space in the teaching work. That's the only time I really see them, but her power is different from his power. She has very loving, nurturing, beautiful energy. He has more...he's a really clear teacher and a very empowered man. His energy is just different from hers and they seem to compliment each other.

RANDAL: Could you imagine being in a relationship that would be something like that? It happens in this case that she has a loving energy and he's more of a clear teacher. Do you associate this relationship that you're seeing now as similar to how you might be balanced in the same way or do you see yourself as more the teacher and your partner might be more loving?

JACQUIE: It could go either way but I definitely know it would be a dream for me to have a relationship that is similar. I don't see that much of their life but I really admire their relationship. I could see myself as the teacher. I do have a lot of masculine energy so I could be the one who is the clear teacher, and maybe he would be like she is.

RANDAL: Okay, you can open your eyes. There are several big related issues around relationships that you've mentioned. There is the power struggle you were just talking about, there is the availability issue, there is the issue of men engulfing you, and the issue of you being stuck in this mother role. Between those different aspects of your relationships with men is there something that stands out as being the most frustrating?

JACQUIE: Like what would be my greatest desire to work out right now?

RANDAL: Yes, at least for starters. Sometimes we start with one thing and go in a different direction. I'm just wondering if something really stands out, especially regarding last night. The timing is perfect. What's your feeling about what happened last night?

JACQUIE: Well, my protections came up gigantically. I have a lot of ways that I protect myself, but one big way is that I start picking him apart.

RANDAL: Out loud?

JACQUIE: No, no, no. (laughter from the group)

RANDAL: So you start picking him apart in your thoughts. At the time or since then?

JACQUIE: It started in my thoughts when I was with him and ever since. As in not sleeping. Oh, I'm exhausted, and I care about this class.

RANDAL: Do you think he is someone who is appropriate for you or do you feel that he is really coming on too strongly and showing you that this would be a serious problem if you continue to see him?

JACQUIE: Part of me wants to say he really listens to me. I thought he listened to what I said but when I think about last night, I told him before that I really have to go real slow and he's coming on strong, so I didn't get heard. He acted like he heard me but that wasn't the result. Part of me wants so much to believe that there is someone who isn't two thousand miles away that can hear what I'm saying and can really work through some stuff. I must say that this is the first mainstream guy I've been with. My husband was a real powerhouse and I have avoided those guys like the plague. I've flipped over to the hippie side and I've trusted those guys because they hear me, they're sensitive and everything. But it didn't work with the hippie guys because they couldn't take my lifestyle. It's hard having two sides. So I think part of me wants to believe this guy. He does have a job and he is sensitive.

RANDAL: There's a guy out there who both has a job and is sensitive. (laughter) Great. I don't know, I think you should hang on to this guy, whatever it takes! (more laughter) I'm just kidding.

JACQUIE: But part of me is like that, thinking, my God, this is the last chance so just keep working with it! There is part of me that thinks if I run away from this it is just one of the ways that I protect myself. I either get totally hooked in or I run because things always seem to get intense. Part of me says don't run this time and don't get hooked in. It isn't like this guy is the one but hang in here and

practice. This is perfect to learn some new skills. You're not really getting hurt and he's saying all the right things.
RANDAL: Good. Are you ready for some hypnosis?
JACQUIE: Yes.
RANDAL: Do you want to lie down on the mat here? Does that feel okay? (Jacquie nods and gets comfortable on the mat)
JACQUIE: (laughing) Put me out.
RANDAL: Would you like a blanket? (Jacquie nods and Randal covers her with a blanket) It's nice to be taken care of. (this is a suggestion for Jacquie, the giver, to be open to and enjoy receiving) Okay, stare at a spot on the ceiling. (Randal guides Jacquie through a series of rapid induction methods and she is showing good hypnotic response)

Focus on your hands now. There's a certain finger on your left or right hand that is your "yes" finger. I'd like you to visualize your "yes" finger lifting and rising or making a movement. Keep picturing the word "yes" until your "yes" finger moves. (Jacquie's right index finger lifts) Okay, the index finger on your right hand is your "yes" finger. Now I'd like you to show me your "no" finger. (Jacquie's right thumb rises) Okay, your thumb is your "no" finger. (Randal is able to move quickly and briefly through the establishment of ideomotor signals with Jacquie because of her substantial experience in this modality)

Jacquie, we're going to explore the issues we've been talking about that tie in with feelings of being engulfed, of being in a mother role, of a power struggle, and of availability. Is it safe and appropriate for you to recall any and all memories that have to do with these issues? Keep focusing on that question with your subconscious mind until the proper finger moves. (Jacquie's index finger moves) The answer to the question is yes. I have another question for you, Jacquie. Is it safe and appropriate for you to be open to your emotions as you recall any experiences that have to do with these issues? (Jacquie's thumb moves) All right, the answer to the question is no.

I want to say something about that before we go on. We're really talking about a lot of issues that are related and I'm going to be narrowing my focus for the moment on one issue. It may be that it's okay for you to be open to your emotions in going over some of the issues but not others. There is one that I'm particularly drawn to right now and that is the sense of feeling engulfed by a relationship, feeling that overwhelming feeling that you sometimes feel.

Jacquie's Attraction to Unhealthy Relationships 201

Within the context of that feeling, is it safe and appropriate for you to be open to your emotions as you go back over this issue? (Jacquie's thumb moves) The answer to the question is no.

All right. We're going to look over some memories now, Jacquie, that are tied in with what happened last night and has happened so often in your life. I want you to imagine that you're in a theater and there are certain reels of film down in the basement that are very significant. They are old reels in your subconscious mind that are continuing to affect your life in a profound way. I'd like you to imagine yourself walking down and perhaps opening a door and going into a room with thousands of old reels of film from when you were a child or from a long time ago. Perhaps you could have someone with you. This person is going to be the person who projects the film and you are pointing out certain reels that you want him or her to bring. There may be one or two or several, but you are sensing that certain films stand out for you and asking this person to carry them up for you.

You are going up the stairs now to the projection booth and this person is setting up one of these films. I want you to look down into the theater now. You thought you were up here in the projection booth but you can see yourself down there in the theater all by yourself, about to see this film. You have this detachment about what you are going to see. You can observe it from this perspective. What you are going to observe are certain difficult experiences of a young girl. You might feel to an extent some feelings such as you would feel watching a movie, but it will be as if it's happening to someone else.

There is a brilliant star above you shining down its healing, protecting rays and bathing you from the top of your head all the way down to the tips of your toes. Any darkness, any negativity, is draining out of your body through the palms of your hands and the soles of your feet. It is dissipating into the atmosphere and fading away, until your whole body is surrounded by light. This light of protection not only surrounds you but it's like being in a womb of light. There is an eighteen inch aura of light around you now so that you can watch this scene from that protection. You will be observing it from this room as if you were watching a movie screen. It's as if you're someone else observing. You can have all that protection from what you're about to see.

Now there is an issue that has come up for Jacquie over and over again. It's an issue that she felt last night. I'd like you to watch

Jacquie watch the movie screen, seeing herself focusing on the feeling of being engulfed in this experience, feeling overwhelmed by this relationship with this man. She's going to go back to something about her childhood, something between the time she was born and the age of ten. She's going to go back to some experience where she felt herself being engulfed in some way.

I'm going to count from ten down to one and as I reach the count of one you're observing that experience. Ten, nine, eight, going back in time, back to that experience and observing it on the movie screen now. It's beginning to come on, the movie is beginning to run. Seven, six, you're beginning to see the experience, Jacquie's feeling engulfed in some way. Five, four, three, two, one. (Randal taps Jacquie's forehead) Okay, right there now. You can speak. Is she inside or outside? Pick one.

JACQUIE: Inside.
RANDAL: Is it nighttime or daytime?
JACQUIE: Daytime.
RANDAL: How old is she approximately?
JACQUIE: Six.
RANDAL: Is she with anybody?
JACQUIE: Yes.
RANDAL: Who is she with?
JACQUIE: I'm with Mr. Biles.
RANDAL: Now remember, you are detached from this experience. You are observing this six year old girl having this experience. Watching the film. Is there anybody there besides you at age six and Mr. Biles?
JACQUIE: Maybe my younger sister.
RANDAL: When you said you were inside, are you in his house or your house or where?
JACQUIE: His house.
RANDAL: So that's the scene. What room in the house are you in?
JACQUIE: It's like an attic in the top story. It's a small room.
RANDAL: What's happening in this attic-like room right now?
JACQUIE: I feel his energy coming on to me. He's saying nice things to me. He's winning me somehow by saying all these nice things.
RANDAL: How do you feel as he's saying all these nice things to you?
JACQUIE: I'm scared and he's bigger.

Jacquie's Attraction to Unhealthy Relationships 203

RANDAL: What is it about him saying nice things to you and yet his being older and bigger? Are you scared of him because he's older and bigger?

JACQUIE: I know he wants something from me.

RANDAL: You sense that.

JACQUIE: I'm very sensitive.

RANDAL: So you're picking it up intuitively that he wants something from you. Do you have an idea or a guess yet what he wants or do you just know he wants something?

JACQUIE: Right now it feels like I don't know but I definitely know it's not good.

RANDAL: So you know that.

JACQUIE: I'm scared of being alone with him.

RANDAL: Is that the only feeling you're feeling about that?

JACQUIE: Confused.

RANDAL: Okay, you're scared and confused. That's plenty but I'm just checking. Is there any other feeling you're having or is that pretty much it at this point?

JACQUIE: I think that's it.

RANDAL: Now remember, you're watching this on a screen. Does it feel like you're watching it on a screen now or that you're looking at it as a hidden observer in the room? Which feels more accurate for you?

JACQUIE: Like I'm in the room.

RANDAL: Okay, but you're seeing this happening to you as the six year old over there, is that correct?

JACQUIE: Yes.

RANDAL: Okay, I want you to continue seeing it that way. It's important for now that you have that dissociation, that detachment. You have that distance and protection as the hidden observer. You might sense angels protecting you and six year old Jacquie, or in whatever ways, you have some protection. Are you ready to continue on in this scene?

JACQUIE: Yes.

RANDAL: Okay, let's have the film go forward now. It's a few minutes later. What, if anything, happens next? (as a reminder, it is extremely important to be neutral during regression, not directly or indirectly hinting at or implying or expecting anything)

JACQUIE: There is a table and I'm on the table.

RANDAL: Take a look at that little girl over there. How is she feeling?

JACQUIE: She's numbed out and she's left her body. She's terrified.

RANDAL: (because of the heightened suggestibility of the subconscious, it is important to approach negative possibilities at first with questions asked in a positive way) At this time is he physically completely apart from her?

JACQUIE: No.

RANDAL: Is this current physical contact platonic?

JACQUIE: No.

RANDAL: At this time is he physically contacting her in some kind of sexual way?

JACQUIE: Yes.

RANDAL: Has he done something like this before?

JACQUIE: I don't think so.

RANDAL: Do you have a sense as to whether your sister is there? You weren't sure before whether she was there or not.

JACQUIE: I don't see her but I sense her. I don't know if it's from another time.

RANDAL: I'm about to take you away from that experience for now and help you get further detachment, Jacquie, but I want to know first if there is anything else you need to see or learn from that experience. Is there anything significant that happens further? Take a look or get a sense within your subconscious mind. "Yes, there is something more," or "No, this is the essence of what happened."

JACQUIE: There is something but I'm having trouble...

RANDAL: Are you talking about something further having to do with your feelings or something further that happens, other than Jacquie being on this table and what you observed him doing?

JACQUIE: I feel there's a connection that I'm missing.

RANDAL: Let's go to this connection. There is a certain connection.

JACQUIE: I got it, I got it, I got it.

RANDAL: What is it?

JACQUIE: I think I'm really confused because this man is a very loving and gentle man and I don't understand. What's he doing if he is a loving man?

RANDAL: Okay, I want you to leave that room now and come to a safe place for adult Jacquie to be with six year old Jacquie. Did you go by the name Jacquie when you were six years old?

JACQUIE: I went by Jacqueline.

RANDAL: Okay, so adult Jacquie is with six year old Jacqueline. I'd like you to have a safe place now where you are away from that experience and you can bring that little girl here. I'd like you to have a talk with her about that experience because she is terrified and confused. Maybe the first thing you could do is hold her. (Randal gets a pillow and puts it on Jacquie's chest, placing her arms around it) Here she is now. You can say something to her or you can just hold her for now.

JACQUIE: I want to tell her that wasn't normal.

RANDAL: Say, "That wasn't normal," and go on from there.

JACQUIE: (Jacquie's voice is slightly muffled into the pillow) That wasn't normal. That's not how men and women are. (speaking haltingly and slowly) That wasn't healthy. That man took advantage of you. He took your innocence. He used your vulnerability. He abused his power. He didn't respect you. He acted like he honored you because he flattered you and made you feel special but he wasn't truly honoring you. You deserve to be truly honored and respected. I know he gave you attention and he saw you and that felt good. I know you deserve to be seen and you never got seen by your own daddy. You are a beautiful child. You don't have to do this to be seen. It was your father's inability, it wasn't something that you did wrong that you didn't get seen.

RANDAL: Say something to this little girl who up until now has tried so hard to do something to be seen by her daddy. What do you want to tell her about that feeling of not being good enough?

JACQUIE: You don't have to do anything to be loved. You're lovable just exactly as you are. And I want you to hear me because you don't know that.

RANDAL: Become six year old Jacqueline now. Adult Jacquie is saying beautiful truths to you. Are you hearing them?

JACQUIE: I hear the words but...(Jacquie's voice drops)

RANDAL: Okay, you hear the words but you haven't as yet been able to take them in. Switch and be Jacquie. How can you get it across to her? (Jacquie starts to cry) It's okay. We're away from that experience so you can go ahead and cry. You can feel any emotions now.

JACQUIE: (crying, voice barely audible) She can't hear me really. I don't know how to get through to her.

RANDAL: Instead of saying she can't, let's just say she won't. There is some way she can do it, you just haven't found it yet. Stay with it. You're just about there. She is such a beautiful girl. She's been wounded. How can you reach her?

JACQUIE: She is so protected nothing can come in. She doesn't believe anybody. She doesn't trust anybody.

RANDAL: She doesn't trust or believe anybody. She doesn't believe you. There are a number of possibilities here, Jacquie, as there always are. One possibility, since you have reached this temporary stuck place, may be to do a dialogue between her and that man. What is your feeling about that? We can do it in such a way that she has some protection, some distance, perhaps some detachment. You can be there with her or I can be there with her.

JACQUIE: In a way I feel like that's okay but then it might be good to be her and me.

RANDAL: Let's start by paying attention to Jacqueline. I'd like to check your finger signals again. Is it okay for six year old Jacqueline to now get in touch with her feelings and emotions? Any answer is fine, just answer whatever the truth is. (Jacquie's index finger moves) The answer to the question is yes.

Become six year old Jacqueline. Adult Jacquie just told me that you feel really closed off, that you're unwilling or unable to hear or listen. How are you blocking yourself? Go inside your body and feel what you're feeling. I'm going to take this away now (Randal takes the pillow) and you can put your arms down. You are six year old Jacqueline who has been sexually abused and you have been abused in other ways. Your father has neglected you. You've been in so much pain. Go inside your body and tell me what you feel.

JACQUIE: (in a little voice) Cold.

RANDAL: Do you feel cold all over or somewhere in particular?

JACQUIE: My hands.

RANDAL: Okay, feel the coldness in your hands. Is there anything else you notice?

JACQUIE: I'm shaking.

RANDAL: What else do you feel?

JACQUIE: Rigid and kind of numb.

RANDAL: Where do you feel that rigidity?

JACQUIE: In my legs.

RANDAL: Feel that rigidity in your legs.

JACQUIE: And in my hips.

RANDAL: Okay, you're going to get some movement in that area now. (Randal moves to Jacquie's feet and picks up one foot in his hands) This leg really is stiff. I'm going to have you kick by bending your knees and kicking out here. Is it okay if I take your

Jacquie's Attraction to Unhealthy Relationships 207

shoes off? (Jacquie nods and Randal takes off her shoes and puts them on the floor) Keep breathing down into your stomach. Okay, let's lift up your legs like this. (Randal pushes Jacquie's feet toward her body so her legs are bent and holds a large pillow between himself and her feet) I want you to start kicking out here at the pillow and say, "Get away from me!" (Randal places her right foot on the pillow to start and holds onto the pillow)

JACQUIE: Get away from me! Get away from me! (Jacquie kicks forcefully at the pillow with her right foot several times) Get away from me!

RANDAL: (loudly) Good! Now say it louder!

JACQUIE: (loudly) Get away from me! Get away from me! (in a whisper) Get away from me.

RANDAL: Now kick with your left leg too. Let's alternate back and forth. (Jacquie, crying, puts her hands over her face and sobs and Randal drops the pillow and goes back to her side)

JACQUIE: It's no use. It's no use.

RANDAL: Feel your feelings. Feel in your body. What do you feel?

JACQUIE: (still crying) It's no use.

RANDAL: I understand what you're saying. I understand what you're feeling emotionally. Go inside your body. What do you feel inside your body right now?

JACQUIE: Hopeless.

RANDAL: Stay with that. I want you to do it one more time now. (Randal moves back down to Jacquie's feet and holds the pillow up) You say it's hopeless but it won't hurt to try. Maybe you're right and maybe you're wrong. Just try it out a few times. Do some kicking alternating your feet and say, "Get away from me!"

JACQUIE: (Jacquie starts kicking) Get away from me!

RANDAL: Louder.

JACQUIE: Get away from me! (louder) Get away from me!

RANDAL: (shouting) That's good! Say it again!

JACQUIE: Get away from me!

RANDAL: Good!

JACQUIE: (slowing down) Get away from me.

RANDAL: (putting down the pillow and moving back to Jacquie's side) Good, good. You're doing great. Go inside your body and breathe into your stomach. Breathe all the way down into your pelvis. (pause) What do you feel in your body, Jacqueline?

JACQUIE: I'm still a little shaky.

RANDAL: Still shaky, that's fine. What else?

JACQUIE: I'm still cold in my hands.

RANDAL: (Randal feels Jacquie's right hand) Still cold in your hands, yes. What else?

JACQUIE: I feel a lot of strong energy in my body.

RANDAL: Feel that strong energy, that life force in your body. Do you feel it all throughout your body? Do you feel it down in your legs and your hips?

JACQUIE: Less there but some.

RANDAL: You're getting that energy going. Good. How do your legs feel now? Are they starting to wake up?

JACQUIE: Some.

RANDAL: Good, good.

JACQUIE: It's confusing again. I feel a lot of confusion. What I feel is good and bad and that was true with the abuse, too. It felt good and bad.

RANDAL: We're going to use a different pillow now. (Randal gets another pillow and gives it to Jacquie to hold) I want adult Jacquie to talk to six year old Jacqueline. Say something about feeling good and bad during that experience. I want you to give her some insight into that.

JACQUIE: Well, sexuality does feel good, Jacqueline. It's very normal.

RANDAL: It's very normal that you partly felt good because sexuality can feel good.

JACQUIE: And that was your aliveness that you felt, your sexual energy. You have a lot of it and that's good. It's your life force. Don't apologize for that.

RANDAL: She felt those good feelings despite the fact that there was something very wrong and very bad that happened to her. Can you explain to her something further about that experience now? About how that happened and how she reacted to that?

JACQUIE: The bad part about that is you didn't go in with full choice. Somehow you felt like you had to do it. That's the only reason you feel disempowered from it.

RANDAL: That's good. Become six year old Jacqueline now. Does that make sense to you, what adult Jacquie said?

JACQUIE: I think I did do it because I thought I had to. And I did want to do it.

RANDAL: There was a part of you that wanted to do it, especially as lonely as you were feeling.

JACQUIE: (in a soft voice) This man acted like he loved me. He did a lot more for me than my daddy did. It felt at the time like I had to. I felt like I owed it to him because he paid attention to me.

RANDAL: Now let's switch places. What do you want to say to six year old Jacqueline about that?

JACQUIE: (in a strong voice) You do not owe anybody anything.

RANDAL: Say that again.

JACQUIE: You do not owe anybody anything. Nothing. You are a beautiful, loving, radiant child and you don't have to give anybody anything ever again.

RANDAL: Good. Become the six year old.

JACQUIE: (softly) He was so nice to me. I had to give him something back. He needed me. It was so little for me to do.

RANDAL: Switch and be adult Jacquie.

JACQUIE: Jacqueline, you deserve to be loved just for who you are. You are love. You are a loving, lovable child. You don't owe anybody anything for loving you. They love you because you've already given them something, something you're not even aware of because you are it.

RANDAL: Beautiful.

JACQUIE: You've already given them a gift. You don't owe them anything.

RANDAL: That's very good. As you're holding onto six year old Jacqueline feel her softening, beginning to open up. She's becoming more receptive to what you're saying. Feel her beginning to realize at a deeper level, despite how much inattention she had before, that that was the limitation of her father, not her own limitation. That is so true that she is a beautiful, lovable little girl who deserves all kinds of good attention and nice things and compliments just for who she is.

Now become that six year old and take that in. Start experiencing deep down that you are this beautiful little girl who brings joy to people's lives. You had a good daddy in some ways but he was really limited. I would like you to imagine if you could have a daddy who was a healthy, normal, loving daddy, what he would look like and what he would be like. Imagine him coming here now and totally being here with you and cuddling you and giving you all kinds of appropriate love. The kind of love a good daddy wants to give to his beautiful little girl. Now six year old Jacqueline, I want you to tell me what your ideal daddy looks like. He might look the same as your daddy looked or he might look like someone famous or he might look like someone you've never seen before. Does anybody come to your mind or is there any description you can give about what your ideal daddy looks like?

JACQUIE: I have a very hard time getting any picture.

RANDAL: We can get help from adult Jacquie now. Can you think of somebody you know who is a good, loving daddy?

JACQUIE: It's the hardest thing. Everybody that runs through my mind, no.

RANDAL: Well, keep working on it. You know that you grew up not having a good, loving daddy so it's harder for you to see that when he comes along. But they're out there.

JACQUIE: The only people I thought were good, loving daddies turned out to...(her voice becomes inaudible).

RANDAL: Just keep imagining. It could be a fictional character, someone you saw in a movie or a television show. It's wide open here. Just for example, in the movie *Kramer versus Kramer*, that daddy really loved his little child and it broke his heart that he had to leave him.

JACQUIE: I think I found someone.

RANDAL: Is this someone you know? An acquaintance or a friend of yours?

JACQUIE: Yes.

RANDAL: Can you imagine him being the ideal father for the six year old within you? Six year old Jacqueline?

JACQUIE: Uh huh.

RANDAL: Okay, be six year old Jacqueline and this is your new daddy. You can have him whenever you want. (Randal strokes Jacquie's hands) You deserve him now and you deserved him all along. Unfortunately life isn't always fair. You were a good girl all along. You didn't have to prove anything and you didn't need to do anything. You are wonderful just the way you are and just the way you were. You always deserved to have this good daddy with you. And maybe he can't be with you all the time but he will sure make it a point to spend quality time with his beautiful little girl every day. Maybe he wishes he could be with you all day because he loves you so much, but he could be with you a lot.

He loves you and he's so proud of you just the way you are. You don't have to prove anything to this ideal daddy. You don't have to do anything for him. Maybe you like to do some things just because you love him but you don't owe it to him. You do things for him because you want to sometimes. He loves being with you and he loves doing fun things with you. He's a good daddy and he's not sick like that other man was. He's a caring daddy and he loves you in all the appropriate ways.

You were confused because the only man who loved you was also sick and he did some bad things with you. What you learned was that you thought you should perform if somebody was nice to you, that you should do what they wanted you to do and that's not true. A man can be nice to you whether he's your daddy or your boyfriend and you don't owe him anything. You are learning that more every day as it becomes a natural part of who you are, that you can just be yourself. If a man asks you to do something maybe you could do it or maybe not. You can say yes or you can say no, and it's fine for you to say no. If you say no, you know that if he's really a good man he can respect that. In fact he wants you to say no if it's not right for you.

You're learning in your life to have that dance be a lighter and more joyful dance. It's a more playful dance. Life involves contact and withdrawal. Whether it's with an acquaintance or friend or lover, you make some contact and then you back off. You'll reach out and then you'll withdraw and that's normal and healthy. You're learning that now more deeply, down to your core. You're finding out that six year old Jacqueline is warming up to the joys that are here for her, and the friendships and the love. What a joyful feeling.

Every night before you go to bed, for the time being, Jacqueline, I'd like you to picture this ideal daddy being with you. You can be this six year old girl and get all the love and affection that is right and healthy from this very loving daddy who is so proud of his girl. And you can fantasize anything you want. You can fantasize going to the circus together or having him watch you when you're playing with friends, just making sure everything's fine. You know you can come running back to that daddy and cuddle him and he can be there anytime you want. And since this is your daddy within, this is someone who really can be there whenever you need him and you deserve that. Take it in. Every day you're opening up your heart more and every day that armor is breaking apart. Whatever is left of it is just melting away.

I want you to imagine your ideal daddy asking you if you want to do something and if you don't want to, you can say no. And imagine him giving you a big hug and saying, "Good for you. I'm so proud of my little girl. You're tapping into what's best for you. That's what I want you to do. I want you to grow up and be a strong, healthy woman. You deserve to have just what you want. It's all there for you. Eventually you'll have a true love and he'll just love you so much."

Your ideal daddy respects you. The fact that you can say no to him helps him respect you more. It even helps him to open up more because he knows that he can ask for what he wants and that you are only going to do what feels right at the time for you. He appreciates your honesty and your integrity. He appreciates the fact that you are a beautiful, healthy, intelligent, fascinating, loving girl, and he accepts you just for who you are. Is six year old Jacqueline feeling good?

JACQUIE: She hears and she's still protecting but it's seeping in.

RANDAL: And you know what? It's like there is a big dam and the water that's been held in all this time is seeping through the cracks now. That dam is beginning to break down until it starts gushing out like waterfalls. It's happening in the days and weeks ahead as you are opening up to the love that is around you. Of course it takes some time because it's been a habit and there have been certain expectations throughout your whole life, but it's finally starting to leave in earnest now and it's an accelerating process.

You may be amazed at how fast your heart opens and your receptivity and your life. Of course you will find a balance where if you really love someone there will be times when you want to reach out and get immersed in a loving interaction, and other times you really want to back off and that's fine. You just need to say no. It's going to take some practice but you're on a whole new plane now. Is there anything else that six year old Jacqueline would like to ask or to say at this time?

JACQUIE: The thing that she doesn't trust is that that man will stay strong enough. Eventually he'll get weak. He'll be like all the other men.

RANDAL: When you say that man, what man are you referring to?

JACQUIE: The man that I finally found to be a role model for a loving father. I just feel like in time he'll be like all the others. He won't be strong enough.

RANDAL: Well, this is an ideal father so he will be strong enough. It's natural for you, six year old Jacqueline, to worry that he'll be like all the others. But you see, you had this way of being in which you expected and felt obligated because of the neglect of your father and the terrible thing that happened to you with Mr. Biles. There were many ways in which you were not nurtured properly and in which you were abused. You got in these continuums where you created the same thing over and over again because you felt obligated. But now that feeling is fading away.

You're finding that you're allowing a whole different kind of person into your life, a whole new ideal father. He doesn't need anything. He just wants to be able to see you and be with you. He wants to love you and be loved by you but that's all he wants. You'll discover as the days and the months go by that he's stronger than ever. And he's had loving parents, a loving mommy and daddy, so there's no reason for him to feel needy. He just loves you. He knows that you need time to yourself sometimes.

JACQUIE: Will he go away? He won't go away will he?

RANDAL: No, he won't go away. He might have to go off to work at some point but he'll be back and he'll make sure that you're taken care of when he's away for a little while. He'll always come back because he wants to. He loves you so very much. Of course you may still have some doubts sometimes but you're opening up and becoming more receptive to the truth. And that feels pretty good, doesn't it?

JACQUIE: Uh huh. Very nice.

RANDAL: Great. Now in a moment I'm going to begin to count you out to help you come back to your fully alert, awake state and then we're going to be taking a break. If you want I can announce the break first and you can have a couple of minutes to just take some more time to come back.

JACQUIE: I'd kind of like to stay here.

RANDAL: Well, you can take plenty of time. I'm going to announce a ten minute break for the people in the class now.

RANDAL: (after the break Jacque is out of hypnosis and sitting in a chair beside Randal) Look at this beautiful woman. (applause)

JACQUIE: Thank you very much, all of you. First of all, I hate to cry in front of anybody. Thank you, thank you, thank you, for this godsend here on my right. (holding onto Randal's hand) This has been a pain I've had all my life. It's been an underlying driving force.

RANDAL: Thank you for opening up and allowing me to be a godsend. My purpose is to be a guide to help get all that stuff out of the way of who you are. It's you doing it and me helping the process.

JACQUIE: I was really ready.

RANDAL: You said some very wise things in the hypnosis. Is there anything else you would like to say about six year old Jacqueline or about the process?

JACQUIE: Well, I was surprised to see how protected she still was because I've done about seven years of body work to try to open myself up. But when I got down there in the beginning nothing could get through. Nothing. And I consider it an absolute miracle that I could become as calm as I was at the end.

RANDAL: Yes, you felt incredibly calm.

JACQUIE: I don't have a clear memory but you said some things when you were talking to me about the father that were precisely what I needed to hear. And there was one thing that I asked for when I said, "But you won't leave me?" That was a very big issue for me.

RANDAL: Yes, an abandonment issue. Your father always left.

JACQUIE: Another thing I did not connect with until today, well, I did intellectually but not on as deep a level, is the fear that there is no man out there who is powerful enough to be a loving father to me. I really had this conception that all men are innately weak and that somehow I always have to be there to heal their weakness. I have never been able to trust that any man could truly be there for me.

The man that I envisioned as an ideal father is someone who lives in Sedona. He's been like a spiritual guide for me and I don't know why this man really sees me. He calls and says these phenomenal things to me and I want to trust him but always in the back of my mind is the question, "What does he really want? He must be needy and he's going to go like this to me." (Jacquie makes a grabbing gesture) I visited him a couple of months ago and I purposely could only stay with him for two hours because I was so terrified that his loving goodness would turn to sexuality. He called later and said, "I was really sad that you left because I just wanted to be with you." Even here as you were speaking of him there was a similar thought and I finally did work through it, but it was like, "It's just a matter of time before he'll let you down, too."

RANDAL: Of course this image of him is as your ideal father, this part of him, whether the actual person would eventually disappoint you or not is not even relevant. What is relevant is that you have an image of an ideal inner father who is totally there no matter what. This absolute Rock of Gibraltar for you to come back to, so be sure to include that imagery in your follow-up self-hypnosis processes in the days and weeks ahead.

JACQUIE: Definitely. It was a very profound experience.

RANDAL: You look beautiful. We can see it.

JACQUIE: Oh no, I'm a mess.

RANDAL: You're not a mess at all. And a lot less of a mess than you were inside.

JACQUIE: Oh, my insides feel great.

RANDAL: In wrapping this up is there any positive feedback for Jacquie?

ROGER: It seemed really empowering when you were kicking and moving that energy. It looked difficult but it felt powerful.

JACQUIE: It didn't feel that powerful to me.

RANDAL: It got a lot more powerful as you went on.

JACQUIE: I think the fact that this was such a gentle, loving man made it hard for me. It's always been hard for me to get up any true anger around it.

RANDAL: Well, that's the irony. On the one hand he was this very gentle man but he also really abused you and there is a part of you that inevitably had to feel anger about the way he abused you.

WENDY: I just want to acknowledge your strength and courage.

CATHY: It's interesting that now that you have this prototype of the ideal father inside you can give to yourself without looking outside of yourself. I think that's wonderful.

JACQUIE: (to Randal) You know, you mentioned cuddling and often, looking back, I ended up in sexual experiences when really what I wanted was that cuddling. And now that I can give that to myself I won't have to look for it and end up with something that I don't want.

RANDAL: Well, you can certainly give it to yourself and also let's reframe this a little. You might be with a man you're attracted to and maybe all he would want is cuddling and you can understand the appropriateness of you backing off. In the same way you can be in a situation in which the man might want more and it's okay for you to be clear that what you want is cuddling. Maybe sometime in the future it could be different and maybe not, depending on the relationship. But there is a shift that is taking place and your subconscious is just beginning to understand it more.

PATRICK: I was fascinated by the process in which at times her reaction was, "No, don't intrude." Actually a number of times.

RANDAL: Six year old Jacqueline had a strong barrier against letting anything in. And no wonder, considering her experience of neglect and abuse. She was so closed up and there was so much tension in her body. I really had tried up to that point in every way that I could, for her to get it. So many good things had happened but there was still this energy that she needed to kick and get out of her. (to Jacquie) Do you know what he's talking about? You signaled that you didn't want to be open to your feelings and so we started with a lot of detachment for you. Then it came around full circle to the beautiful things you were telling the six year old but she wasn't willing to listen. It felt like there were such big blocks that really needed to get out in a physical way so she could open up. How did that feel for you?

JACQUIE: I think that was the only way to go. I was so protective of her that it wouldn't have mattered if you spent another two hours with it, nothing was going to happen.

RANDAL: Sometimes when someone signals, like Jacquie did, that she wasn't ready to feel her feelings, that doesn't mean that the subconscious won't feel differently later. It eventually felt that her body was saying, "Hey, I need to get through this and I need to move on." I will always do my best to be receptive to subconscious communication. As Jacquie said, there didn't seem to be any other way at that point and we really needed to break through. That really made a difference. Let's give a hand to Jacquie. (applause)

Interview Five Years Later

RANDAL: (a class of hypnotherapists has just watched the video of the session with Jacquie, who is visiting this class and now calls herself Joy or Jacqueline Joy) Some of you, including those who have experienced such a tragedy, may be well aware of some of the effects of molestation but may not be aware of others. It's a very important issue. Hypnotherapy to work through the great difficulty of the experience can have a profound impact in various ways. There was an added complexity to this session that Joy's father was not there for her while this man who was there was very nice in many ways and yet also very sick. The confusion and guilt that resulted from that was inevitable. Joy, would you like to say something about the session?

JACQUELINE JOY: After that session I really opened up like I've never opened up in my life. For a year and a half I didn't have anyone in my life sexually but many men came into my life in a loving way, which was really amazing. Five or six men came into my life just to, I don't know, let me experience men who weren't asking anything of me.

That session was at the end of 1993 and then in 1995 I met my partner, who I've been with now for three years. He's the most nurturing human being I've ever met and he loves it when I say no to him. He encourages me to say no to him because I do still have a bit of that pattern. I tend to be over-giving, although not in obvious ways anymore. It's purely energetic now. If I'm really in my joy, for example, which I am way more now than I ever was, and I walk into the room and he's depressed, I feel his depression and I will immediately lose my joy. It's like my energy goes out to him and I don't even know what happens.

So it still occurs on more subtle levels but I'm working with it. It feels like in the last four months or so it's really improved as I've gained more and more awareness. It's about learning to keep my own good energy. It's always been that. How do I keep my own great energy on my end instead of giving it away for whatever reason? So I really noticed that everything Randal said in the session, I manifested. (to Randal) I'm very excited and thankful to you for implanting that. You're absolutely right, though, that the effects are pervasive in my life. They still are. There's been a huge improvement but when Randal called about four months ago to ask if I would like to be here, it was interesting because it was just coming up again. It comes up on different levels constantly. I've done an enormous amount of work even since the session and have so much more joy in my life. My middle name really is Joy.

RANDAL: So you were born with it.

JOY: And I know that that's what I'm really here to bring but I also brought in a lot of wounding to work through. What's amazing to me is that eighty percent of my clients and people who know me or don't even know me but meet me for the first time, call me Joy as a first name. That really shows me how impactful this work is.

RANDAL: I remember in 1993 you were just radiant in class afterwards, then you sent a fantastic letter about how great you were doing. Then I bumped into you in town a month later and you were absolutely, and you continue to be, radiant. I just look at you and think joy. And you put together some literature six months or a year after the session calling yourself Joy.

JOY: (laughing) I started the Joy Company.

RANDAL: All right! You have wonderful energy. I'm so delighted that you are continuing to move forward. Obviously that was a big step along the way, and it's what you do with that step that counts the most. You've made choices and decisions all along to allow this energy, your vital energy, your sexuality, your love, your joy, all of your feelings to manifest more and more.

I wonder if you'd like to tell the class something about how you remembered the molestation experiences? I asked you once whether this was a memory that you'd always been aware of or just recalled in the process of your life or that you suddenly had as a flashback, and your answer was very interesting.

JOY: What happened is that I had a couple of therapy sessions and it hadn't even been brought up. Then on the way home after the second one I had this very slight, maybe for half a second, vision or memory that had something to do with sexual abuse. I was thinking, wow, what's going on? It was coming out of nowhere. I was thirty eight years old and I'd never had a memory about that, which shows how we can block ourselves so strongly. Many years ago, I'd say seven or eight years before this ever occurred, my younger sister had gone to my mother and told her about being sexually abused. My mother had told me but I didn't remember it being true for me when she brought it up. I still didn't remember anything for the next seven years. When the memory did come up, that little whiff of a memory, I still didn't make a connection.

Then I went to a massage therapist and she told me that I could go into meditation and ask to remember, but only if there was something to remember. So I did that. I went up into the hills and sat down and called spirit to help me remember anything I needed to and the memories came in vivid detail. And one of those things that was sort of surprising is that I did remember my sister being there and what was crazy is that there was a very pleasant feeling about it. The man that came back in the memory was very gentle, so it was not an aggressive thing. It didn't match up as sexual abuse. What was this gentle man?

Then my sister called two days later and asked if I could come to Dallas to be with her for awhile because she was having a hard time. When I got there we started talking and I told her that I had had some memories come back of some sexual abuse and I asked her if she remembered anything. And she's always had a great memory and she said, oh yeah, and rattled off all the details. The age, the time, the place, the man. The same experiences I'd had. Even the thing of saying that he was really a gentle man. It was amazing because I hadn't opened my mouth to give any facts about what was given to me in the meditation. I just listened to her and they matched up perfectly.

RANDAL: And, in fact, when you'd heard years earlier that she'd been abused you hadn't heard the details.

JOY: No, I had not.

RANDAL: So what a validation that you remembered all of these specific and unique details. The way you were abused was unusual. And all those memories came back. It's normal when recovering memories of abuse to think, this is crazy. Could this really have happened? And you got that validation because your sister gave the same details that you remembered.

JOY: Actually, without her validation I could really have discounted the whole thing. That's also amazing because I don't see my sister that often. Maybe once every two or three years. But for her to call me and to say come, and come now, was pretty synchronistic.

RANDAL: See how powerful you are in the things you create in your life?

JOY: Well, thank you. I was thinking how powerfully I'm protected and guided and taken care of.

RANDAL: And that experience was some years before the session we had five years ago.

JOY: Yes. It was eleven years ago. By the time I did that session with you I'd done all kinds of work with the sexual abuse but never hypnosis.

RANDAL: The appropriate use of hypnosis, in which the therapist is neutral and careful not to lead and so forth, can be so powerful. (to class) Any questions?

JAMIE: Was that the only session you had with Randal or with dealing with that issue at the time?

JOY: I never had a hypnotherapy session before or after.

JAMIE: That was it, just the one time. Amazing.

RANDAL: She's a powerful lady.

MADELINE: When you were doing the ideomotor technique and there was the issue of not being safe to be open to her emotions around engulfment, I was wondering if what you did explore was not engulfment per se, but an area that felt safe for her to be open to her emotions?

RANDAL: It was an interesting challenge. I did something unique by repeatedly encouraging detachment while attempting to gently bring in an affect bridge. But the feeling I encouraged, as she was dissociated from the experience and seeing it on the screen, was specifically that fear of engulfment. It worked and she was able to link to the initial sensitizing event while keeping a fair measure of emotional detachment as a "hidden observer."

MADELINE: I remember that but then after awhile she really got into it.

RANDAL: That was after I helped her go away from the scene to a safe place where she could have a supportive dialogue with adult Jacquie. She spontaneously began crying and I encouraged it, since the previous ideomotor signal to avoid feelings was specifically referring to the regression. Then after she signaled that it was safe to now get in touch with her emotions I had her explore what she was doing internally, which eventually led to the kicking and shouting. Do you want to add anything, Joy?

JOY: I just thought when I said no, it's not all right to feel my emotions, that when Randal had me do it neutrally, or watching it, it seemed like it was okay. And after that we weren't in the situation anymore and that's when I could open up to the feelings. And maybe it was the fact that I said no and he found another way that then I could say yes. Oftentimes that's the way it is.

RANDAL: Yes. Once she was away from the scene, it was the nurturing adult Jacquie and the child Jacqueline and the child needed to open up in this safe and supportive environment. And it is particularly interesting, considering her issues, that having complete support for saying no may have helped her subconscious become ready to open up to that option.

ROBERT: I was curious that after she said it wasn't safe you actually went right into it and all of that came up. I thought it was brilliant how that was handled. I found myself unsure of how I would have handled that if I was told two or three times in no uncertain terms that this is not a safe area to go into and yet this is the primary issue. I was just amazed at how that unfolded.

RANDAL: It was fascinating to me how it evolved, too. Eventually we went away from the regression "film" scene and still this young girl was so blocked in receiving the beautiful truths from adult Jacquie. One thing led into another and after she signaled she was open to her feelings I had her go inside her body. And there were blocks from her pelvis on down and the logical step to me was to do the kicking.

It was interesting because in a way it tied back to that scene in which I had not wanted to have her be in touch with her emotions because of her signal, but this was a couple of steps removed from that. I was telling her to kick and say, "get away from me," but it was in the context of her being there within a supportive environment. She was away from that scene but still getting into it. I felt that the energy that was still in her body from that scene would manifest in many ways in her life, including in terms of her ability to say no, for example. This kicking and saying, "Get away!" was a way for her to tune into her ability to say no. So it related to the original scene and at that point it felt perfectly appropriate to do that.

MARY: When you get a signal like that, "No, this is not safe," is that usually a signal to you that this is a very powerful issue, and do you try to go in that direction but find a different way to get there?

RANDAL: Actually this was somewhat unusual. The "no" answer will happen, but it doesn't happen that often. Sometimes people have had terrible abuse issues and will still, in many cases, be ready to go right for it. I'm not tremendously surprised in either direction under any circumstance. Once I get a "no" answer I do not expect to end up going where we went. I thought it was very interesting how that happened. I had her look at the scene from a detached place and I gave her multiple levels of detachment. She was in the theater so she was watching the screen, and furthermore she was watching herself watching that, and furthermore if after all that she was drawn to be closer to the incident she could become the hidden observer in the room. She had all these different ways to choose what worked best for her. After we got to the initial sensitizing event that had to do with her feeling of being engulfed we went on to the lessons from that.

In this particular case I felt that there was all of this internal stuff with the inner child that I wanted to work with. It evolved in that unexpected direction because the girl had been so terribly traumatized by that event that in spite of how far Joy had come in her life and the wonderful insights she was giving, this terrified girl was still understandably having a hard time letting things in. That led to going inside the body. The body never lies. What are you feeling inside your body? I'm not looking for any particular thing to feel, I just want to know what she's feeling.

Boy, I could feel that blocked energy in the pelvis when I went to move her legs. To me, that stiffness was tied in with anger energy. It could also have been tied in with blocked sexual energy as well, but she had a lot to be angry about and the kicking would take her where she needed to go. Both, if necessary, would be dealt with by the energy of her kicking. I didn't want to skirt around it. I usually will not deal with the emotions when someone says no, but sometimes the circumstances shift.

LORIS: It seemed like once you got to that point in the trauma where you named it sexual abuse, that you moved on from that without exploring the details. Are there some instances when you would get more details of the incident itself or do you usually just name it and move on?

RANDAL: I will often go into a whole lot of detail about an incident. I got out of that incident as soon as I was clear that we had what we needed. The reason for that was because she had signaled that she did not want to get in touch with her emotions. My feeling was to go to the scene of the crime, get what we need to get from that, and get the heck out. Get her away from that so she doesn't have to see any more details than she needs to see. What she needed was to know the essence of what happened and that's all. If her signal had been yes, I would have been very thorough in that scene, at least in the feelings, as we may not have needed to explore many details of the molestation itself. But we would have dealt very thoroughly at that point in a Gestalt process with the details of her feelings, her responses, her rage, her grief, her betrayal or whatever came up from that experience.

REYA: My question is about the ideomotor responses. When you get a, "No, it doesn't feel safe or appropriate to go there," where do you go? After that you narrowed it down to a more specific question and she still said no. Then you went right into it because you intuited that there was still a way to get there. I'd like to know what you would have done if it didn't present itself to move on in some way?

RANDAL: I want to specifically mention that the first answer was yes, that it was safe and appropriate to be open to all memories, so that was acknowledged first. Then the "no" responses came up exclusively with the association of her feelings when she went back to those experiences. So she had given complete permission to go wherever she needed to go to look at what happened. That was fine and safe and appropriate for her.

If she had signaled no to that first question, then I would not have had her consciously look at the experience. I could still have very carefully detached her, grounded her, all of that, and then told her subconscious mind to go back, observe what happened but keep it blocked from the conscious mind, and bring back the understanding of what she needed to know about how that experience was continuing to affect her without consciously finding out the details of that experience.

JAMIE: When you got her to the point where she was beginning to experience the emotional connection with the abuse, where she was kicking and so on, you jumped out of that relatively quick. It seemed to me that she rose up like she was ready to make another breakthrough. If you were able to perceive it, would you suggest to her that maybe you should do another session or a couple of sessions outside of the classroom?

RANDAL: She was doing some kicking and she got into a lot of feelings and then I had her come back. Then it felt unfinished and I had her do more. She was still kicking but she was starting to slow down and I felt that this might be enough. I had her go into her body to see how she was doing and her voice was starting to come out really strong and her physical feelings were shifting, and it felt to me that it might really be enough.

There are times when it can go on for a shorter period. A person just kicks a couple of times and they did what they needed to do and at other times they just keep going and maybe it develops into primal screams and/or a deluge of violent kicking. Joy's response was that she was still feeling some coldness and that tingling, but the energy we were dealing with was gone. It had dissipated and she was feeling a lot of aliveness. To me it seemed complete with that particular issue but I'd like to see what Joy feels about that. (to Joy) I know it was five years ago but I'm wondering if you have any thoughts?

JOY: Well, the thing is that I had already been in a lot of anger groups and molestation stuff and done a lot of that. It was much more important to get in touch with what was going on on the inner levels because a lot of times anger is just a cover anyway for what's really going on.

RANDAL: Yes, and beneath anger there will very often be another feeling, such as grief or loss or whatever. But a lot of times you have to go through it to move on. So it was complete for you in this case and that's the key.

Watching the video I realized there wasn't a lot of kicking, but it felt powerful. It felt like she was really bringing more energy into it. Some strong emotions eventually appropriately came up even though she initially said no to being open to her feelings. It was interesting how that ended up manifesting itself. Regarding how much is enough, you can have your client communicate internal awareness. In this case I was helping her move her energy through and liven up that area. When the feeling has shifted or changed, and hers had changed in a dramatic way, then we may be complete in that part of the process.

Note: Joy has a powerful follow-up session with Randal at this point, which will be included as part of a forthcoming book on the healing of molestation with hypnotherapy.

CHAPTER 14

Recovered Memories
Reclaiming Logic on Both Sides of the Controversy

The Recovery of Memories

The subconscious, "the other 90% of the mind," has a variety of major functions including the storage of memories. Accessing the subconscious through hypnosis can bring back long-forgotten memories or recover further details of recent or distant memories. There are many ways hypnotic access of memories can be beneficial, and not just in a therapeutic context. For example, many people have successfully used hypnosis to help solve a mystery or to find lost valuables.

Whether or not the details of our memories have been hypnotically enhanced, our memories do not work as some kind of exact movie or snapshot of events. Even witnesses of the same very recent event will often recall key aspects of the event in different ways from each other. Memories of childhood experiences recalled decades later, in or out of hypnosis, can be influenced by other memories, and influenced by dreams and various expectations, perspectives, projections and fantasies. Fritz Perls told a story about a fight between Pride and Memory. Pride won.

Within this context of our imperfect memory and recall abilities, hypnosis used properly can significantly heighten recall. The phenomenon of hypnotic memory enhancement is called hypermnesia. The most comprehensive book on the recall of forgotten memories and related ramifications is the mammoth, extremely well-researched, *Memory, Trauma, Treatment and the Law,* by Brown, Scheflin and Hammond. It gives thorough coverage of major voices on all sides of the recovered memories debate, and in the process documents a large amount of research demonstrating that "hypnotic procedures combined with free recall and appropriate warnings result in a significant increase in the total amount of information recollected about a meaningful target event without a corresponding significant increase in the memory error rate."

There are various tools we can use to hypnotically increase recall. One especially important key to increasing recall of experiences in ways that will produce greater detail with a minimum of inaccuracies, is for the therapist and client to approach the recall of memories from a truly neutral position.

The Controversy

Controversies around recovered memories exploded in the 1990's. The fires were stoked by extremists on both sides of the debate. On one far end of the spectrum were therapists who used exceptionally inappropriate methods in a highly suggestive environment. On the other were so-called "experts" who in some cases weren't even experienced therapists. The radical positions taken by some on both sides of the debate were exceptionally naive and misinformed. At one extreme there was an assumption that any apparent memory that ever occurs under even highly suggestive circumstances in hypnosis or therapy is completely true, and on the other that neither hypnosis nor any other technique can ever recover a real memory.

Two key factors in the controversy are science and politics. "The political portion of the debate is relatively simple to understand, the science is relatively complex," state Brown, Scheflin and Hammond. "Because of zealotry, science has taken a back seat. In its place have been wild and inaccurate articulations...that have served, not as science, but as emotional sound bites for a gullible media."

There have always been logical, balanced voices in the debate, some of which emphasized a particular point of view. One example is Michael Yapko, author of *Suggestions of Abuse.* He recognizes the reality and importance of recovered memories, but emphasizes great concern regarding the dangers of suggestive therapists. Unfortunately, concern from the more balanced voices of true experts were sometimes ignored, especially in the years the controversy unfolded.

There are very important issues on both sides, and I am particularly disturbed by influential voices in the debate who always take one side. For example, Sociologist Richard Ofshe, an eloquent writer but not an experienced therapist, has been rejected more than once as an expert witness in court. He co-authored the book *Making Monsters,* which attempts to repudiate the very idea of recovered memories, tarnishing the good points he does make. "Recovered memories is the psychiatric, psychological quackery of the 20th century," Ofshe proclaimed on *Dateline* in 1995. "It is an utter fantasy without one shred of scientific support." Logically and in reality, such radical points of view make no sense. "Forgetting and remembering are universal experiences," says Neuroscientist Rawn Joseph. "We may go through an old photo album and be triggered with childhood memories." The media, at times, has been drawn to promoting such simplistic points of view incontroverted, eager to make a proponent such as Ofshe out as a hero and leading expert, thereby promoting a complete rejection of recovered memories without rebuttal.

The term "false memory" is strange, often being used in contexts that connote either a memory is entirely true or entirely false. Memories, especially from long ago, previously recalled or not, are usually more complex than that. However, inappropriate counseling and therapy techniques can sometimes yield "memories" that are mostly or entirely fabricated, and for that matter, many people have false non recovered "memories" as well.

Since concern regarding false memories has been used in such a one-sided and frequently biased way, let's focus on this phenomenon from another perspective. Psychiatrist Lenore Terr, author of *Unchained Memories: True Stories of Traumatic Memories, Lost and Found,* has worked for 30 years with battered and traumatized children and their parents. In an interview with Patricia Holt of the San Francisco Chronicle she discusses therapy sessions she has had with parents who were recognized perpetrators of abuse. "When I first started out in this field, I used to get the most horrible headaches after long sessions with parents who would deny they ever injured their child. I would have proof - photos and medical examinations - but they would simply deny it anyway, and I finally came to realize we had to go in another direction or I would just die of headaches." Regarding returning memories of childhood trauma, she believes the number of false-memory "victims" is a "drop in the bucket" compared to the number of people coping with true repressed memories.

Ross Cheit's experience served as a rebuttal to the kind of proclamation ("not a shred of evidence of recovered memories") propagated by Ofshe and others and sometimes eagerly disseminated by the media. He had been a member of the San Francisco Boy's chorus at the age of twelve. When entering therapy more than two decades later he began to recover memories, to his shock, about having been molested by Bill Farmer, the chorus' summer camp administer. Cheit taped a phone call to Farmer in which he identified himself and got a confirmation that Farmer remembered him. He stated he was one of many young boys whom he had molested, and he had located other chorus members who said Farmer had molested them. Farmer's voice is heard in response, confirming the allegation but stating "that was a long way back." Cheit went on to sue Farmer and won a $450,000 judgment.

There has been a tremendous variety of documentation of recovered memories, and of the value of therapy in that context, throughout the past century. Before legal restrictions against many uses of forensic hypnosis in California (and most other states), the Los Angeles Police Department solved hundreds of crimes by using hypnotically enhanced memories as leads. In the famous Chowchilla kidnapping case, bus driver Ed Ray was able to remember a license plate number during hypnosis with William Kroger, which led police to the kidnappers, including the irrefutable evidence of fingerprints. Thousands of people have refreshed memories or found lost items through hypnosis. Examples go on and on.

It is easy for most of us to understand how a memory of a consequential event from early childhood may be forgotten from the sheer length of time and youth of the experience, then later recalled upon focus of an issue or event, with or without hypnosis. What is surprising for some, however, is the way major traumas can be dissociated and blocked that occurred later in childhood, and in particular in adult years. But this is not a new discovery and has been well-documented, which refutes the contention of Ofshe and Singer that "neither amnesia nor robust repression was implicated in post traumatic stress disorder" literature until recently. For example, during each of the World Wars, there are hundreds of cases of soldiers who responded to intense battle and war trauma by developing amnesia. Using hypnosis for recall, abreaction, reassociation, and reintegration of amnestic memories was used very effectively with many "shell shock" victims during World War I, and for trauma during and after subsequent wars.

Terr states that instances of overwhelming terror disrupt the normal process of memory encoding. Sensations and images can be recorded without a story in discreet, hard-to-reach areas of the brain. She explains that when children are repeatedly abused they learn to put themselves into trance states. Afterward, telling no one what has happened, some of the memories may never get transferred to the part of the brain where stories dwell.

Rawn Joseph further explains how victims can forget and then remember terrifying trauma. "Repressed memories have been validated, then repudiated by the courts - but the essential truth has not changed. Recovered memories, blocked for years because of trauma, do exist." He explains that under stress the part of the brain that stores long-term memory may shut down, leading to a loss of memory. Under repetitive trauma and fear this same part of the brain, the hippocampus, can be so overwhelmed that it is actually damaged by the chemicals that are released by the body as part of the "fight or flight" response. As a result, individuals who have undergone repeated abuse in childhood often recall very little. Yet even after severe trauma, lost memories may be recovered. Joseph calls this process "shrinking retrograde amnesia," in which over time traumatic details may begin to appear.

Science News published the findings of the UCLA Medical Center's study in which a 54-item trauma questionnaire was administered to children ages 8 to 15. Among those who had documented evidence of sexual abuse, such as physical signs and recovery of pornographic pictures taken of the child, 7 percent made no mention of sexual abuse and another 5 percent recanted past reports of abuse. Children who did not cite their abuse exhibited virtually no traumatic symptoms, according to the study, in stark contrast to those who disclosed their abuse. Dennis Alsop, a hypnotherapist with extensive experience working with childhood trauma, responded in a later issue of *Science News*, "Aren't amnesia and denial traumatic symptoms? The fact that the children who seemed least affected by evidenced abuse had no memory of their abuse tells us something important, doesn't it?" That is that the ability to dissociate from the memory of the experience may help a trauma victim cope.

David Cheek writes in *Hypnosis: The Application of Ideomotor Techniques*, "It has not been generally recognized that there might be a phylogenetic need for such amnesia throughout the animal kingdom. Human survivors of a serious accident, a fire, or an earthquake may have vividly clear memories for details during the next few hours. Their memory will then rapidly fade from consciousness but will remain to haunt the victim's unconscious mind during sleep, during similar time of day, or when entering a similar location. The triggering stimulus may come into the brainstem reticular activating system (RAS) by way of any sensory channel. Epinephrine, the adrenal hormone released during stress, seems to be the cause of imprint type of learning as well as of the forgetfulness that is associated with trauma (Weinberger et al. 1984)." He points out that this relationship has been observed clinically and is supported by recent research with animals. After herd animals of the plains of Africa rush wildly to escape from predators, behavior changes rapidly upon reaching safety. Within seconds, they are grazing as if nothing happened. He believes that evolutionary adaptive factors have encouraged conscious forgetfulness of a recent danger and that crisis amnesia serves a biological purpose. Amnesia supports the survival of animals, helping release them from periods of constant worried alarm after crises, which could diminish feeding, sleeping, nursing and procreation.

The Power of Suggestion

Some of the backlash to recovered memories has come from horror stories resulting from improper therapy procedures, which in some cases have involved hypnosis. The most famous aspect of hypnosis is its inherent suggestibility, but that fact seems have been lost on a small percentage of therapists. It must be spelled out that therapists need to be extremely careful to avoid leading their clients regarding memories, even when there has been no formal induction of hypnosis.

To fully appreciate the power of suggestion we can look beyond the suggestibility of individuals in therapy and hypnosis to focus on the effectiveness of the placebo, which is also a suggestion. Many dramatic examples of its potency have been documented. Dr. Shapiro, in the *American Journal of Psychotherapy* wrote, "Placebos can have profound effects on organic illnesses, including incurable malignancies." In a study on postoperative pain by Beecher and Lasagna, patients who had undergone surgery were given alternating doses of morphine and placebos. Those who had been given morphine immediately following surgery reported a 52 percent decrease in pain, while those given a placebo reported a 40 percent decrease. Not only was the placebo almost as effective (77 percent), but the more severe the pain the more effective the placebo was. Another doctor, A. Leslie, reported that morphine addicts given placebos (saline injections) did not suffer withdrawal symptoms until the injections were stopped.

Our knowledge of the power of the placebo is nothing new. Beecher stressed back in 1955 in the *Journal of the American Medical Association* that placebos can have serious toxic effects and produce physiological damage. He was referring to documentation that patients given placebos would also in many cases develop expected negative side effects associated with the medication that was being replaced.

In his extended studies, Dr. H. Gold documented the correlation between high suggestibility and high intelligence. The greater the intelligence, the more susceptible the individual was to placebo therapy and the greater the potential benefit. Placebo studies show us how easily people can be influenced by an authority figure such as a doctor or therapist, even when there has been no formal hypnotic induction. The important corollary here is that these studies are exciting because they show just how powerful the subconscious mind can be, even to the point, in many cases, of physical transformations. We have the capability for tremendous achievements through understanding and using the power of our subconscious minds, without needing to project our power onto authority figures.

Individuals struggling with physical, mental or emotional health issues can be exceptionally suggestible with an authority figure who is assisting in the recovery process. Even without a formal hypnotic induction, we need to be very careful. Many clients are working on issues that began as a result of trauma from an early age. There can be a dangerous receptivity to a therapist who probes the past while having an expectancy, or even seeming to have an expectancy, of what the client may have experienced or repressed.

When hypnosis is used properly it works to bring up memories, by and large, accurately and effectively. A caveat is that sometimes when memories come up, in or out of hypnosis or therapy, two memories can partly merge together, or a dream, fear or fantasy can influence some memories. Greater overall details and accuracy tend to be consistent when a session is approached from a neutral place, using effective techniques such as those in these volumes.

Some Therapists in Denial

Some people, in a suggestible state, can be manipulated into creating a memory. I had a new client who described her experience of an initial session with a previous therapist she had been referred to. The therapist, who called herself an expert in molestation issues, had noted the client's difficulties with low self esteem, sensitivity to criticism, and eating control, along with previous struggles at times with alcoholism and drug abuse, and said, "Those are all signs of having been sexually molested as a child." The client responded that she hadn't been. The therapist explained to her that memories can be repressed and said, "Let's use hypnosis and find out if you were molested." She entered hypnosis and sure enough, seemed to recall a molestation memory.

This is an exceptional example of a therapist's illogical reasoning and insensitivity to the potential effect of suggestion. For starters, even calling oneself a specialist in molestation issues is in itself a suggestion. Of course, just because certain symptoms can be found in some people who have been molested, that doesn't mean that anyone with any of those symptoms was probably molested. My client, affected by the apparent expertise of an authority figure and the seeming documentation provided by the alleged memory, was still somewhat skeptical. In my discussion with her, I could not say that the memory was certainly false. But she was thrilled when I told her about a television interview I had recently taped about musician Judy Collins. Collins had been quite open about how harshly her father had treated her and what a perfectionist he had been in wanting her to succeed. She developed all of my client's symptoms and more, including having had suicidal feelings at times in her life. It would seem to be an obvious truism that there are many kinds of traumatic experiences that a child can have that can produce similar ongoing life difficulties. A therapist's obsession with one particular possibility does not yield proper procedures.

A student once described to me having been in a women's therapy group, led by a therapist who would take turns hypnotizing different group members. In a very suggestive environment, she eventually coaxed "repressed memories" of molestation out of every group member. When my student had approached her questioning the consistency of such experiences with all of them, the therapist said there was a "synchronicity" that attracted women to her who had been molested.

There is an irony in that some of those who care most deeply about issues of child abuse, and molestation in particular, have been well-meaning therapists who have sometimes traumatized clients, and who have been instrumental in helping create the intensity of the backlash that has occurred regarding repressed memories.

It is essential when working with memory in therapy, in and out of hypnosis, to keep absolutely neutral in any work that is being done. One of Trudeau's Doonesbury comic strip characters was hypnotized and regressed on his radio station. "You see something, don't you? It's an alien, right?" the doctor asks. He responds that he doesn't think so. "Then it's your mother. She's holding a knife, isn't she?" Unfortunately, there have been a small minority of therapists for which this isn't much of an exaggeration. One hypnotherapy instructor told his students that 90% of the women he does regression work with report molestation, and we can be very concerned about the effects such statements have had on his therapy sessions, including class demonstrations and prospective hypnotherapists.

I'll describe a unique experience I had with a student I'll call Nancy, who worked as a psychic. She was in the same class as Pat, who's sessions are transcribed in Chapter 17. As is described at the beginning of that chapter, Pat developed intense fear after we did a session for preparing to quit smoking. Her reaction was so strong that I stopped the session right there and encouraged her to consider having a session later in class to work on these deeper issues. Nancy approached me at the break, after I halted the session, and quietly mentioned she'd tuned in and discovered that Pat's reaction was caused by molestation by her uncle. Two weeks later, as will be seen in Chapter 17, Pat described the horrible beatings she experienced as a baby by her father, including the broken leg that had never completely healed. None of our work together brought up any recall of a molestation.

Right after that session, I found out that Nancy had given psychic readings for two class members outside of class, and both were about discovery of a molestation. I carefully and thoroughly got details from each person so that I could talk to her about it. While we had barely begun to touch upon regression at that early stage of class (and my lecture on recovered memories hadn't occurred yet), in one of the sessions she had already incorporated hypnosis and a simple regression. She asked the man about any problems from childhood, and he described that he had been told his long-passed childhood stutter had developed after he came home from his first day at a day care center. She took him into hypnosis and regressed him to the scene. He described that he was outside in the yard feeling lonely and scared, surrounded by kids who were mostly bigger than him, and a big kid came over and started pushing him. Nancy said, "Are you sure it was a big kid? Could it have been a small adult?" He paused and said, "Well, I guess so. Maybe it was a small woman?" "Oh, good, yes," she responded. "Now, are you sure she was pushing you, or was she doing something else?" He paused again, and felt he sensed the kind of thing Nancy meant. "Well, maybe she was fondling me?" She responded with obvious satisfaction and relief, "Yes, very good. You got it!"

Nancy's projections were reflecting her own issues. Luckily, he was disturbed by her methods and had serious doubts about that "memory" which is why he informed me about the experience. Such manipulation is dangerous and unnecessary. Intuition can be used appropriately in sessions to help decide what direction to move in, or what kinds of neutral questions to ask, or to focus on energy that the person may not be consciously aware of. It is not appropriate to "give" information no matter how certain one might be. It is critically important to avoid leading a client. Even if such information proves to be true, the only person who will ever really know what they have experienced is the client. The therapeutic goal is to help individuals find out for themselves, which is often more about working with process than discovering a memory.

The case of Laura Deck provides an example of the dangers of manipulative and leading procedures. Deck had been referred to a mental health counselor by her family doctor when she reported symptoms of depression and insomnia. In her first session with psychologist John Laughlin she described her difficulties growing up in a broken home, and informed him she had a history of depression, alcoholism and suicide attempts, and had depression following the birth of her third child. In written notes after that consultation he stated that he would use hypnosis to get at "what is really going on."

When Deck said she did not remember ever being sexually abused as a child, Laughlin told her to read a book that included a discussion of repressed memories. Two weeks later he was getting subconscious "memories" of her getting hit over the head with a baseball bat by her uncle and raped. A year later the same counselor was encouraging Deck to remember her mother placing her in a satanic cult that murdered babies on alters in the forest.

In 147 therapy sessions over 2 1/2 years, Laughlin's own notes showed that Deck resisted him at least 62 times. "Basically, she wants to be who she is but doesn't want to tell the truth, doesn't want to give information, doesn't want to do things that people could be hurt about," he wrote. Eventually a very traumatized Deck went into treatment with other therapists who concluded that the many "memories" of rape and satanic abuse had been manufactured by Laughlin. Deck sued Laughlin and in 1995 won a large monetary settlement.

These are extreme examples, and to the vast majority of us such improprieties are obvious. What we have to be diligent in is avoiding the much more subtle ways of leading our very suggestible clients.

Toward a Balanced Perspective

There are still vocal extremists. The False Memory Syndrome Foundation took a scientific position in the very beginning that was moderate and sensible, as stated in 1992 in their first newsletter. From there most members of the Scientific Advisory Board quickly took increasingly aggressive and controversial positions, such as recovered memories being necessarily inaccurate.

The False Memory Syndrome Foundation has generally been treated reverently by the media. It is worth noting that Ralph Underwager, who coined the term "false memory syndrome" and who co-founded the False Memory Syndrome Foundation in the U.S., was forced to resign from the FMSF board in 1993 after giving an interview to a pedophile magazine in which he stated that having sex with children could be a responsible choice. His wife, who participated with him in the interview, remained on the FMSF board. Since that occurred, one book highly recommended by the FMSF quotes studies that purport to show that adult-child sex can be harmless, and the author states that childhood sexual abuse is basically only a cultural taboo. Most members of the FMSF are parents accused of molestation, and the extent that some prominent members of this organization have sometimes gone to defend adult-child sex has especially disturbing implications.

The FMSF has succeeded in getting much public and media acceptance of a "false memory syndrome," but this term has not come close to receiving general professional acceptance. Hovdestad & Kristiansen say the idea of a false memory syndrome has little discriminant validity, pointing out, "False memory advocates have no data in support of a false memory syndrome as a valid scientific construct." Psychiatrist Richard J. Lowenstein states, "Although writings by FMS board members tout the foundation's 'scientific' approach, I know of no clinical research or tradition of clinical description that empirically validates or supports that such a clinical condition exists as such. FMS is a syndome without signs and symptoms (the defining characteristics of a syndrome)."

In spite of some continued uncompromising positions, such as found in the FMSF, Christine Courtois, author of *Recollections of Sexual Abuse: Treatment Principles and Guidelines,* has noted a recent shifting of tone and a more collaborative and less adversarial approach taking place in professional circles. "By and large, (professional task forces) support aspects of each side of the controversy (i.e., recovered and delayed memories are possible, as are the creation of false memories) and urge clinicians...to practice conservatively.... All caution that the current controversy must not be used to obscure or deny the reality, prevalence, and seriousness of child abuse as a social issue but also indicate concern for the seriousness and destructiveness of false accusations."

Kalichman reports that even with massive under reporting, a few million cases of child abuse and neglect are reported in the United States each year. "The majority of reports involve neglect (45%), but physical abuse accounts for 25% of reports, sexual abuse for 15%, and emotional maltreatment for 6% of reports." Child abuse is a serious, widespread problem, repression of memories can occur, and recovery of memories can occur within or outside of therapy. We need to approach these issues carefully and realistically.

Effective Procedures for Recovering, Revivifying and Enhancing Accurate Memories

No method, in or out of therapy, provides perfect recall. However, a law review article concluded that psychodynamic psychotherapies that attempt to uncover the past are slower than hypnosis and no more likely to be more reliable. Kanovitz concurs, saying, "Talking psychotherapies are as capable of implanting false memories...as hypnotic ones," and "There is as much opportunity for memory alteration to occur in non hypnotic psychotherapies as hypnotic ones." This is true outside of therapy as well.

Some psychotherapists inappropriately push a client in session after session to try to dredge up a possibly repressed memory. Marriage counselor Marche Isabella did this in the Holly Ramona case, which has various complexities and will be worthy of further discussion in Volume II. But the subconscious mind is the seat of the memories and with the valuable and appropriate use of hypnosis, if a significant memory is buried and needs to come forward, it often will if the subconscious feels trusting of and supported by the practitioner. There are examples of jogging memories throughout these volumes, such as the affect bridge followed by quick neutral questioning techniques. This section, however, is not primarily about techniques to bring forth memories which may be beneath the conscious awareness. The emphasis here is on how to proceed with the greatest likelihood of *accurate* recall.

Using correct procedures, hypnotically enhanced recall involves maximizing hypnotic memory enhancement, or hypermnesia, while minimizing inaccuracy. In this chapter and throughout these two volumes, there is information about the recall of subconscious memories that can help guide us in directions to take and directions to avoid in eliciting memories and details of memories.

It is abundantly clear that the therapeutic context is rife with suggestibility, even when there is no hypnotic induction. The language employed when I use ideomotor questioning, especially in the early establishment of responses, gives good examples of careful neutrality in requesting information from the subconscious. It isn't simply a matter of not asking leading questions. There are various ways we can unknowingly lead if we're not paying attention, and we must be careful not to communicate, or seem to communicate, a particular opinion or expectation. In fact, hypnosis is typically effective in revivifying memories if the therapist is neutral not only in words, but in tone and in the manner and kind of questioning and other procedures used.

When I am working with ideomotor responses I repeat the answer I have observed, in part because the person may not be consciously aware of the movement that has occurred. One of the beauties of ideomotor methods is that often the subconscious mind can help out with memories, realizations and self-discovery before the conscious mind even becomes aware of it. Repeating the answer provides good feedback to the person who is getting the answer through the signals of the subconscious, and can reinforce the validity of the answer even when it was already recognized and understood by the conscious. I might also summarize after a few answers, using the present tense, "Okay, it's inside now and it's daytime. There are two other persons present and you're in your house." I can encourage that it may start to get more clear now, and that may help the details come forth from the subconscious.

Helping a client find lost items, while valuable in itself, is a good way for hypnotherapists to initially develop skills in bringing back details of memories and is also good practice for being non-leading in preparation for the increased complexity and intensity of working with emotionally charged issues. Brown, Scheflin and Hammond believe scientific literature indicates that "hypnosis is especially more likely to assist someone in recalling personally meaningful, affect-laden events, than non-meaningful information about which the person is indifferent." Efforts to recall the last place the client left something of value hardly ever include the advantage of connecting to the key memory via an affect bridge, but the importance of the lost item(s) helps motivate the focus. Patient use of appropriate hypnotic techniques can often lead to solving the mystery, as is demonstrated in detail in my forthcoming book, *Ideomotor Magic*.

There will be times when memories or associated feelings are beginning to surface and the best choice may be to encourage getting more in touch with the feelings. Such techniques often lead to more specific, detailed memories, although the main reason for getting more in touch with feelings at such a time is for the intrinsic value of processing those feelings at that stage. Usually questions will not need to be suggestive, specific or leading in initial opening or further details of a memory. Are you inside or outside? Is it nighttime or daytime? When questions of possibilities are needed to get more details, start with a more positive or less negative possibility. If a vague memory is developing of being afraid as a child, you can encourage fully feeling the fear (if the subconscious has given the green light for feelings), then you can ask, "What are you afraid of?" as opposed to a leading question like, "Who are you afraid of?" If the client doesn't know what the fear is about, the question might be asked, "Do you feel safe?" The answer might be, "Yes, I just woke up from a bad dream." Then that might possibly lead to an issue about what the dream was about, or about a significant recurring childhood feeling, perhaps one of alienation or loneliness or not having anyone to confide in.

Another example would be to have the person stay with whatever the feeling is and direct the awareness into the body, then intensify that feeling even more. Working with that feeling will often bring up specific issues and memories, and/or will give the feeling an opportunity to be experienced, released and dissipated. Or a suggestion can be given, like, "Now this could have to do with something or someone. What comes to your mind right off the top of your head?" In some selective cases during regression, a well-timed very light tapping on the forehead with the index finger, a kind of startle technique, may help bring up some specific memory. Or you could just work with that and do some Gestalt dialogue with the feeling. Memories may begin to arise as a Gestalt process develops, or you may not necessarily need to get back to various aspects of the memory. In some cases, it may be something you can work with in context to the energy itself. We're discussing various procedures that can heighten recall, but that is only a step in regression therapy, one aspect of a comprehensive process.

What about removing an alleged recovered memory that arose in very suggestive circumstances with a well-meaning but overzealous therapist? It is challenging to work in this context because it is sometimes possible to bring up accurate memories even under these conditions, and because inaccurate memories implanted in such conditions often seem so real, and are sometimes mixed with real memories. The therapist needs to have a thorough discussion with the client about issues of recovered memories and only proceed if there is an open mind on the part of both therapist and client to get to the truth, whatever that may be. The best hope is to include work with ideomotor methods in identifying inaccurate memories and releasing them. Identifying and releasing a false memory is not a perfect science, but I have had success with good certainty and powerful healing, as will be demonstrated, in part, through a transcript and commentary in my forthcoming book on the healing of molestation.

The Purpose of therapy

As shown by the sessions in these volumes, most regression therapy sessions cannot be easily broken down into some kind of construct regarding whether the session is or is not about recovered memories. Sometimes among a series of familiar memories, a memory arises that the subject hasn't thought about in years, but remembers having thought about at times in years past. Often added details arise during a revivification of a familiar memory. The subject may remember them just as details that were not thought of for some time, or may not remember ever recalling them since the incident. Sometimes in a single session we work with a series of memories, including various combinations of the above possibilities. And especially significant, the memories themselves are usually parenthetical, of secondary importance, to the various primary aspects of comprehensive regression therapy.

If a regression is a self-exploration as described in Chapter 2, or to find a missing object of value, or being facilitated in forensic hypnosis to help solve a crime, then the regression can be about the possibility of recovering a memory. The object in regression *therapy* is not to assume there could be or is some lost or blocked memory and try to find it. The purpose of regression therapy is to transform challenging issues that are continuing to have an effect in the present. Sometimes there are surprises regarding memories during regression. Very often the surprises have to do with just how powerful and deep the effects have been of experiences that *the client was well-aware of all along*.

Good therapy leads to maturation (as per the Gestalt definition of moving toward self-support), self-expression, inner strength and acceptance, self-actualization, peace and sometimes forgiveness. Good therapy does not lead to suing one's parents.

Regression therapy is not about recovering memories. The elicitation of reasonably accurate heightened memory recall is sometimes a secondary effect of therapy which is demonstrated throughout the sessions of these volumes. In addition, a chapter in Volume II will be devoted to further elaboration of this important topic.

CHAPTER 15

Christine's Overwhelming Responsibilities
The Breech Birth: "I Can't Do It"

The title gives away a dramatic development that will occur early in the regression. However, knowing in advance that Christine's issues spawn from her birth lend insight and an interesting context to the study of the pre-induction interview.

RANDAL: What would you like to work on?

CHRISTINE: It's a recurring problem that has been with me most of my life and causes me a great deal of anxiety. It's a very deep belief that surfaces that I can't do something. It really holds me back from progressing in many areas of my life and causes me an overwhelming anxiety at times. It's strong and I don't know where it's coming from.

RANDAL: Have you noticed this more in recent years in your life or has this been significant throughout much of your life?

CHRISTINE: It's happened more as I've done more work on myself, but I can recall even as a child going to my mother and saying, "I can't do this." She would have to encourage and push me to get out and do things. But it's becoming a real issue at the moment, with the school my partner and I are starting up, for example. It's causing me a lot of problems. In my head I know I can do things, I know I've been successful. But I have trouble believing or tapping into the resources of those past successes, if that makes sense. And it's like the emotional content of the anxiety overwhelms the logical thinking.

RANDAL: Right. Subconscious fears overcoming conscious knowledge.

CHRISTINE: And it is a fear.

RANDAL: Describe it some more in your own words. What is it that happens?

CHRISTINE: What tends to happen is that I find myself through circumstances with a tremendous amount of responsibility. I enter into something thinking this is going to be shared by two or more people, then circumstances change and I find that I have 90 percent of the work load and responsibility. I can handle 50 percent of it if I have that support or that sharing, but suddenly to be doing most of it on my own is scary.

RANDAL: When you say you end up having 90 percent, are you talking about between you and your business partner or you and your staff or other people?

CHRISTINE: Usually my business partner. Circumstances change and he has to go elsewhere and I find I'm carrying the load.

RANDAL: I'd like to look at the whole picture as we go through this discovery process. There could be some resentment because you're having to carry so much. We can check whether you really have to carry that much or whether your partner could do more when he's gone or could be doing more to catch up before he goes and after he comes back. This could possibly have to do with an issue of speaking up, of taking charge, of expressing your needs and being confrontive. Does that seem to be part of the issue here?

CHRISTINE: To a small degree it may be, and that's an issue that I have addressed recently. I do find to a certain extent that some things are resolved if I speak out. But there's still a fear, an anxiety that I don't feel should be there.

RANDAL: That's clear. While we're on the subject I'd like to encourage you to do some positive suggestions in self–hypnosis on the issues of recognizing the importance of not taking on much more than your share and of speaking up. (Randal emphasizes options for the future at various points during this session, within the context that this will be a single session with no direct follow-up for Christine, who has come from Australia to this International Hypnotherapy Conference) If you find down the road that there is still an issue that is a barrier for you, then you can consider possibly doing regression work on that, too. But I understand what you're saying. There is definitely a core issue here regarding how you end up with a lot of responsibilities and you feel overwhelmed.

CHRISTINE: Yes, overwhelmed, and it seems to be issues that are new for me. Something I'm doing for the first time. It's the unknown. Fear of the unknown comes up.

RANDAL: Is it primarily the responsibility you feel combined with having major decisions to make, or do you think it's more a fear of the unknown?

CHRISTINE: It's the responsibility and it seems to be doing it on my own. This lack of confidence comes up. "Am I doing it right? Is this okay?" It comes back to the fear. Self–doubt.

RANDAL: Let's focus on your childhood. Do you recall being in situations where you felt self–doubt and a lack of confidence? Like, "Am I doing this right?"

CHRISTINE: Yes.

RANDAL: Can you give me an example of that?

CHRISTINE: One classic example that comes to mind was at an athletic meeting. I started at a running club.

RANDAL: And you were how old?

CHRISTINE: Seven.

RANDAL: You started taking on responsibilities a little bit on the early side, didn't you? Good for you. Okay, you started at a running club.

CHRISTINE: And I remember having this fear of running through the tape. It was like I'd run up to the tape and stop and my father actually had to run with me and take me through the tape. Once I'd done it, I was fine.

RANDAL: I realize that was a long time ago but do you have any memory of what you were afraid of with the tape?

CHRISTINE: I didn't realize that the tape was going to just move away. I thought the tape was going to hurt me in some way.

RANDAL: All right. Can you give me another example of feeling this lack of confidence or wondering if you were doing something right?

CHRISTINE: Oh, there's been lot's of... (Christine's voice fades) Piano examinations. I went through piano examinations every year and I'd come up against the same obstacles - a new grade, a new material, a new examiner. Terrible fear.

RANDAL: At what ages?

CHRISTINE: From the age of ten right through to my twenties. It's the same with my work.

RANDAL: You refer to the examination itself, but also meeting a new teacher and going to a new level or a new grade. At every new level there was a feeling when you were just starting out or just taking the examination. Would you call it fear or what would the feeling be?

CHRISTINE: A fear, a lack of confidence. It didn't seem to matter that I'd done well on the previous examination. When the next stage came up I still had the same feelings of lack of confidence, fear, worry. Would I do well? Would I fail?

RANDAL: It sounds like there are many examples. Give me one more example of a time when you were a child and you felt some difficulty in getting to the next level or doing something.

CHRISTINE: All that comes to mind is going to a new school. I had lots of changes of schools. New schools, new friends, new experiences.

RANDAL: That happened on several occasions?

CHRISTINE: Many times.

RANDAL: That would be normal, of course, for a child to feel nervous going to a new school. One thing that makes it significant in your case is that this has been such a pattern in so many ways for you. When you went to a new school do you remember feeling particularly traumatized? Did you cry or anything like that?

CHRISTINE: No, not really.

RANDAL: And did you get over it fairly quickly?

CHRISTINE: I would say so.

RANDAL: You mentioned you're just starting a school. What kind of a school is it?

CHRISTINE: A hypnosis school.

RANDAL: Is this the first time you've done that?

CHRISTINE: Yes.

RANDAL: So is that the main reason these feelings are coming up now?

CHRISTINE: It's the most recent. It's been coming up strongly recently. Usually I wake up at night with quite a lot of fear and mental activity, thinking of all the things I need to be doing or should be doing or just worrying about, "Is it going to be okay?"

RANDAL: I'd like to address the group for a minute. If my client's issue is a lack of confidence, in some cases I would begin with several sessions of positive post-hypnotic suggestions, including visualizing getting organized, setting goals, and achieving those goals. As the sessions move on I'll check to see how the person is progressing and further explore whether there is some significant issue from the past that would make it useful or valuable to go into regression. The decision for each individual about the methods to use and their order within the sessions can be interesting, and is based partly on current goals and recent emotional responses to those goals, the seriousness and length of an issue or block, and the apparent possibility of a major trauma as cause.

I have a sense that Christine is a good candidate for immediate regression work. I would suggest that she follow this up with some self–hypnosis for strengthening confidence. In doing regression work, often in one session you can deal with a major aspect of the issue. Then, say after this session, Christine can take some more time to fully integrate it into her life. Some people are even at a point in their lives that they can do really well with a single comprehensive session. It's like a process of breaking up ice that then just naturally begins to go down stream and continue to break up. (Randal uses his communication to the group in part to increase Christine's mental expectancy via direct and indirect suggestions)

(to Christine) Can you describe something about your fear regarding this new school? What could go wrong?

CHRISTINE: I don't know. I haven't even worked that one out. It's just a fear.

RANDAL: So it's just a vague fear. Is it a fear that it's not going to succeed or that you're going to end up doing something wrong or that nobody's going to come to the classes? Can you narrow it down a little bit?

CHRISTINE: One thing that comes up is a fear of something going wrong or many things going wrong.

RANDAL: Something going wrong in the administration or the teaching?

CHRISTINE: Yes. Running out of time. By that I mean running out of time to prepare what needs to be prepared ahead of time.

RANDAL: And such fears sometimes wake you up at night. Are you generally a fairly organized person?

CHRISTINE: Yes. I like to be and if I haven't organized sufficiently, then I worry.

RANDAL: And one of the things that has helped you to come a long way in your life is being well organized in general. Has it been in the last few weeks that you've been waking up at night?

CHRISTINE: Yes.

RANDAL: Does this also happen to be one of those times when you're taking on ninety or eighty percent instead of fifty percent of the work?

CHRISTINE: Yes. It's always when that's happening.

RANDAL: Have you talked to your partner about this?

CHRISTINE: Yes.

RANDAL: And does that issue seem to be getting handled now?

CHRISTINE: It will resolve itself for awhile but the pattern will still recur later on.

RANDAL: When the pattern recurs do you feel like it's partly you and partly your partner that causes that to happen?

CHRISTINE: Yes.

RANDAL: What is it about you that causes that pattern to recur?

CHRISTINE: Self–doubt, a need for reassurance, and that's not always possible. It's like my partner can often be busy with other things or other responsibilities and my head says, hey, I shouldn't be needing the reassurance or input from him at the times when I do, or as much as I do. Does that make sense?

RANDAL: Yes, it does. Now for the sake of time, why don't you just show me which is your "yes" finger during ideomotor questioning. (Christine moves the index finger of her right hand) Okay, the index finger on your right hand is your "yes" finger. And your "no" finger? (Christine moves the index finger of her left hand) It's the index finger on your left hand, so you use the index finger on your right and left hands. Do you have an "I don't know" finger that sometimes responds?

CHRISTINE: At times. It has, I'm not sure which one it is now.

RANDAL: Well, if another finger rises we'll explore that then. Is there anything else that you would like to say that you think might be useful or important before we do the hypnosis?

CHRISTINE: The only thing, which I've mentioned, is that when I tune in or listen to myself there is a deep belief or something that says I can't do this. Everything seems so difficult and I become aware of an obstacle. It makes me quite sad because something is there blocking or making life so difficult.

RANDAL: So when you get in touch with the fear you come up to this obstacle and that makes you sad.

CHRISTINE: Yes.

RANDAL: Close your eyes now and go into your body. Breathe down into your stomach. Feel that sadness that comes up because of some obstacle. Describe what you feel in your body.

CHRISTINE: I feel it in my stomach and solar plexus. Mostly in my stomach and a little bit up through the heart and chest area.

RANDAL: Okay, you can open your eyes now. Please lay down here and put this pillow under your knees to take a little pressure off your stomach. (Christine gets comfortable) All right, Christine, do you want to put your arms at your sides here? Does that feel comfortable for you? (Christine nods) I'd like you to look up at my little finger. (Randal leads Christine into hypnosis through a series of rapid induction methods)

Now I want you to focus your attention on your hands. I'm going to ask you some questions. The questions are for your subconscious mind to respond to, so you can signal with the correct answer. (Randal asks Christine a couple of sample questions to which the answers are obviously "yes" and "no" and she responds appropriately) Very good. Most or all of the questions that I ask your subconscious mind will be able to be answered in a "yes" or "no" manner. If I were to ever ask you a question that your subconscious could not answer for some reason with yes or no, then you could signal with another finger of your subconscious mind's choosing.

What I want to draw your attention to now, Christine, is the general subject matter we've been discussing. We talked about feeling that sadness, and about getting in touch with an obstacle having to do with a lack of confidence that sometimes happens with you. A feeling of self–doubt, worrying about whether you're doing things right, a fear of the unknown, a need for reassurance, these feelings that sometimes come up for you when you're wanting to achieve something. In some way or other, depending on your answers to my questions, I'll help take you back to some earlier experience when you strongly felt these feelings.

The question I have for you now, Christine, and you can signal with the appropriate finger, is regarding these feelings such as a fear of the unknown, some obstacle, self–doubt, sadness. Is it safe and appropriate for you to consciously remember any and all memories having to do with these feelings of yours? (Christine's right index finger moves) The answer to the question is yes. The next question is, as you recall earlier experiences in which you had these kinds of feelings, is it appropriate and safe for you to be open to your feelings and to your emotions? (Christine's right index finger moves) And the signal is yes. Okay.

Continue focusing on your breathing. Let your breathing be slow and steady, deep and continuous. I'm going to count from one to ten. As I count upward, Christine, I'd like you to become more aware of that feeling that you were just feeling a few minutes ago, that sadness that sometimes comes up when you reach a certain obstacle. There are many ways in which you have a lot of confidence, but lately there have been times when you've been sad and afraid. It's affected you very strongly. And you've sometimes woken up, as you mentioned, feeling fearful, feeling worried.

I'm going to count from one to ten and as I count upwards you can become more and more aware of those feelings. Perhaps you'll feel the fear more strongly, perhaps you'll feel the sadness more strongly. Whatever your subconscious taps into now is fine. Number one, two and three, becoming more and more aware of that sad feeling or that fearful feeling. Number four, five and six, that fear of the unknown. Seven, eight, feeling the feelings more strongly now. Feeling them in your body. Feeling that fear, feeling that sadness. Number nine, on the next number I count you're right there with that feeling. Number ten.

Stay with that feeling as I count down from ten to one. I'm going to count quickly. You're going to go back to an earlier time in your life. Way back to an earlier time when you felt that same kind of feeling, that fear or that sadness. Going back now, number ten, nine, eight, going back in time quickly. Seven, six, getting younger, getting smaller. Five, four, getting younger. Three, two, on the next number I count you're right there now. Number one, you're right there. Stay with the feeling. Keep breathing into your stomach. Are you inside or outside? Pick one.

CHRISTINE: Inside.

RANDAL: Is it nighttime or daytime?

CHRISTINE: Daytime.

RANDAL: It's daytime and you're inside. Are you alone or with other people?

CHRISTINE: With other people.

RANDAL: Are you under ten years old? Yes or no.
CHRISTINE: Yes.
RANDAL: Are you under seven years old? Yes or no.
CHRISTINE: Yes.
RANDAL: Are you under four years old? Yes or no.
CHRISTINE: Yes.
RANDAL: Are you under two years old? Yes or no.
CHRISTINE: Yes
RANDAL: Are you an infant?
CHRISTINE: I'm sensing it's before I'm born.
RANDAL: Are you in the womb?
CHRISTINE: Yes.
RANDAL: Okay, you're in the womb. What is the feeling? What's happening?
CHRISTINE: All this feeling of spiraling and feeling almost dizzy and just great anxiety.
RANDAL: All right. Have you ever felt this feeling before?
CHRISTINE: The anxiety, yes.
RANDAL: When I say have you ever felt this anxiety before, I mean have you felt this anxiety before in the womb?
CHRISTINE: No.
RANDAL: Okay, finger signals. Is this the first time that you've felt this kind of spiraling, dizzy feeling while in the womb? (Christine's left index finger moves) The answer is no. Okay, this is a feeling you have felt before in the womb. So you're feeling this spiraling, dizzy feeling. How does that make you feel?
CHRISTINE: Insecure.
RANDAL: Let's go ahead a few minutes. You've been feeling this spiraling, dizzy feeling. It's now ten, fifteen, twenty minutes later. Are you still feeling that?
CHRISTINE: It's past.
RANDAL: Is this something that comes and goes?
CHRISTINE: Yes.
RANDAL: It's come and gone for you while you've been in the womb. How do you usually feel in the womb? Is there a usual feeling of some kind?
CHRISTINE: No.
RANDAL: I'm going to ask your finger signals, this feeling of feeling dizzy, this spiraling in the womb, this uncomfortable feeling, is this a feeling that you often feel in the womb? (Christine's

right index finger moves) The answer is yes. (Randal's next question is an example of avoiding asking an initial leading question negatively in hypnosis) This spiraling, dizzy feeling, is it usually a pleasant feeling? (Christine's left index finger moves) The answer is no. Is it always an unpleasant feeling? (Christine's right index finger moves) The answer is yes. Spiraling, dizzy feeling. Stay with that feeling now. Where do you feel it?

CHRISTINE: My head and my chest and the upper part of my body, but also my legs.

RANDAL: Your head, your chest, the upper part of your body and your legs. Okay, stay with that spiraling, dizzy feeling. That's right, stay with it. (pause) Can you describe the feeling now? Is it exactly the same or is it more or less intense? Has it changed?

CHRISTINE: I feel nauseous. There's a sick feeling in my stomach.

RANDAL: Stay with that feeling and breathe down into your stomach. Feel that feeling.

CHRISTINE: I'm feeling a fear.

RANDAL: What are you afraid of?

CHRISTINE: (Christine begins to cry) Feeling of being alone.

RANDAL: Uh huh. Stay with the feelings. It's okay to cry.

CHRISTINE: It's a feeling of being stuck. I can't go back and I don't want to go forward.

RANDAL: You're stuck. You can't go back and you don't want to go forward.

CHRISTINE: (crying and sounding scared) And I have no support.

RANDAL: Now feel that feeling of having no support. Stay with it, you're doing great. You need to stay with your feelings.

CHRISTINE: I'm aware of my heart and my chest. I'm feeling a pressure and a fear and a trembling.

RANDAL: A feeling of fear and trembling. Feel that in your chest. Become the feeling.

CHRISTINE: I feel dizzy.

RANDAL: Okay, feel that dizziness. That's good. (pause) What are you feeling right now?

CHRISTINE: (body and voice shaking) The dizziness. A fear. My body trembling. Very uncomfortable.

RANDAL: Okay, exaggerate that trembling. Let your body tremble more. Become that trembling. (Christine right hand is especially trembling) That's right, tremble. Repeat after me, "I'm afraid."

CHRISTINE: I'm afraid
RANDAL: "I'm scared."
CHRISTINE: (crying) I'm scared.
RANDAL: Okay. Feel the trembling, especially in your right hand. If you could talk to your right hand now, what would you say to it?
CHRISTINE: Be calm.
RANDAL: Become your right hand. What do you want to say in response?
CHRISTINE: I can't.
RANDAL: Say, "I won't".
CHRISTINE: I won't.
RANDAL: Okay, what do you want to say to your right hand? Your right hand is saying, "I won't be calm."
CHRISTINE: I need you to be calm.
RANDAL: Be your right hand. What does your right hand say?
CHRISTINE: It's difficult. I don't know how.
RANDAL: What do you want to say to your right hand?
CHRISTINE: I need you to have control. I want you to have control.
RANDAL: Good. Be your right hand.
CHRISTINE: I need to find control.
RANDAL: So where's your control? You're the right hand now. You're out of control.
CHRISTINE: Somewhere ahead of me.
RANDAL: What is there somewhere ahead of you?
CHRISTINE: I don't know.
RANDAL: Is that what's frightening you, that you don't know?
CHRISTINE: Yes.
RANDAL: Okay, there's something ahead of you. Are you ready to go find out what's ahead of you?
CHRISTINE: Yes.
RANDAL: Good for you. Let's go ahead. Going forward now to the unknown that's ahead of you. It's coming up now. I'm going to count from five down to one. At the count of one you're going to be right there with what's ahead of you. Five, four, three, two, one. Okay, what's happening right now?
CHRISTINE: It's my life. (sobs)
RANDAL: It's your life. Your life is ahead of you, that's right. You're going to be born. Stay with your feelings and breathe into

your stomach. It's okay to cry. It's so good to cry. Get it out of your system. It's okay to be scared. Keep breathing into your stomach. What do you feel right now?

CHRISTINE: Dizzy.

RANDAL: What do you feel in your body right now?

CHRISTINE: (still crying) Calmer. A tingling.

RANDAL: A tingling, good. It's good to cry, good to get that feeling out. Sure, it's scary. It's a profound new experience. You've been in the womb all this time. Your whole life is ahead of you. Feel your body. What do you feel in your body right now?

CHRISTINE: I feel tension in my back.

RANDAL: What else do you feel?

CHRISTINE: A trembling.

RANDAL: And where are you trembling?

CHRISTINE: My back.

RANDAL: So you can say, "I am trembling my back."

CHRISTINE: I am trembling in my back and my hands.

RANDAL: Are you ready to be born?

CHRISTINE: Yes.

RANDAL: Okay. The process is happening now. This time you're going to go through it and make it to the other side and it's going to be great. Right now though, what you need to do is stay with the feeling. Stay with your body. You're getting to be born now. That's right, let your hand tremble. Let your body tremble. Feel yourself. You're beginning to go through the birth canal. You already signaled that it's appropriate and safe for you to go through whatever feelings come up, and this is what we're doing. Beginning to go through that birth canal now. You can hear the heart beat of your mother. Feel the pressure as you're going through the birth canal. Are you going head first or otherwise?

CHRISTINE: Otherwise.

RANDAL: Is it a breech birth?

CHRISTINE: Yes.

RANDAL: Where do you feel the pressure?

CHRISTINE: My back and my lower body.

RANDAL: Yes, feel that pressure in your back and your lower body. Can you feel it in this position or do you need to get into a different position?

CHRISTINE: This position is okay.

RANDAL: Okay, good. Feel the pressure in your lower body and your back. You don't know what's out there but you somehow subconsciously know your life is out there. It's a whole new, spectacular, amazing world that you can only dream of now. What are you feeling as you're going through the birth canal?

CHRISTINE: A pressure.

RANDAL: Where do you feel the pressure?

CHRISTINE: In my back.

RANDAL: What about your emotions? What are you feeling emotionally now?

CHRISTINE: I feel okay but I feel I'm doing this alone.

RANDAL: Do you feel any help from your mother?

CHRISTINE: No. I'm not aware of my mother.

RANDAL: You're not aware of your mother and you feel you're doing this alone. How does it feel to be doing this alone?

CHRISTINE: Difficult.

RANDAL: Feel that difficulty. Do you sense if your mother is helping the process by pushing?

CHRISTINE: No, she's not.

RANDAL: Then you may have to be born by yourself. We come into this world on our own and we die on our own. And you're going to have to be on your own many times in between.

CHRISTINE: Yes.

RANDAL: You just have to accept that. It's part of life. You may have to do this particular very challenging process mostly by yourself.

CHRISTINE: Uh huh.

RANDAL: Okay, feel yourself going through the birth canal. Breathe down into your stomach. Feel the pressure. Feel the trembling. Feel the tension. Tense yourself. Tingle. That's right. Trying to find your way through there. Push your way through. You're advancing. That's right.

CHRISTINE: A sensing of my body turning. (her whole body is intensely shaking)

RANDAL: Are you in the birth canal now or are you just entering it? Go with it, let your whole body shake. Your thumbs are cramping, being turned inward. Classic birthing experience. The fingers contracting. That's good, just let your body go. What you're doing is letting all this tension move through and out of your body.

That's great. Shaking it out. Letting go of that tension. As you let go of that tension you're going to feel so free. Getting all that fear out of your system. Just releasing it. Letting those arms go. Breathing down into your stomach. There's a shifting in your body, a turning. That's right. Letting your body go. It's a safe place and time to just let your body go. It's going to be all right. What are you feeling in your body right now?

CHRISTINE: My head is dizzy. (Christine is moving her head and her face looks distressed)

RANDAL: Yes, I'm noticing your head. What else do you feel in your head?

CHRISTINE: Pressure.

RANDAL: Where do you feel the pressure?

CHRISTINE: Feels like the temples, the side of my head.

RANDAL: Is this the experience of your head going through the birth canal or is it something else? What is your sense of it?

CHRISTINE: I'm midway somewhere.

RANDAL: You're midway somewhere. And maybe on some level you have some idea but on another level you don't. You know you're going through a whole new adventure, a whole new experience. This time as you go through it, it's going to be a different perspective because there's some part of you inside that knows it's going to be okay. It's going to work out okay. This is something that you need to do. Maybe there's still some fear there but there's some part of you deep down that knows this is going to take you somewhere very special and very beautiful.

You're somewhere midway through this process. Keep going. Let your body do what it needs to do. Keep breathing into your stomach. Your body can move whatever way it needs to. Your arms and your body are moving, that's right. Letting go of the tension. This time it's different. Feeling the tension but also letting go of the tension, moving through it. Your body is shifting and dancing. Be aware of all the different feelings happening in your body, the release of energy, the movement of your feet now. (Christine's movements continue to intensify) That's good. Letting go. Going through it. Going forward. You're most of the way through this experience now. As you exhale make some kind of noise. Let some noise out of your mouth.

CHRISTINE: Ahhhhh!

RANDAL: That's right. Keep breathing and as you exhale let more sound out of your mouth.

CHRISTINE: (louder) Ahhhhhhhh!

RANDAL: Keep doing that now.

CHRISTINE: Ahhhhhhhh!

RANDAL: That's good. (Christine continues breathing deeply and making noise) Letting go of that tension. Let's get it out of your system. It's good that you're releasing it. You're beginning to feel more confidence. You're going to make it through. You're alone and you're not alone. You weren't aware of it until now but you are getting support. You're getting support on some level from your mother. You're getting support from a spiritual force around you, an energy, a life force there that's supporting you.

CHRISTINE: Yes.

RANDAL: It's a great initiation that's taking place and we're all with you. Go into your body. What are you feeling?

CHRISTINE: It feels good.

RANDAL: It's good this time around.

CHRISTINE: Yes.

RANDAL: That's great. It's going to work out even better than you dreamed it would work out. And you had no idea of all the wonderful things that are in store for you. The thing that was unknown turns out to be something very special and very beautiful. There's a whole great big beautiful world. You're going to have a tremendous variety of experiences. And even those experiences that are difficult or challenging are actually opportunities to grow and expand and learn. That's what life is about. You've chosen life, you've chosen this body, you've chosen your spirit. You're going to take full advantage of it. You have the full use of all of your tremendous resources. You're looking forward to each new opportunity and being very present and powerful.

You'll find with each opportunity, Christine, with each new situation in which you find yourself, a core of confidence that is building within you. You have a tremendous sense of power and confidence and wisdom within you that is a driving force to propel you forward to new and exciting adventures and achievements. The more you give, the more you receive. The more you put out your energy, the more you receive in return. You're receiving the love, the approval, the affection, the appreciation, the success, the prosperity, the generosity of those around you. What was fear is transforming into excitement and joy and aliveness.

Anxiety is defined as the gap between what is happening and what we fear could happen in the future. What you are doing now is learning more than ever before to be in the present. In the present there is no anxiety. Being right here, staying with your feelings and trusting that it's all going to work out. You can trust universal consciousness and wisdom out there and your intuition within. You can trust your beautiful intelligence and awareness to take you in directions that are good for you and good for those around you.

It's good and appropriate to express various feelings including anger, grief, sexual feelings, joy. You can express frustration, you can express loneliness, you can express happiness. There is a wonderful array of feelings that are valid. And there are times when it might be appropriate to not communicate your feelings at that particular moment but know you can find a constructive and appropriate outlet for them. You're feeling more and more in touch with a power and energy to express and direct yourself. Breathing into your stomach. I'd like you to describe what you're feeling right now.

CHRISTINE: I feel peace. I feel happy. That everything's okay. That now I can do it. It's a good feeling.

RANDAL: It's a very good feeling. You had the courage to stay with your experience and to follow through, and it has brought you to this other side. You made it. You're born. Happy birthday.

CHRISTINE: Thank you.

RANDAL: Feel your body. Feel the aliveness from your head to your toes.

CHRISTINE: It feels great!

RANDAL: Just stay here. You don't have to do anything or go anywhere right now. Just feel your body. Keep breathing down into your stomach and feel that clear, good, relaxed, serene feeling. Feel at rest. Sometimes there's no place you have to go, nothing you have to do. You can just be. It's nice to stop sometimes and experience your body, your spirit, your mind, your feelings. Feel all of you. You're a beautiful, spiritual being. There's never been anybody like you and there never will be anybody like you again.

Something else very special is happening right now and that is that you're beginning to find that there is an ease, a swiftness, a smoothness, a grace of movement within you, that moves you through new experiences in your life with ease and freedom. Almost effortless. There may be a feeling sometimes of fear but you'll just go through it and each time you go through it and get to the other side you feel even more confident, even more accepting. And in fact even in a way appreciating the feeling of fear if it comes up at times, recognizing that this is leading you toward something new and special and good. The challenge helps you to get even stronger, more alive and more aware. This challenging birth you just took charge of has made you so powerful. Everything now becomes easier. Just like this experience, you stay with it, you breathe into it, and you get through it. You feel all the more that you come to a whole new level.

You are feeling the joy and excitement of starting a new hypnosis training center and you find that it has all kinds of benefits for you and for your students. You find it's a joy to do because you know that hypnotherapy is really helping to transform the world. You're doing your part to help make this world a more beautiful place. You're doing your healing and you're training other people to be fine healers. Some of them will just do work on themselves and their families and friends, and others will go on to do major work in hypnosis. Some will do it for personal growth. Others, even though they're going to go on to do hypnosis work, may discover that they've begun to use the principles you've taught them in valuable, useful ways that are not directly hypnotic.

Take in all the appreciation and all the thanks, the approval, the good compensation, the joy that people have for the good work you do and the good teaching you do. Just being who you are, being yourself and giving that special energy that only you have, to your classes. There's a whole wide range, from teaching to administrative work, to doing therapy. There are many different things involved and you keep moving forward, experiencing a fluid movement, an ease in which what might have been a barrier before is like butter now. You just slice right through it with ease and grace and style.

You can easily visualize your excitement in your own self–hypnosis processes as you move forward and are successful and prosperous. The more you give the more you receive in so many ways. You handle each situation that comes with cool and positive assurance, looking forward from one success to another and enjoying yourself along the way. Taking charge and also taking care of yourself to have a balance in your life. Having time for your rest, your recreation, your personal life, your social life. You make time for it all.

You continue to develop your communication and your efficiency with your partner and anyone else that you work with, so that you are getting better and better at delegating authority. It's a wonderful learning process that is helping you to be balanced in your life. You have certain responsibilities and you delegate certain responsibilities. It feels good because you're in charge, you're doing the choosing and you're choosing to handle each situation in constructive and positive ways.

Is there anything you would like to say or ask before I bring you out of the hypnosis?

CHRISTINE: A while back I became aware of my mother. It was like a wonderful meeting that felt very joyful and wonderful. A real connection with her and a feeling that even though I did this on my own, I had her strength and support.

RANDAL: Yes. Absolutely, you did do it on your own. Only you could take yourself through that. And also you did have the strength and support of others, especially your mother. Were you talking about a while ago in this session or was there some other experience you had prior to this session?

CHRISTINE: No, just a few minutes ago.

RANDAL: Feel that connection with your mother, knowing that on one hand you absolutely did it on your own and you had to accept that. On the other hand she was doing everything she could do. She's your mother. She brought you into this world. She loved you and cared for you and did her best. You can appreciate the love from her and the love you have toward her. If she was right here would there be anything further you'd like to say to her?

CHRISTINE: Just thanks, Mom.

RANDAL: Great. Is there anything further she would say to you if she was right here?

CHRISTINE: Just the words, "I love you," and I see her looking at me so proudly.

RANDAL: Good, good. It's great to complete this connection for now and you can connect with her any time you want. Say goodbye to her for the moment. Is there anything further that you would like me to say before I bring you out of the hypnosis?

CHRISTINE: No.

RANDAL: All right, feel your body. Feel the clarity and aliveness in your body, all the way down to your toes. Feel the peace and relaxation. Feel how free your chest feels, how free your stomach and pelvis feel, as you breathe in deeply. Breathe in that life force. I'm going to count from one to five, Christine, and with each number that I count you become more and more rested, refreshed and invigorated. At the count of five you open your eyes and you are then fully alert, rested, refreshed and feeling good. Noticing also, as you open your eyes, that there is a wonderful world with a room full of beautiful people in it. Notice that colors seem to be brighter.

I encourage you later today or early this evening to take a period of time to just rest and feel yourself. Relax, do a little hypnosis or meditation, and just nurture yourself. Get a good night's sleep tonight and have some healing dreams. You're going to have a great conference and a great trip and a lot of exciting things happening when you get home.

Number one, slowly and calmly begin returning to your full awareness. On number two, more and more alert, awake and aware with each number that I count. Number three, hearing the sounds around you and feeling your body resting comfortably. Feeling more and more invigorated and rested and refreshed. Number four, getting ready to open your eyes. On the next number opening your eyes, feeling fully alert, awake and aware. Coming back, number five. Open your eyes gradually and take a deep breath. You can stretch if you like.

CHRISTINE: Thank you. Thank you very much.

RANDAL: You're very welcome. Do you want to sit up? (Randal helps her sit up) I want you to look around. Look at people in the room. Make some eye contact. Who would like to say something to Christine?

SEVERAL PEOPLE IN UNISON: Happy birthday.

AUDIENCE MEMBER: This is the first day of your new life.

RANDAL: I'd like to acknowledge you for having the courage to go through your fear of the unknown here in front of everybody, and being willing to go through all of those difficult feelings. You did a great job.

CHRISTINE: Thank you.

RANDAL: (to the audience) We can take some questions now.

AUDIENCE MEMBER: Would you say something about the sequence of your induction? Was that for deepening purposes?

RANDAL: My induction was a series of rapid techniques. Some people associate rapid with authoritarian, but these were mostly done in a rather directive but gentle style. There was a moderately directive eye catalepsy. I usually tend toward using rapid techniques, pyramiding with statements like, "As your foot drops you feel yourself go deeper," and so forth. I included a bit of shoulder massage because that can be a brief, effective addition. I can get better results with a series of rapid techniques in three or four minutes than what might take fifteen minutes for some traditional inductions, like a progressive relaxation. And these methods feel good. People report regularly how much they enjoy them.

AUDIENCE MEMBER: Just out of curiosity, if Christine's mother is still living would it be important or even satisfying to touch base with her to reinforce her experience? Maybe to ask her if this was an accurate presentation or enactment of what really happened?

RANDAL: I would leave that to Christine's intuition. If she feels like she'd like to do that, then she can. Or if she feels this is something that is complete within herself, then that's fine. (to Christine) Do you have any feelings about that at this point?

CHRISTINE: Well, my mother is no longer alive but I do know my birth was difficult. It was actually a forceps delivery and that was the pressure I felt on my temples, but this time I did it without forceps. My body had to be turned and I was aware of going in a circle at a certain point. Another point is that I know they actually gave my mother far too much medication and she was not present.

RANDAL: Yes, that's what happens so often.

CHRISTINE: And she didn't even know she'd given birth to me, so hence the forceps.

RANDAL: So she wasn't able to do the pushing or any breathing techniques. And that affected you, too. I felt it was important for you to feel both the feeling of doing it alone on one level, but also the feeling that your mother was there. Only on the most primitive level, subconsciously, could your mother be there at that particular time. That experience imprinted a feeling and expectancy of fear, of being alone and having to do it yourself, but you have transformed that to a successful birth yielding accomplishment, wonder, wisdom and confidence.

AUDIENCE MEMBER: Christine, I was curious about why you didn't ask, "Is something wrong?" in the womb. Were you aware of knowing that something was wrong before you started to be born?

CHRISTINE: All I felt was that I didn't want to be born and then it changed to, was I going to be born?

RANDAL: There were a number of different things going on, and her description of her experience was very much in touch with reality. She was becoming aware of her intense physical feelings, a sense that she was entering a major transformation, and she sensed the increasing difficulty and very important issue of being alone. Part of that issue was the breech birth becoming even more difficult because her mother was given too much medication. And there was also, naturally, a growing a fear of the unknown.

(to Christine) It was also interesting to me that you signaled you often felt a dizzy feeling in the womb. Do you recall if you had a sense that this was normal during that stage in the birth process, or whether that was something you had felt at different times previously when you were in the womb?

CHRISTINE: No, I couldn't really relate to the timing at all. All I was aware of was just feeling dizzy and spiraling.

RANDAL: So you were just so much in the present that that's all there was at that particular time.

SAME AUDIENCE MEMBER: I'm also wondering if there was more going on than came up at this time. You described it was too late to go back and you felt stuck about going forward. Were there deeper issues about coming into this world, into the situation you were coming into, that made you reluctant?

CHRISTINE: It was more a feeling that things had been far more comfortable and I had support. Suddenly I was in the situation of being very uncomfortable and out of control. That sense of spiraling, I felt I was going to faint. It was very uncomfortable and I felt totally unsupported. And because I didn't have that support I didn't like going forward. It was like, "Hey, I don't want to go anywhere without feeling comfortable and without support." That was the feeling.

RANDAL: Well said. (to the audience) Rather than intellectually projecting about even more possibilities, we can stay present with Christine and recognize the profoundness of such a trauma for an unborn infant. Her response was normal and natural. The important thing is that this feeling did come up and it became an all encompassing feeling. It was tied in with the fear of the unknown. It got Christine psychically off balance and the overwhelming experience created a core imprint. Even though Christine has obviously been very successful in many ways, this was a barrier.

(to Christine) I'll be looking forward to hearing from you at some point how great it feels to be really clear and fully alive now.

Letter from Christine Ten Years Later

Reading the script of our session continually amazes me. Some aspects of it I vividly remember in detail; other parts I have no recollection. It is certainly interesting to read after ten years. I had no idea ten years had gone by.

I have given considerable thought to the results of that session. It is interesting to note the feelings and beliefs I had back then, i.e. "I can't do it", "overwhelming anxiety", "feeling stuck", "a trembling feeling". These are all most significant. A trembling feeling had plagued me in my body, all of my life - for as long as I can remember. That has disappeared completely. I no longer feel "stuck". While at times I still worry about things or experience tension, the "overwhelming anxiety" has gone. When I feel nervous or apprehensive about anything, I resolve my problems much more quickly and effectively than before. Interestingly, I no longer think, "I can't do something". I face the challenges of new beginnings with much more confidence.

I would have to say that the Regression was most successful. I went on to complete the teaching material for the Hypnotherapy School, we commenced classes and they rapidly grew from there - going from strength to strength. Initially, the administration work was my responsibility, ensuring everything ran smoothly and to a timetable. However, that soon changed, and I found myself thrown in at the deep end, teaching classes as well. To begin with, I was nervous, but I did it and I enjoyed the interaction with the students. What helped me tremendously was the positive feedback I received from the students, for without that I would not have known if I was doing my job well or not. I learned a great deal from teaching and from the sharing and input from students; overall finding it a most rewarding and humbling experience. I feel most grateful for the opportunity.

Randal, it was a pleasure being your client. I felt incredibly safe and cared for during the Regression, and thank you most sincerely for giving me this opportunity. It has been an added bonus, reading the script word for word, and realizing just how many changes were made that day. I felt incredibly light and free after the regression, as though a huge burden was lifted off me.

Again, thank you so much. I wish you every success with all that you are doing, and hope that someday our paths will once again cross. Take care and lots of love.

CHAPTER 16

Ron's Mysterious Heartache
Discovering the Source of His Sadness

After the induction, the next step of this session will be a series of ideomotor questions to discover the source of Ron's sadness. The realization, which comes very quickly in this case, regresses him back to the feelings and memories of the unfinished incident. The relatively brief questioning sequence gives a hint of some procedures that can be used in ideomotor explorations, which can be combined very effectively with regression. This extremely important subject will be the focus of my forthcoming book, Ideomotor Magic.

RANDAL: I'm looking for a volunteer who would like to work on an issue in which there seems to be some subconscious resistance. Maybe you understand part of it, yet feel stuck in some way. (looking for a raised hand) Okay, Ron, come on up. (Ron sits beside Randal) Can you describe what your issue is?

RON: Well, a few years ago I used to be very angry and that had built up over ten or fifteen years. I realize that I wasn't angry at other people, I was just pretty much angry at myself. I worked on getting rid of the anger and I got rid of a large part of it, but now it seems like I tend to be very sensitive. I've always been sensitive to other people and I'm fairly insightful except that before, with my anger, I didn't react so emotionally. Now whenever I hear a touching story or someone is having problems I get caught up in their emotions. When I'm working with a client though, I can step back a bit.

RANDAL: Do you mean that when you're actually doing therapy work with someone you're able to get some detachment?

RON: Yes, I'm able to get a little detachment. But it seems that with half the stories in these class demonstrations I get really emotional. I don't want to take that sensitivity away, I just want to...I'm wondering if there is some way that I can still experience having empathy and insight, but maybe stand back a little without getting so sucked in. Maybe centering myself, or maybe I over-compensated in getting rid of that anger, or maybe there is still something there with that anger. I never felt guilty so much, other than normal feelings like, "I should have done this or that."

RANDAL: Our problems can be solutions to previous problems. You had a lot of anger and you've gotten rid of most of that, and now you're feeling a lot of empathy for people, which seems to be a lot less of a problem overall. Having so much empathy is really an aspect of a very good quality that you have. A person who has strong empathy is tuned in to caring, to being a healer and a good therapist. Of course if it feels too intense at times, then one way you can handle that is to do some grounding and centering techniques. Visualizations like having a grounding cord and imagining an aura of protection around you, and so on, can help you to be present with more detachment than you've had. That's a partial solution that you were hinting at yourself.

RON: I've tried, I mean I actually work at doing that.

RANDAL: Does it help?

RON: It does a little bit but like right now I'm still a little emotional (eyes watering and voice shaking slightly) and...I can't see any reason for it.

RANDAL: You're still a little emotional about what? Is there something that happened from a recent session?

RON: No, it's not about...it's not for anything in particular. That's the thing I want to explore. Why do I feel this way right now?

RANDAL: What's the problem with feeling emotional right now?

RON: I just feel...not free of something, or not letting go.

RANDAL: When you say emotional can you be more specific? Is it like feeling sad or a sense of longing or loss or fear, or what would you say?

RON: It's not a fear and it's...not an anger. It feels like there is something inside that I just haven't been able to let go of.

RANDAL: Does it feel like a sadness or a grief that you're not letting go of? Something like that?

RON: (pause) It's more of a sadness. It's not a grief. And it's right in here. (motioning to his chest)

RANDAL: (because getting in touch with his feelings is leading Ron into a light state of hypnosis, Randal immediately begins the hypnotic induction) Would you like to move into this reclining chair? (Ron sits in the chair) Stay with that feeling. I'd like you to look at my outer two fingers as I move my hand toward your face and down. Just follow those fingers until your eyelids close. (Ron's eye's close) Turn those muscles loose as I count from three down to one. At the count of one your eyelids are locked tightly closed. The harder you try to open them the tighter they lock and seal and the deeper into hypnosis you go. Number three, stuck tighter and tighter together. Two, sealing as though they were glued. Number one, go ahead and try but it's as though they were stuck together. (Ron attempts to open his eyes) Now just relax, stop trying and go deeper. That's good.

I'm going to lift up your right hand by the thumb. Just let your hand hang loosely and limply. I'm going to drop your hand into mine and when I do send a wave of relaxation down your body. (as Ron exhales Randal drops his hand) We'll do the same thing with your left hand. I'm going to drop it into mine and you send a wave of relaxation down your body and go even deeper. (Randal drops the hand) That's good. Deeper with every breath that you take.

In a moment I'm going to count from three down to one and only your eyelids open. When your eyelids open I'll snap my fingers in front of your face like this (snap) and on the finger snap you'll immediately close your eyes and go deeper, even deeper than you are at this very moment. Getting ready now. Three, two, one, opening. (snap) Close your eyes and go deeper. I'm going to use the phrase "sleep now" which is not referring to the kind of sleep you sleep at night but to hypnotic sleep, sleep of the nervous system. We're going to do that again. Three, two, one, opening. (snap) Sleep now, close your eyes and go deeper. That's good. And again, three, two, one. (snap) Sleep now, close your eyes and go deeper. That's your signal. Whenever I snap my fingers and say, "sleep now" you close your eyes and go deeper.

I'm going to come around and push down on your shoulders in a moment. Take a nice, deep breath and fill up your lungs. On the exhale as I push down send a wave of relaxation down your body and feel yourself go much deeper. As I rub your shoulders feel yourself going deeper and deeper relaxed.

Now I'd like you to put your attention on the hand that you like to do ideomotor signals with. (Ron's ideomotor responses are established with his left index finger signaling "yes," his left thumb signaling "no," and his left little finger signaling "I don't know") If I ask you a question that your subconscious mind does not want to answer or doesn't know how to properly answer, then you could lift the middle finger here. (tapping the finger)

I'm going to do a couple of practice questions now. Are we on the seventeenth floor of the building that we're in? (Ron's thumb moves) The answer is no. You signaled correctly with your thumb. Would you consider this to be the second floor of the building? (Ron's index finger moves) The answer is correct, as you've signaled with your "yes" finger.

Now, Ron, you've been communicating about a sadness that you've been feeling inside. Is your subconscious mind willing to explore this issue of sadness that you sometimes feel? (Ron's index finger moves) The answer to the question is yes. Does this sadness have to do with something that would be good for your conscious mind to find out about in the process of helping you with this? (Ron's little finger moves) I see an "I don't know" response, and that was fairly quick. Let me ask you the question again and maybe that will be the best answer but maybe your subconscious mind might know the answer to that. Regarding the sadness that you were describing and you were even feeling a few moments ago, would it be good for your conscious mind to find out what that sadness is about? (after a pause Ron's index finger moves) The answer to the question is yes.

I'm going to say something to the group, Ron, and you can just relax for a moment. (to the group) Some of you may have noticed a movement from Ron's finger for a few seconds before I actually acknowledged it. Once I get the slightest quiver of movement I like to see if it's going to continue to move and once in awhile I might get a mixed signal. I want to get a definitive sense of that finger movement or a repeated movement, to see if that happens. There is no rush with this and sometimes we may get additional or alternative information.

(to Ron) All right, you're doing fine, Ron. You've just signaled that it would be good for the conscious mind to be aware of what this sadness has to do with.

There can be many different reasons for sadness so I'll be asking you some questions to help your subconscious mind bring forth some understanding of what this is about. You were saying a few minutes ago that this feeling is not grief, but it is sadness. I don't know what that sadness has to do with. As I ask you questions I'm not trying to imply a "yes" answer or a "no" answer. I'm just checking out different possibilities. I'd like your conscious mind to remain neutral with me and to allow your subconscious mind to come up with the truth about this issue.

The question is, does the sadness have primarily to do with someone other than yourself? (after a pause Ron's index finger moves) The answer to the question is yes. Is there more than one person other than yourself? (Ron's thumb moves) The answer to the question is no. Good, you're doing fine.

Is this person that this sadness has to do with, Ron, someone that you are related to? (Ron's thumb moves) The answer to the question is no. Is this person someone who you would have characterized for at least a time in your life as a significant friend? (after a pause Ron's index finger moves) The answer to the question is yes. Is this person someone who you would currently characterize as a significant friend in your life? (after a pause Ron's thumb moves) Okay, after a pause I'm getting a "no" answer to that.

Now this person that you're feeling sadness about, is your conscious mind aware right now of who this person is? (Ron begins to cry softly and his index finger moves) The answer to the question is yes. It's okay to cry. Breathe down into your belly and let out any sounds that need to come out. (Ron sobs quietly) Feel your sadness. It's good to feel your sadness and it's good to get your sadness out. (pause while Ron cries quietly and takes some deep breaths) Okay, when I touch your shoulder you'll be able to tell me the name of this person. Three, two and one. (Randal touches Ron's shoulder and he begins to sob more)

RON: (struggling with the words) Its...our little dog.

RANDAL: It's good to cry. Many of us have very strong feelings for and about our pets. They can be like a member of the family. What is the reason that you're feeling so sad about your little dog?

RON: (sobs quietly for a moment and then takes a deep breath) He...a big thing is that when he died...(breaking into sobs) I wasn't with him. (pause while Ron cries softly and struggles with the words) When he was a little puppy I was kind of mean to him. I wasn't like...I didn't beat him or anything like that...he wasn't completely house broken and maybe he would make a mess on the floor and I would really get mad at him...and I knew that he was only a puppy. It was just a reflex. (crying softly) We forgave each other for that.

RANDAL: That's good.

RON: He lived for seventeen or eighteen years.

RANDAL: How wonderful that you got to have him that long. He had a very long life for a dog, and I would imagine he was generally healthy.

RON: He was always very healthy.

RANDAL: And while he was just a puppy and you were still training him you forgave him for making a mess and he forgave you for being mad, and you had a real special bond for all those years.

RON: (softly) Oh, yes. (crying) The thing that I really...(sobbing quietly) feel so bad about...he was only sick about the last week of his life. Of course he was with us all that time and we were good friends and played together and loved each other. What happened is that he had renal kidney failure.

RANDAL: How long ago was this?

RON: About three years ago. (crying softly)

RANDAL: So he had renal kidney failure and that was what caused him to be sick that last week of his life.

RON: We took him to the vet, of course, and he told us that they could do some blood tests to see what was wrong. We knew he was an old dog. He had lived many years in his body so we knew he...(pausing to sob) wasn't going to be with us long.

RANDAL: You knew he was dying.

RON: Yes, and he knew he was dying...so we were just loving him and taking care of him. (sobbing) He couldn't go upstairs or anything anymore and I just pretty much stayed with him and slept with him...the last two or three days. (sobbing) And we were very close.

RANDAL: You stayed with him, you slept with him, and you spent a lot of time with him. That's very good.

RON: When we took him in again, because he just kept getting worse, like the last couple of days he stopped eating and just drank water...he could still walk but you could tell...he wasn't a happy camper. They tested his urine and confirmed that he wasn't going to live more than a short time. A couple of days at most...(choking up and unable to talk for a moment) The part that was hard...(whispering) I get kind of angry at myself and sad at the same time. My wife and I were there with him and we left him for a couple of hours while they were doing some tests.

RANDAL: You left him at the vet's?

RON: Yes, we left because I needed a little time to analyze things and so we decided that what was good for him...(crying quietly) was to put him down. (sobbing) We knew that was good because that would put him out of his misery. There was no question but that we were going to do the best thing for him...so that was okay.

They brought him out to us...and we were together for awhile...and that was good. (sobbing) That was real good. And they asked us if we wanted to be with him when they put him down...and my wife just didn't think she could take it...so she stayed in the waiting room. They asked me if I wanted to be with him and I didn't answer them. I forget what the words were. They were loving and caring and he didn't seem frightened...and (sobbing) they explained what they were going to do, what the procedure would be...and that it wouldn't be painful. It would be very tranquil and he would just go off to sleep very quickly.

I don't know what I was thinking but I just kind of stood there as they were taking him away...(sobbing and talking haltingly) He kind of looked back at me...it wasn't anything bad or anything...I just wish I would have gone in there with him...to just be there with him while they were putting him down.

RANDAL: (picking up a stack of pillows) How big was he?

RON: He was a little silky terrier so he was very small.

RANDAL: (Randal puts a small, soft pillow in Ron's arms) Go back in time to when Flash has just passed away. Imagine he's here with you now. You can talk to him and he can hear you. What do you want to tell him?

RON: (sobbing) I just want to thank Flash. (holding the pillow close and stroking it gently) You know that we love you so much. I know that you know that and...I wanted to be with you when you took your last breath and...I could see your eyes as they were taking you away...I want you to know that I was there with you and I've always been with you and I always will. You taught us so much. You were such a wise spirit in a little animal...and I don't ask for forgiveness because I don't think that's what I need. I just want you to know that we were really there with you and...you're still with us in spirit. It's a good feeling...(voice cracking) a joyous, beautiful feeling...your presence.

RANDAL: Very good. Be Flash. If he could talk, what would he say in response?

RON: I was just saying goodbye to you both.

RANDAL: Do you mean when he looked back at you?

RON: Yes.

RANDAL: Good.

RON: You gave me a wonderful life. I'm glad I was able to help and be part of your family and all of the love that was there. That was just my body. The energy and the love and the spirit that was in that body is always going to be there with you.

RANDAL: Thank you, Flash. Switch and be Ron. What do you want to say to Flash?

RON: Thank you for touching our lives. We...me and the rest of the family...understand that that was just the physical body...that your spirit and your energy and your love will always be with us. We will always be family and you can take comfort in that.

RANDAL: Is there anything you want from Flash or want Flash to know?

RON: There's nothing that I want from Flash.

RANDAL: Is there anything more you want to say to him?

RON: Nothing specific because he knows.

RANDAL: Yes, he knows. Is there anything else you want to say to him?

RON: (sobbing) Thank you...and may you rest in peace. We miss you...but you know that. (whispers) Thank you.

RANDAL: Very good. Switch and be Flash. What do you want to say in response to Ron?

RON: I'm always here to help you and other wonderful people with their love. It's okay.

RANDAL: Very good. Is there anything else you want to say to Ron or does that feel complete?

RON: It feels complete.

RANDAL: Switch and be Ron. Does it feel complete for you now, too?

RON: It feels complete in the sense that we've let each other go physically and I...I and my family are just so fortunate that we had the experience of this wonderful little animal. You'll always be with us.

RANDAL: So when you say goodbye now you know that he is always with you.

RON: Yes, I got to tell him...I got to tell Flash how I felt even though he knew...I just had to tell you again to free myself.

RANDAL: Just for now you're going to complete your communication with him and say goodbye. He can be with you again whenever you want. (Randal reaches for the pillow but Ron hangs on) Feel yourself say goodbye. Is there anything more you want to put into words?

RON: No.

RANDAL: Be Flash and feel yourself saying goodbye to Ron now, from the context of everything you've shared together and knowing that you'll still be here. (pause) Now switch and be Ron and take some time to let go when you're ready. (Ron takes a deep breath and Randal takes the pillow) That's right. Feel that love. Breathe down into your belly. Checking with your finger signals, do you feel at peace now? (Ron's index finger moves) The answer to the question is yes.

It feels so good and it's such a relief to be able to get in touch with your sadness, to feel it and have a chance to communicate and say goodbye. It's such a peace of mind and such a peace in your body and your heart now. Where you were feeling that sadness before, now you can feel that radiant loving energy. You can truly feel that you have said goodbye in peace, knowing that the love is there both ways. You know that Flash really loves you and appreciates you and you completely love and appreciate Flash. You feel very lucky, very fortunate to have had such a wonderful relationship. You had one very lucky and happy dog there, with a very loving family. That was mutual and you can carry that bond with you forever.

To recognize and understand this is a sign of your wonderful empathy and compassion. How good it feels to be capable of having the very special loving friendship you had with Flash for so many years. You can extend your loving energy to those that you want to, recognizing that you have a tremendous amount of heart energy, Ron. It's a part of who you are. In fact, as a result of completing this process, you feel a lot more complete yourself. You feel that something very important has been finished so that when you're with people you can feel present and open and receptive and grounded.

As a therapist you can feel your compassion but in a detached way, which can be of greater service to your client and to you. With this completion you can also be with people and when someone is feeling a strong feeling it won't trigger something in you that feels unfinished. You can truly rest in peace in your own way, knowing that Flash is resting in peace. Is there anything further that you'd like to say or to ask before I bring you out of hypnosis?

RON: No.

RANDAL: Get in touch with your body now. Feel how good, how clear you feel. What a burden has been lifted. What a sense of freedom and peace that you feel now. What a sense of relief. It's time for you to come back to your full conscious awareness, but it's a more complete, more whole consciousness as you come back. When I reach the count of five you come back feeling rested, invigorated, refreshed. Getting ready now. (Randal brings Ron out of hypnosis, giving suggestions with each number that he counts) Taking your time. (Ron takes a deep breath and opens his eyes)

RON: Whew. That feels much better.

RANDAL: I don't think you were the only one with tears in the class. (laughter) A lot of us could very strongly identify with you. My eyes were certainly very watery.

RON: Thank you. Thank you so much. (Ron and Randal hug)

RANDAL: (to the class) Each situation is different when discovering information through ideomotor responses and this was an example of not needing to ask many questions. We got down to the issue very quickly. I asked if the sadness had to do with himself and he said no. When I asked if it was someone else it turned out to be not a person, but his dog. They had a very special relationship and many of us can relate to a pet being part of the family. I grew up with a dog that I felt that way about.

Sometimes ideomotor can be much more involved because there is more that's been buried, or it's harder to get to or more complex, and we may need to work with that for some time. In this case I suspected that this would switch to something like Gestalt dialogue before too long. Ron was feeling emotional and emotions are good to work with. I was even concerned about taking him away from his feelings to get in touch with the finger signals, but I felt the ideomotor would be a good way to get to the bottom of it. It worked out really well, and then he spontaneously came back to his feelings.

There was such a beautiful relationship between Ron and his dog that it's not surprising to see how well and how easily this worked out with the communication. There wasn't any conflict but a deep understanding there. Is there anything that anyone would like to say to Ron now?

CHORUS OF VOICES (with applause): Good job!

Interview Two Days Later

RANDAL: The session with Ron two days ago started out as an exploration with ideomotor questions to get down to an unfinished issue that Ron did not understand. With very few questions we got right down to the mystery of his heartache. There was no resistance and it wasn't complicated.

When he began to feel some emotions I asked him if he was now aware of who it was he felt this sadness about. He signaled yes, and I told him to go ahead and verbalize. It turned out that it was his beloved dog, Flash, who had been with him since he was a puppy. There was a painful unfinished feeling for Ron that he wasn't with him when he died, but it was worked out beautifully. While doing the Gestalt the very strong bond between them was obvious. Gestalt dialogue doesn't have to be limited to human beings.

I have a question for you, Ron. You were feeling such a strong sadness for a few years now and you didn't know what it was about. When I was asking those very few questions, I asked you if it was about just one person or more than one person. Did you already start to know what the issue was about at that point or was it after the end of all the questions that you started to get that realization?

RON: It was kind of strange because when I came up here I told you that there was this feeling and I didn't know what the feeling was. You started giving examples so I had something more tangible to check off. "No, it isn't that," and when you came to sadness it just clicked. It was sadness, but I still didn't know what the sadness related to. I feel very fortunate in my life that I haven't had a lot of tragedy so I couldn't imagine what it was. Even when you were asking me about a person, that didn't register yet.

RANDAL: So you didn't consciously realize it until near the end of the questioning.

RON: It came to me about three quarters of the way through the questions that I don't think it's a person. Then I knew it was Flash.

RANDAL: I wonder if it happened around the time I asked, "Is this someone you would consider a significant friend?"

RON: Yes, right around there. And the reason for the long hesitation on the next question, is he still a friend? Well, he's not currently a friend in the here and now but in my mind he's still a friend, he's still a part of me, so it was difficult to answer.

RANDAL: I asked the question in that way because there was a lot of sadness regarding someone who used to be a significant friend. I just didn't know if this was a loss of a relationship or a dear friend with whom you'd parted in a bitter way or what, but at that point you got really clear about what it was and we could talk about it. I think this is a splendid example of how ideomotor responses can be so effective for solving a mystery. When you were getting those initial answers did you have an idea what finger would move or were you following the communication of your fingers like the rest of us were?

RON: I wasn't actually making the decision to move my fingers so most of it was just coming from inside but I was aware of which finger was raising. I knew what was going on but I knew I was in a deep trance because I wasn't aware of anything except for you and me. At the end it seemed like only ten minutes.

RANDAL: So you weren't necessarily aware of what finger was going to come up until it came up, is that correct?

RON: Yes, and the other thing is that I knew who it was before I knew what it was about. I knew it was Flash and you kept asking the questions about a person. I thought about that for a minute but it didn't really bother me. I thought it wasn't that important. Then all of a sudden I got emotional when I realized what it was about that relationship. That's when you asked me what was going on and I told you it was Flash.

RANDAL: So you were able to answer the questions for Flash even though I was asking about a person because you understood the context of what I was looking for.

RON: Right, because I knew you didn't have any idea and you had to have some term to ask the question.

RANDAL: Also, when I was asking about various kinds of emotions, I picked out several possibilities. I used the word grief as well as the word sadness. You said, well, it's not grief, it's sadness. Some people might consider them to be the same but for you it was something distinctly different.

RON: Yes, to me grief is real deep and maybe has negative connotations. Sadness to me is having empathy for the situation and love and it's a sad sort of thing, but positive. You know, Flash that I love. It was unfortunate that things went the way they went and I wasn't there at the time. That's how I differentiate between grief and sadness. It was something that I knew I could work through.

RANDAL: I appreciate the subtleties of the differences there. Does anyone have a question for Ron?

LISA: When you became aware that it was about a dog were you content to go along with the ideomotor questions and wait for that to come out or did you at any point feel like you would like to speak out?

RON: After I knew that it wasn't a person, that it was Flash, there were a couple of more questions directed to me about a person and I was almost going to come out and say, "It's not a person," and then I just thought I will in a minute. It progressed another one or two questions and then it came out. When I had all that emotion he asked me what was going on or something like that, and then I told him it was my little dog. So I really didn't feel a need to say it wasn't a person.

LISA: And that's my follow-up question to Randal. Do people sometimes speak out in ideomotor or do they wait for you to ask about something they already have a sense of?

RANDAL: Sometimes someone will spontaneously speak out but not very often. I'm careful enough with the ideomotor that I don't stray so far off that a person will usually feel a need to say something. Buried subconscious information can be hard to get to and to switch to verbalization can be distracting. But an exception might occur, for example, in which we've gotten to the point of realizing something valuable was left in a container and I ask, "Is it a metal container? Is it a box? Is it plastic?" If the answers continue to be no, the person eventually may become conscious of the answer. I may ask, "Is your conscious mind right now aware of what kind of container it is?" If the signal is yes, I just have the person tell me. The feeling that came up with Ron in that situation may sometimes occur. The person starts to feel a desire to say something but it's not important enough yet, and then it usually gets resolved rather quickly, such as through an ideomotor question and answer.

LISA: So you don't feel that people feel constrained from speaking?

RANDAL: No, because to some degree the person is trying to cooperate with the process, and there is generally a disinclination to move or to speak unless asked directly. But if a person really needs to speak, he or she will.

LOIS: (to Ron) Is there a difference between how you feel today versus how you felt before the session?

RON: I do feel differently. When I left here there was still some emotion and I wanted to do some reframing, to go through the experience with Flash and accept it and be joyful for both of us that he's no longer in pain. I realized that everyone has their time and he'd given me plenty. Immediately when I left I went home and I wrote a tribute...(Ron's voice gets emotional and he pauses) to Flash. I read it several times aloud, which helped a lot. Writing and then reading it so I could hear it. Then I did another session in my dreams. I've dealt with most of it now but there's a little more that I'm going to be working with through time. What's left is real small.

RANDAL: That's great. So when you said you did the reframing, what I understand is that because you weren't able to be with Flash when he died you felt a completion with that by imagining being there with him as he died?

RON: Yes, in addition to writing the tribute and reading it. That helped me to express a lot of things that Flash taught me...(pausing with emotion) so that was part of it. The other part was working on the reframing a second time to really take in that gift.

RANDAL: I remember at the end of the class when we talked before you left, you felt like you were just flying. I guess what happened was that you were feeling that way but your intuition kicked in and said there's something more here.

RON: Yes, I was feeling great afterwards but I was aware that I still had more to do. I felt so good because I could let go of...guilt, maybe. No, it wasn't really guilt. It was a sense of letting Flash down that I wanted to work with more. He was, and still is, such a wise spirit. I don't have to carry his load.

RANDAL: (to the class) If Ron were seeing me for private work, the normal situation after doing regression is to have at least one follow-up session. So if Ron hadn't done this work on himself, we'd naturally get straight to the unfinished stuff early on in the first follow-up session. You don't have to get everything done at once. That's what subsequent sessions are for. And people will process and integrate in their lives to some degree between sessions.

Maybe you'll see a hypnotherapist for seven sessions, which can often be more effective than the seventy sessions in some kinds of traditional therapy. You take things a step at a time. Ron has done good work with himself before and during the class in self-hypnosis, so he was already able to do a lot of good things for himself since the session. (to Ron) Are you feeling pretty complete now?

RON: Yes. I'm probably going to work a little bit more on it and it's going to be totally liberating. If I were a lay person, as Randal was saying, I would have needed more help. I wouldn't know what to do with it on my own.

RANDAL: Absolutely. I don't normally even reach the point of doing hypnosis in a first session in private practice. If you had come in for a first session as a referral we would have had a much longer interview, getting a lot more background information. I would have also taken time to explore any previous experiences you might have had with hypnosis and explain procedures and methods we might use in the hypnotherapy.

SARA: How has this solved the original problem?

RON: The original problem was that I used to be very angry and I got rid of the anger, but there was still something like a veil or a fog, something that was keeping me from clarity in what I was doing. I didn't know what it was. I thought maybe I went overboard with getting rid of the anger and was being overly sensitive. There was this fog that felt like unhappiness. Now that I've recognized and worked through that, it's gone. It feels so good and so liberating. It's wonderful.

RANDAL: Is there anything more you would like to say about your session, Ron?

RON: Just thank you very much, and the class as well. (applause)

Note from Ron a Week Later

This is just a quick note to send you the "Tribute to Flash" I wrote after the session. Writing and reading this aloud periodically has helped me move toward complete resolution of issues surrounding Flash.

TRIBUTE TO FLASH

Oh Flash, I love you so much - your chipper personality, the way you carry your self: proud, with dignity, such a positive outlook on life. Happy, healthy, scampering around in total abandon, truly enjoying life. The unconditional love you give so freely, asking for naught. Like a star beaming out in every direction, illuminating everyone and everything with so much love, wisdom and compassion. A peerless role model. You give me so much more than anyone will ever know.

You teach me so much that I still cannot comprehend it all. New wisdoms constantly enlighten me. I understand only now, the best I can, the patience you had with me. The way you cocked your head, calling me softly, sternly, to look into your eyes. Waiting motionless till our eyes lock together in a gaze so that you can pass along directly to my soul, soul to soul, those gems, the higher aspects of life that words cannot express. Like a wise master, knowing that I will not understand just yet. But you beam information in, a treasure, a legacy, that will all be there intact and available at a future time when I have progressed far enough to comprehend your teachings.

I used to think that if I could just talk to you for five minutes you would understand. Little did I know when all the while, like the wise master that you truly are, you held your ground with dignity and patience until the naive spirit in me turned and locked into your gaze. Flash, you are truly wise beyond your years. I am only now just beginning to realize the priceless gift you have given me and all those you touch. Even now I feel it unfolding, blooming, flowering into compassion, humility, love, courage, wisdom, and strength. These qualities and more I will pass on, to and through all things. You have taught me well. I will always strive to honorably conduct myself in ways respectful and sacred to your teachings. Thank you, Flash.

Note from Ron Two Years Later

While I was in trance and you were inquiring about a person when I knew it was a dog, it did not bother me nor did I feel the need to correct you. I consider living organisms to be marvelous gifts of creation. Therefore, I considered Flash a marvelous energetic being that just happened to manifest itself in the form of a "dog". By not having the sense of a specific person, dog, or thing, I understood the context of what you were having me get in touch with.

After that session I have never had that aching feeling in my chest. I feel that session has strengthened my ability to create a healing, nurturing space for clients without triggering my own stuff. Thank you Randal.

CHAPTER 17

Pat's Struggles From Abuse
The Baby Who Didn't Dare Cry

RANDAL: Pat developed intense fear after we did a session for preparing to quit smoking. At the beginning of our second session, she started to describe what had been coming up for her. Her reaction was so strong that I halted the session right there and encouraged her to consider having a session to work on these deeper issues. So here we are. Pat, would you say something about that feeling?

PAT: It's a lot of fear over getting to whatever this is. I've had it for a long time so it's normal for me, even though I know it's not normal. I'm accustomed to it and I don't like it so I'd like to get rid of it. My fear right now is double sided. On the one hand I'm afraid to get to what's causing it and on the other hand I'm afraid I'll resist so much that I won't respond.

RANDAL: Has this fear been consciously with you or in the back of your mind?

PAT: You could say it's in the back of my mind but I'd say it's present in my life.

RANDAL: When do you notice its presence?

PAT: Well, right now I really notice it in making the decision to quit smoking.

RANDAL: Can you describe the fear?

PAT: It looks like death to me, to quit smoking. Like I'm going to lose something that is so much a part of me that I won't be here anymore.

RANDAL: But you noticed this happening at other times in your life, too. Is there another recent time when you've felt this same kind of fear come up?

PAT: If something happens in my life that is very emotional it automatically comes up. Or even situations that are medium emotional, like if my mother calls and there's a certain pattern of negativity. It's not so bad now, I've broken a lot of that. But when she puts me on the spot I can feel that same fear of death.

RANDAL: You experienced some great difficulty when you were a very young girl and you started to say something about that in class last week. Can you tell us about that experience now?

PAT: When I was nine months old my parents drove to Tennessee. My biological father hated crying so he pretty much beat me all the way there and all the way back, and when they stopped at restaurants he'd make my mother leave me in the car. They took me to a friend's when they got back to California and the friend found all the bruises on me and told my grandparents. That started an issue at that point. And then later when I was a year and a half old he broke my leg.

RANDAL: Whew. I remembered there was severe abuse and I was so overwhelmed I didn't remember all the details. It's coming back to me now.

PAT: In fact I think the feeling is still so intense, even though I can't remember the incident, that in the leg he broke I have a cyst. When I do a lot of walking it starts affecting me.

RANDAL: The abuse wasn't just regarding these two incidents. Was your biological father with your mother for the first few years of your life or was he just with her part of the time?

PAT: My parents lived with my grandparents a lot of the time and after my leg was broken my grandfather told my mother that she had to choose between my dad and me or he was going to seek custody of me and disown her. Then my parents moved to Colorado and my mother told me that at one point, I think it might have been after my leg was broken, they were trying to work things out and she went back and forth. She was pregnant with my younger sister when she divorced and then she married my step-father when I was two.

RANDAL: The roots of your fear of death obviously begin very early.

PAT: When I found out all these details I also felt a lot of resentment towards my mother. I mean, I have kids and I don't care how much I loved a man I could not allow anybody to do that to my kids.

RANDAL: And she was there when your father abused you.

PAT: She drove two thousand miles with him while it went on. And one thing that comes to my mind is that when I was a baby he would smoke and my mother would put her head under the covers to get away from it and he'd lift them up and blow smoke underneath. My grandmother told me that he used to do that to my mother a lot. It was one of his ways of torturing her. So maybe I associated something out of thin air but maybe there's an association of power because he was definitely the power source.

RANDAL: Those specific acts could be a strong association or a lesser association with your current issues. And your father was around not only on these trips, but at least on and off in your first two years. Or was he there the whole time?

PAT: From what I understand he was there a lot of the time and part of that time they lived with my grandparents.

RANDAL: Didn't you say something about sitting quietly being too afraid to cry?

PAT: I remember just crying silently without making any noise because he was standing in the doorway while I was on the kitchen floor playing with pots and pans.

RANDAL: Do you know how old you were?

PAT: Probably about a year old. But I can remember. I mean, I can't see him in detail, I don't know what he looks like, but I can remember. It's real to me, let's put it that way.

RANDAL: Some of what you know is because you've been told what happened, but that particular scene really struck a cord with you.

PAT: Well, the trip at nine months old and the broken leg experience are like they happened to somebody else.

RANDAL: That's distant to you.

PAT: Yes, but the one about being in the kitchen, that was real to me. I connected with that, that it is not okay to make a sound. It's kind of interesting that my kids are real quiet and I'm irritated by noise. I think maybe to me that was the truth. That was the way it was supposed to be. From my experience I learned that to live I had to obey that.

RANDAL: You've been able to communicate with your kids, without beating them of course, that you're upset by loud noise.

PAT: Yes, they know. We live on two acres. If they want to make noise they can go outside and that's fine.

RANDAL: Have you done therapy on any of this before?

PAT: Matthew and I went to some counseling in our first year of marriage.

RANDAL: Was it directly or indirectly about this?

PAT: I was having a lot of problems with my mother at the time.

RANDAL: All right. Is there anything else that you would like to add about these issues?

PAT: I notice that I'm not real comfortable with men. Even with my husband, and I can trust him with my life. I know he loves me more than anything but I'm really afraid to show any vulnerability with him because I'm scared to death that he'll take some of my power away or use that against me. Even though I know he never would. I mean, for nine years he's never been in any way abusive or emotionally harsh or anything, so he's had to suffer through that.

RANDAL: What would be a way of showing vulnerability?

PAT: I just have to do everything perfectly. Everything is taken care of, everything is organized. I don't make mistakes.

RANDAL: If you don't do everything perfectly you are afraid you could get clobbered by a man in some way or other?

PAT: It's more that I bottle my emotions. I don't really let them out that often. I do at times, but I have a tendency to keep a lot of stuff inside or when I process it at all with Matthew it's very left brain and analytical.

RANDAL: Okay. Is there anything else?

PAT: No.

RANDAL: I want to repeat what I told you briefly during the break. We'll only move as far as what feels appropriate and comfortable to your subconscious mind. We'll see where it goes today and we could consider another session later this week. I know you've been preparing to quit smoking and I have no idea as yet as to whether our work on this will take you directly to that step. What I want to say is that this is more important. At the end of our work on this you may feel like quitting smoking immediately or you may want to take time to integrate your healing of this core issue, and you can quit in several weeks or at some later time. You can put that off. I don't want you to feel the pressure that you are supposed to quit smoking today.

PAT: So if I come out and I want to have a cigarette I can do that.

Pat's Struggles from Abuse 285

RANDAL: Of course. There is no pressure about cigarettes. If you spontaneously really feel like staying away from cigarettes after this session, fine, but you can always deal with that later on. Okay?

PAT: Yes.

RANDAL: Why don't you lie down and get comfortable on the mat. (Pat adjusts herself on the mat and Randal sits beside her) Let's get the pillows just right for you. (Randal leads Pat into hypnosis and preparation is made for ideomotor questioning)

I'm going to ask you a question that has to do with this issue we've been talking about, Pat, that you could describe as a fear of death. The question is for your subconscious mind. Is it appropriate for us to help you to bring these issues to your conscious mind at this time? (Pat's index finger moves) The answer to the question is yes.

As we look back over the initial onset of the development of your fear of death, is it appropriate and safe for you to be open to your emotions around this issue? (Pat's index finger moves) The answer is yes. All right. Now I have another question for you along these lines. We talked about the memories and we talked about the emotions. Is it appropriate, if it were to happen during this process, for you to get in touch with some physical feelings that you felt? (Pat's thumb moves) The answer is no.

What I will do then, Pat, is help you to get in touch with certain memories and certain feelings regarding those memories, but to encourage your subconscious mind to help you have some detachment from the physical feelings that were occurring then. When I refer to physical feelings I'm talking about possible bodily injury or hurt. I want to encourage your subconscious mind to distance yourself from that part of it, but to encourage you whenever appropriate to be open to whatever emotions you feel. You have every capability of doing that.

You may, for example, choose to observe some of these experiences as if you're seeing them on a movie screen. You can identify with and feel for the character that you know is you on the screen, but you are detached from the physical sensations of it. At the same time you may feel yourself being aware of the emotions that she, you, are going through.

In a moment I'm going to begin to count from one to ten. With each number that I count you become more and more aware of an unpleasant emotion that you sometimes feel. I want you to stay with that feeling and I just want to remind you that the reason we're doing this is to help you to get this out of your system. To help you get it out, you are first going into it. With each number that I count you're going to become more aware of that feeling that has to do with the fear of death.

Pat, I want you to know we're with you. We're supporting you in going through this. You'll do fine. As I count from one to ten you'll become more aware of this fear of death, this panic that you sometimes feel. Number one, two and three. Becoming aware of that feeling. Perhaps you get certain sensations, perhaps you're noticing your heart beating faster. Four, five. More and more aware of that feeling, that emotion, that fear of death that you sometimes feel. It goes way back in your life. You felt it many times. Six, seven, and eight. Feeling that feeling now more and more intensely with each number. On the number nine, like the flood gates of a dam, feeling that more and more intensely, that fear of death. That feeling like you're going to die, like you're going to get hurt very badly. Number ten, you're right there with that feeling.

I'm going to count quickly from ten to one. As I do, you go back to an earlier time in your life when you felt that same feeling. Ten, nine, eight, going back in time quickly. Stay with that feeling. Seven, six, five. Stay with the feeling. This fear of death. You're going back to some time when you were a child when you felt this fear of death. Sometime between the time you were born and a young age. Stay with the feeling. Four, three, two, with the next number I count you're right there with the feeling. An earlier time in your life. Number one. You're right there with the feeling. I'm going to be talking to you now. You can answer my next questions verbally. Are you inside or outside? Pick one.

PAT: Inside.

RANDAL: Is it nighttime or daytime?

PAT: Morning.

RANDAL: It's morning and you're inside. Are you alone or with others?

PAT: My mother.

RANDAL: Your mother is there. Is anybody there besides your mother?

PAT: No.

RANDAL: Are you under six years old?

PAT: Six.

RANDAL: You're six years old, you're inside, it's morning. What room are you in?

PAT: My bedroom.

RANDAL: What's going on?

PAT: (Pat sobs) I want to go live with my grandparents. (breathing rapidly and crying)

RANDAL: Is this something you're telling your mother or just feeling?

PAT: Both.

RANDAL: You want to go live with your grandparents. Are you telling your mom why you want to live with your grandparents?

PAT: (sobbing) Because she hates me.

RANDAL: Stay with your feelings. (Randal pauses as Pat sobs) You're doing fine. You feel that she hates you. You tell her that you think she hates you. What do you call your mother when you're six years old? Do you call her mom, mommy or what?

PAT: Mom.

RANDAL: Okay, what does your mom say when you tell her that she hates you?

PAT: That I'm a spoiled brat.

RANDAL: Do you respond to her when she tells you you're a spoiled brat?

PAT: I don't.

RANDAL: Have you ever told your mother before that you want to go live with your grandparents?

PAT: (sobbing) Yes.

RANDAL: Was it the same kind of reason, that you felt she hated you?

PAT: Uh huh.

RANDAL: Do you tell your mom why you think she hates you?

PAT: No.

RANDAL: Well, tell her now. Just as if she's right here and you're six years old. Go ahead and tell her.

PAT: Because she doesn't want me there. And because my dad and my sister are the family and I don't belong.

RANDAL: Your dad and your sister and your mom are a family but you feel like an outcast.

PAT: But she won't let my grandparents have me.

RANDAL: What makes you feel like an outcast?

PAT: Because she does everything right and I do everything wrong.

RANDAL: How old is your sister when you're six years old?

PAT: Four.

RANDAL: She's four. And that's the way you feel about both of your parents? That both of them treat you different from your sister? They treat her better than you?

PAT: Uh huh.

RANDAL: What are you called when you're six years old? Pat, Patty or what?

PAT: Pat to her.

RANDAL: Okay. Be your mom and talk to Pat. Your daughter has just said that you don't love her and she's an outcast. She says you treat her sister better, that you like her sister but you don't like her. Be Mom and talk to her.

PAT: I don't know how she feels.

RANDAL: Why don't you just make it up? You're just imagining what she might do but imagine as if you really are six years old and you tell her that she's always treating your sister better and she really doesn't love you.

PAT: I don't tell her that.

RANDAL: Why don't you tell her that?

PAT: Because she'd get very angry.

RANDAL: So you do know how she'd feel. She'd get very angry. So be your mom now and get angry about that. Go ahead and talk to Pat. Tell her how you're angry at her.

PAT: I don't want to. I don't want to be my mother.

RANDAL: Well, then, you don't have to. I won't force you. Stay with your feelings and breathe down into your stomach. I'd like you to get in touch with your body now, Pat. It's good to stay with your feelings. It'll help you to go through this. I want you to report to me what you feel in your body right now.

PAT: My stomach.

RANDAL: What about your stomach?

PAT: It hurts.

RANDAL: Describe the hurt in your stomach. The shape, the size. Does it move or stay in the same position or what?

PAT: Right here (motioning to her abdomen), like I could throw up.

RANDAL: It feels like you could throw up. What does that feeling feel like? Is it a hollow feeling or a full feeling or what? How would you describe it?

PAT: It's full, I think. I don't know.

RANDAL: Do you feel tension or a lack of tension?

PAT: Tension.

RANDAL: Does the tension go in a certain direction or does it go inward?

PAT: It goes up and my arms and my legs are getting tingling and numb.

RANDAL: Feel your arms and legs getting tingling and numb. Are you noticing any other feelings that stand out in your body right now?

PAT: My jaw hurts.

RANDAL: Feel the tension in your jaw. You're tensing your jaw. Are you feeling that feeling in your stomach?

PAT: No.

RANDAL: You're not? What do you feel right now?

PAT: Relaxed.

RANDAL: Isn't that interesting, Pat? Instead of running away from your feelings, as you stay with them, they're going away. That's a good lesson for your subconscious mind to learn. Sometimes you can just stay there with something and be with it, give it the chance to express itself, and it'll go away. So right now stay with your feelings. You're doing very well.

I want to say something to the group for a moment. When I talked earlier about avoiding the physical feelings that had to do with the fear of death, that was in relation to any particular thing that could have happened physically to her when she developed this fear. That's far different from the way she is now getting in touch with her physical feelings that are tied in with her emotions. The sensations are coming from the emotions, not from a physical assault. (to Pat) Stay with your body now, Pat. Notice what feelings you feel and where you feel them.

PAT: My shoulders feel a little tense.

RANDAL: Say it this way, "I'm tensing my shoulders."

PAT: I'm tensing my shoulders. And my temples are starting to feel tight.

RANDAL: Say, "I'm tightening my temples."

PAT: I'm tightening my temples.

RANDAL: Good. That way you're taking responsibility. Is there anything else you notice in your body right now?

PAT: No.

RANDAL: How does your stomach feel?

PAT: It's fine.

RANDAL: That's great. You just stayed with that feeling and it went away. I want to draw your attention back to the conversation you were having with your mother when you were six years old and you wanted to leave because you felt she didn't love you. She got very angry at you. You came up with that image when I talked to you about getting in touch with that feeling of the fear of death. Just be aware of that. I want you to focus on your fingers now as I check with your subconscious mind. Is it appropriate for us to continue along these lines, going into emotions and experiences that have to do with your fear of death from the past? (Pat's index finger moves) The answer is yes.

All right. I want you to know that you're doing fine. If you ever feel that you don't want to do something I may encourage you a little bit, but I'm not going to force you to do anything that you don't want to do. I'm not going to insist upon anything. This is your choice. I'm just helping you to go through all this. Fear of death goes very deep for you, Pat. You just got in touch with an experience that had to do with the development of your fear of death.

Now I'm going to help you to go back to a different scene. Some other scene from between the time you were born and the age of six that has to do with your fear of death. Go back to some time that your subconscious mind chooses. You may have no idea where you're going to go and you might have some idea. It doesn't really matter. Your subconscious mind is going to take you back to this feeling you've had at various times when you were a little girl and you were afraid you were going to die. I'm going to count from five to one. At the count of one you're right there at another such experience. Five, four, going back in time. Three, two, on the next number I count you're at another experience, being afraid of death. Number one, you're right there now. Is it nighttime or daytime? Pick one.

PAT: Daytime.

RANDAL: Are you outside or inside?

PAT: Inside.

RANDAL: Are you alone or with others?
PAT: I don't know.
RANDAL: Are you under five years old? Yes or no.
PAT: Yes.
RANDAL: Are you under two years old? Yes or no.
PAT: Um. No.
RANDAL: Get a sense of your age. Two, three, four? How old are you?
PAT: I'm a little over two.
RANDAL: Are you in your house or some other building?
PAT: My grandparents' house.
RANDAL: What room in the house are you in?
PAT: The living room.
RANDAL: You're not sure if there are others present or is it growing more clear to you now?
PAT: I'm in the room by myself.
RANDAL: Are you lying down, sitting up, playing, or what are you doing?
PAT: Sitting on the floor.
RANDAL: And how are you feeling as you're sitting there on the floor?
PAT: Sad.
RANDAL: Do you know what you're feeling sad about?
PAT: I did something I wasn't supposed to do.
RANDAL: What did you do that you weren't supposed to do?
PAT: I touched something
RANDAL: How do you know you weren't supposed to touch it?
PAT: I got in trouble.
RANDAL: Who did you get in trouble with?
PAT: My mother.
RANDAL: Did this just happen earlier today that you got in trouble?
PAT: Uh huh.
RANDAL: What does your mother say or do when she gets angry or upset at you for touching this?
PAT: She spanks me.
RANDAL: How do you feel when she's spanking you?
PAT: Scared.

RANDAL: Are you scared of the physical pain or are you scared of something else? You can talk about it. What are you scared of?

PAT: That it won't stop.

RANDAL: It seems to just go on and on. Has she spanked you often before or is it just once in awhile?

PAT: When my grandparents aren't home.

RANDAL: Are you living with your grandparents right now?

PAT: Uh huh.

RANDAL: Does she spank you often when they're not around or just once in a while?

PAT: Just when she gets mad.

RANDAL: And does she get mad at you for different reasons or if you do something that she says is wrong?

PAT: She's just mad all the time.

RANDAL: It feels like she's mad all the time. I'd like you to bring your mother here. You're two years old and here is the scenario. I'm here with you so you can talk and say whatever you would like to say to your mother and I can help to protect you. If you could really talk to her and just this once really tell her how you feel about the way she treats you, what would you say to her?

PAT: Leave me alone.

RANDAL: And what would your mother say if you were to tell her, "Leave me alone"?

PAT: She'd slap me.

RANDAL: Suppose she tries to slap you and I stop her. What's happening next? Does she say anything?

PAT: That it's none of your business.

RANDAL: What does she say to you?

PAT: I don't know.

RANDAL: Do you want to say anything further to your mother?

PAT: No.

RANDAL: Get in touch with your body right now. What do you feel, Pat?

PAT: Tingling in my arms and legs.

RANDAL: Anything else?

PAT: No.

RANDAL: When your mother spanks you do you sometimes feel a fear that you're going to die?

PAT: I feel panic.

RANDAL: Is that similar to the panic you felt when you thought of quitting smoking?

PAT: Uh huh.

RANDAL: You may have felt this panic even before the age of two. Focus on your finger signals. I'd like to ask your subconscious mind to please give me an answer to this. Did Pat feel any feelings of panic prior to the age of two? (Pat's index finger moves) The answer is yes. Is it safe and appropriate for us to help Pat recall memories and emotions associated with any panic she felt before the age of two? (Pat's index finger moves) The answer is yes.

All right. I'm going to count from one to five. With each number that I count you become more aware of that feeling of panic. I'm helping you to deal with this and get it out of your system. For now you need to stay with it. You're feeling more and more of that feeling of panic with each number. One, two, three, feeling that panicky feeling that you felt when you were just a little girl. (Pat gasps) Four, on the next number that I count you're right there with that feeling. Number five. I'm going to count down to one and you're going to go back to the memory of that panic you felt before the age of two. Five, four, three, two, one. Right there now. Are you inside or outside? Pick one.

PAT: Inside.

RANDAL: Is it nighttime or daytime?

PAT: Nighttime.

RANDAL: Is anyone with you?

PAT: My father.

RANDAL: How old are you?

PAT: And my mother.

RANDAL: You're with your mother and father. How old are you?

PAT: One and a half.

RANDAL: What's happening?

PAT: I got shampoo in my eye. (crying) I couldn't help crying. (Randal hands her a tissue)

RANDAL: What happened when you couldn't help crying?

PAT: He grabbed me from my mother.

RANDAL: What happens when he grabs you?

PAT: He shakes me.

RANDAL: If you could talk to your father and tell him what you really feel, what would you tell him right now?

PAT: I hate you!

RANDAL: Good! Just imagine that you can tell him whatever you want. Say "I hate you!" to him.

PAT: He'll hurt me.

RANDAL: Okay, I'm protecting you now. You're away from him. He can't touch you. Tell him exactly how you feel. Imagine what that would be like if you never had to see him again. You could tell him just how you feel about what he's doing to you. Get in touch with your body. What do you feel?

PAT: I'm trembling.

RANDAL: Where are you trembling? All over or in one place?

PAT: All over.

RANDAL: Okay, keep trembling. Stay with the trembling. What else do you feel in your body?

PAT: My stomach feels tight.

RANDAL: Is there any other place in your body that feels tight?

PAT: My shoulders.

RANDAL: What do you feel in your left hand? Do you feel tightness there, too?

PAT: No, I feel a tissue.

RANDAL: (laughing) And it looks to me like you're holding it very tightly. Okay, here's what I want you to do. Let go of that tissue for a moment and use your hands to put that tightness in my arm. Get that out of your system. And I want you to tell your father, "I hate you!"

(Note: When Pat felt tightness in her stomach and hand, I used the Gestalt method of having her externalize the tension. In this case, and later in the second session when she felt tension again, I directed it into my arm. This work with Pat in 1990 is the earliest transcribed material in this book (1990) and was one of the last times I ever did that. I recommend encouraging the client to use an object, such as a pillow, to direct negative emotional energy.)

PAT: (in a tiny whisper) I'm afraid to.

RANDAL: You're separated from your father. You can tell him that now. Go ahead. This is your chance to get it out of your system once and for all. Say, "I hate you!"

PAT: I hate you.

RANDAL: Now squeeze my arm when you say that. Really squeeze it now. (Pat sobs as she squeezes) Good! Say it again now. "I hate you!"

PAT: (still sobbing) I'm scared.

RANDAL: I know you're scared. Stay with it. He can't hurt you now. I'm going to protect you so go ahead and say it. "I hate you!"

PAT: I hate you.

RANDAL: Good. Say it again. Feel the hatred that you feel toward him.

PAT: I can't.

RANDAL: Okay, relax. You did a lot that you haven't done before. Get in touch with your body. It was good that you had the guts to do that, to think of the terrible things you went through as a little girl. To go back there and just imagine telling your father you hate him. You've just come a long way. What do you feel in your body?

PAT: I feel okay.

RANDAL: You're not trembling any more? (Pat shakes her head) Now I want you to bring in what we can call your higher self here. Whatever higher self means for you, Pat. It's all that you really are, all of you that can and does transcend the terrible experiences you had as a girl. This part of you can be a very loving mother to the child within, this poor little girl that got treated so terribly. Talk to this poor little girl. (handing Pat a pillow) You've got her now. She was starting to get shaken by her father, the kind of thing that happened so often before. What do you want to tell this little girl?

PAT: You'll live through it.

RANDAL: That's true.

PAT: There are safe spaces. Safe people. You'll be okay.

RANDAL: Be the little girl. Be yourself at the age of one and a half. You've got a loving mommy for a change now who's here holding you and comforting you and you can feel that she really does love you. She really is protecting you now. What would you like to say to her?

PAT: Don't let me go.

RANDAL: Okay, switch and be Pat the mother. Your baby said, "Don't let me go." What do you want to say to her?

PAT: I won't.

RANDAL: Be the baby. How does that feel? She says she won't.

PAT: (whispers) Good.

RANDAL: Just feel that. Feel yourself being held by your mommy. You're with someone now who really can care for you well and be very gentle and loving with you. This mother loves you very much. Whenever you want to you can go into hypnosis and become this little girl and become the nurturing mother who loves you very much. And within you, you can have a beautiful, healthy, strong, kind, loving, gentle father who loves you very much. Just know that you can do that.

Now we're going to bring in the part of you that can analyze the situation. Even as you stay with these feelings of love and nurturance, Pat, I would like you to analyze what happened to this little girl and how these things have still been affecting her until now as an adult. There were certain lessons that were learned by this little girl about the world and about herself. Lessons that are misconceptions. Pat has been reacting to the world as the little child learned to react to the world back then. I'd like you to say something about at least one of those misconceptions.

PAT: That you have to be perfect.

RANDAL: What would happen when you were a little girl if you weren't perfect?

PAT: I got in trouble.

RANDAL: And if you got in trouble you could get hurt badly. You got treated terribly so you decided very early on that you would do your best to try to be perfect. That decision goes very deep and has been with you for a long time, but you can let go of it just like that. (Randal snaps his fingers) Can you understand why this little girl would feel like she had to be perfect?

PAT: She couldn't afford not to be.

RANDAL: Right, absolutely. Now here we are in 1990. What is your age?

PAT: Thirty five.

RANDAL: Full grown, thirty five year old Pat, you have been reacting to the world all this time like that little girl because you learned a very hard lesson early on. You'd better do your best to be perfect or you could get hurt very badly.

PAT: But it was confusing because my grandparents loved me unconditionally.

RANDAL: Aren't you lucky that you had grandparents that could love you unconditionally?

PAT: My mother hated it.

RANDAL: Did your mother resent them for loving you unconditionally? Was that maybe even part of the abuse that you got?

PAT: She thought they loved me more than her.

RANDAL: So she was jealous of you and she took it out on you sometimes. That was a terrible thing to do to you.

PAT: (laughing) She still does.

RANDAL: She still does take it out on you sometimes?

PAT: Yes, but I don't take it any more.

RANDAL: That's good. Well, you can be very lucky in spite of the jealousy of your mother. You can thank God for having grandparents who really loved you and helped you to be all that you are today. And you're going to be all that much more from now on. You'll feel breakthroughs right and left from here on because of realizations your subconscious mind is making. I have a question for you, Pat. Looking right now very clearly at these experiences, how the misconceptions developed, how you learned to try to be perfect, getting it all in crystal clear perspective, do you need to continue acting in the same way that you did when you were one and two years old?

PAT: I don't know.

RANDAL: Well, let's check it out. I'm asking your fingers now and talking to your subconscious mind. Does your subconscious mind recognize that the world is a very different place for you now, in terms of how you need to act, than it was when you were a little girl? (Pat's thumb moves) The answer is no. Okay, I'd like you to get some realization of what that's about. How is it that the world isn't different from when you were a year or two old and you need to relate the same to it?

PAT: I guess I don't feel like I've gotten to where I really made the decision in the first place.

RANDAL: What decision?

PAT: About the world.

RANDAL: You made the decision early on that you would try to be perfect. Is that the decision we're talking about now?

PAT: I guess. I don't know.

RANDAL: So there's some lack of clarity about it. Let me check with your fingers. Did you make a decision very early on in this life that you needed to try to be perfect? (Pat's index finger moves) The answer is yes. Has that become an ingrained habit pattern with you?

(Pat's index finger moves) The answer is yes. Do you recognize that you no longer need to have that ingrained habit pattern ? (Pat's index finger moves) The answer is yes. Are you ready now, in an appropriate manner, to begin to change that former habit pattern of always having to try to be perfect under any and all circumstances? (Pat's index finger moves) The answer is yes.

Okay, I'd like you to bring in some wisdom from your higher self. Bring your higher self here now and talk to the part of Pat that's been so used to trying to be perfect and working so hard to please others and not get into trouble. I'd like you to talk to Pat about how she can do some of those things differently. Just take your time and whenever you're ready, talk to Pat about those former patterns of trying to be perfect.

PAT: Don't be everything to everyone. Don't expect more out of yourself than you do out of other people.

RANDAL: This is great wisdom. It's the truth. You've got a smart higher self there. What else?

PAT: Don't take everything personally.

RANDAL: There might be some more but let's stop here for a moment and be the child within you that is alive and well and healing now. How do you feel when your higher self tells you that? Do you recognize the truth of what she's saying?

PAT: Uh huh.

RANDAL: Okay, let's continue. Does your higher self have any other ideas to say to the child within you? That exuberant, wonderful, beautiful girl within you that wants to have fun and play and live life and enjoy herself?

PAT: (laughing) Break a vase.

RANDAL: Well, now that's interesting. It sounds like the adult side of you can be pretty playful. Let's see, I'm going to talk to your little girl now. I'm going to give you an interesting little vase here. (Randal places a pillow in Pat's hands) You can go ahead and break it.

PAT: It doesn't feel like a vase.

RANDAL: It doesn't feel like a vase? (both laughing)

PAT: You can't fool the subconscious.

RANDAL: Let's see. Okay, here is a nice vase. It's even got some water in it. (Randal hands Pat a paper cup with some water still in it) Go ahead and break that.

PAT: That's a good vase. (Pat drops it on the floor with a giggle)

RANDAL: Oh! It's all over! You broke that vase! Well. How does the little girl feel about that?

PAT: I'm fine and I didn't cut myself.

RANDAL: Don't worry, I'll make sure you don't put your hand over there so you don't get cut on any of those pieces. How did it feel to drop that vase and break it?

PAT: Good.

RANDAL: I'll bet there are a lot of ways you can have fun and break vases without hurting anybody, including yourself.

PAT: Uh huh.

RANDAL: Let's talk about different ways to "break vases" in your life. What can you do?

PAT: Um. (laughing) Probably yelling at the top of my lungs sometimes when I feel frustrated.

RANDAL: That sounds great. Who knows, maybe you'll hit the right note and shatter a glass vase with that. That's one of many possibilities. How else can you sometimes "break a vase" in your life?

PAT: Sometimes I do it spending money but I don't think that's a good way.

RANDAL: Well, perhaps once in awhile you can do it spending money up to a point, if it feels appropriate. Give me another way.

PAT: Not fixing dinner sometimes.

RANDAL: Good. You see your subconscious mind is learning right now that you don't have to be perfect. For example, it's okay not to fix dinner sometimes. My sense here from what you've told me about Matthew is that you have a very understanding husband who will recognize that you need to go through some changes here. Most of the time he will be understanding and if on occasion he's not, you're not going to get hurt. You can live through it if you have some disagreements. That may happen sometimes and that's okay, too. If you seem to get in trouble now it will be much different from getting in trouble then. You're not going to get physically hurt.

Of course you want to make sure that you do the necessary things, that you handle responsibilities that really need to be handled. For instance, there are certain responsibilities that are appropriate all the time with your children or when you drive a car, but there's a lot of room for play in many aspects of your life. Not fixing dinner sometimes is a great example of "breaking the vase." You're breaking down these patterns of trying to fit yourself in a certain box and be perfect. You can let go of a lot of trying. Give me another example of how to "break a vase."

PAT: Going to Circle K and getting a gallon of milk instead of going to the grocery store and getting everything I need to get. (both laughing again)

RANDAL: That's great. Just be easy with yourself. Sometimes it's okay to do a little bit and not to do everything with absolute efficiency. You've got five kids, you've got your work, you've got your art. You've got the time and energy it takes to deal with your husband, to deal with yourself, to deal with your friends. There are a lot of aspects to your life.

And it's very important for you to recognize deep down that you deserve to take good care of yourself. You can be a good mother to yourself and allow the child within you to play and allow the mother within you to play, too. See if you can come up with one more example now on how to "break a vase." (whispering) And enjoy it.

PAT: I could not get a project done on time.

RANDAL: Now wouldn't that be nice? To just feel like stopping a project and not finishing on time. That's okay to do sometimes. It'll feel good to do that. And inside let that be okay. You know, some people are really good at that. Some people are too good at that and they need to work on not procrastinating and completing things. They need to learn to follow through. But you have an imbalance in the other direction. You have been such a perfectionist and you have tried too hard.

PAT: (giggling) And Matthew is such a procrastinator.

RANDAL: Interesting. Well, who knows. Maybe as you allow yourself to occasionally procrastinate he'll learn to improve and procrastinate less. Anyway, that doesn't concern you. You'll just take care of yourself on this. You can allow him, unless you really need to express your feelings, to take care of himself.

PAT: As long as he does the cat box.

RANDAL: Right. (laughing) Certain things he has to do. There are limits to this stuff. There are certain absolutely critical responsibilities like driving safely and having Matthew do the cat box.

PAT: That's right.

RANDAL: There are necessary things in the world. That's reasonable. All right, I'm going to talk to the mother and father within you. You are beginning to recognize that you can have more peace of mind, more patience, more acceptance, more trust, more ability to let go and not have to be perfect. You don't always have to make dinner. You don't always have to get other kinds of projects done. You don't have to try to be all things to all people, but just be yourself.

The people that really matter will love you and appreciate you just as you are. You can be yourself and be angry, you can cry, you can express your feelings. You can be upset about certain things and that's all part of life. Just as you can respect that in other people, respect their feelings, you are learning now to become very loving and very accepting of those feelings in yourself. You have some old habits from before that have been very ingrained in you until now, and you are developing new habits. The old habits are falling by the wayside. If you ever catch yourself trying to push yourself too much, just back right off.

I'm going to wrap this up in a moment but I want to touch on the subject of cigarettes momentarily. I wonder if you have any comments about cigarettes at this time?

PAT: It would be nice to have one.

RANDAL: Okay, then enjoy it. You've just gone through a lot and you're continuing to expand and grow and learn and become more loving to yourself. You may come up with a decision later on this month or at some other time in your life to quit. This is something that is up to your own subconscious mind. But I do want to say that if or when you do come up with the decision to quit smoking, you'll find that the former issues having to do with survival have fallen by the wayside. They're just melting away. If you choose at some time in the near or further future to quit cigarettes then you'll have every freedom, every ability to do that easily and mostly effortlessly. There might be some effort in the beginning but you'll have the will and the strength and it will not be such a big deal to you. But for now, during the break, enjoy having your cigarette and give that to yourself. Is there anything further you'd like to say or to ask before I bring you out of the hypnosis?

PAT: No.

RANDAL: Okay, Pat, you've done a terrific job. You've had the courage to go back and deal with some very difficult experiences of severe child abuse. You handled it very well in your life. You handled it with great strength and determination. What you're finding is that it's a different world you're coming into now. It's a world in which you can find a lot more support, a lot more kindness, a lot more acceptance. The physical dangers from the past are no longer there. They are something from the distant past that continue to fade away. What is there for you is a sense of freedom and vitality and trust and love and goodness.

You find yourself more and more easily able to have fun and take chances and make mistakes and not do things perfectly. You can change your mind about things. And you really enjoy this growing sense of freedom and discovery. You are now reliving, in a very healthy and appropriate way, those parts of your childhood that you never got to experience. You are allowing that little girl within you to grow and blossom from this time forward. And that's a very beautiful thing to experience and be a part of, both for you and for many other people around you. It improves your relationships with others as well as your relationship with yourself. People really love that sense of enjoyment and joy and self expression and fun and silliness, etc., that you are tapping into more and more in your life.

(Randal counts from one to five, giving suggestions as he brings Pat out of hypnosis) You don't know this but somebody cleaned up the pieces of the vase so you don't have to worry where you walk in your bare feet. How are you doing?

PAT: Okay.

RANDAL: Are there any other feelings or thoughts you want to share?

PAT: I felt a lot of resistance to really go into...I think the emotional feelings really brought up the physical feelings even though I knew that I wasn't going to feel them. Just a lot of resistance to really going any further into it.

RANDAL: You went quite far, I want you to know. In dealing with this major issue you're not necessarily going to get from A to Z in one fell swoop. And you may find that certain areas where you did come up against your own blocking and chose not to go any further, you may not necessarily need to go further. Those things may not need to be explored or they may get resolved in the process of your life in the days and weeks ahead. I kept encouraging you to go as far as you wanted to. I usually don't even ask the question about physical feelings but I felt that would help you to at least steer away from those feelings. And it may have helped you to back off and not go any further when they came up and you started to feel them.

PAT: It wasn't that I was feeling anything physically. It was more that here it comes and I didn't want to feel it.

RANDAL: You didn't want to and that's what we had decided, that you weren't going to focus on that. I encouraged you to protect yourself and to essentially block yourself in that way. When you were starting to feel those physical feelings come you backed off and that's what your subconscious mind had communicated would be best.

Follow-Up Session One Week Later

PAT: When you were working with Sandy earlier today I felt so much sadness and grief. I really feel like when we did that session last week I didn't get to where a lot of this stuff still is.

RANDAL: We got to a lot but there still is some deeper stuff. It felt like we went up to a barrier and you backed off, and it didn't feel appropriate for you to go beyond that point.

PAT: I think I have assimilated some of what came up from last week to where I'm ready to go for it. I'm scared, but...

RANDAL: It goes very deep for you.

PAT: Uh huh.

RANDAL: It will be important to check again with your subconscious to help us explore this properly. Are you ready to move right into some hypnosis work?

PAT: Yes.

RANDAL: (after doing a hypnotic induction and preparation for ideomotor questions) All right, Pat. We're going to deal with issues of grief that go very deep for you. I want to work on those issues only in ways that are appropriate for you. Is it okay for you to recall and explore memories from childhood and infancy that have to do with grief? (Pat's index finger moves) The answer is yes. Next question. Is it appropriate and safe for you to be open to your emotions as you go back and deal with these memories? (Pat's index finger moves) The answer is yes. Is it appropriate for you to include an awareness of physical pain in those memories? (Pat's thumb moves) The answer is no. I'm going to ask you another question to fine tune this last one. Is it okay for you to choose to be aware of some physical sensations and not others? Would that be appropriate for you? (Pat's index finger moves) The answer is yes.

I want to encourage your subconscious mind to only allow you to feel those unpleasant physical sensations that are safe and useful for your process. You'll find that you can detach yourself from some physical sensations and allow yourself to tap into others. I also want to remind you that any physical sensations that are the direct result of your emotions are okay for you to deal with. You can detach yourself from those physical sensations that are the direct result of physical violence.

I'm going to count from one to ten, Pat. As I count upwards you become more and more aware of a feeling that goes very deep for you. It's a feeling of grief. A feeling of sadness. It goes way back in your life to childhood and infancy. Number one, getting more and more in touch with these feelings. Number two, more and more aware of the feeling of sadness that you sometimes feel. Number three. As I continue to increase the numbers your feelings continue to increase. Stay with those feelings. Four and five. Feeling more and more of that feeling of sadness. Six. More and more aware of that feeling of sadness and grief that came up for you when I was working with Sandy today. Seven. More and more intensely aware of that feeling of sadness. Number eight. Feeling more strongly now that feeling of deep, profound grief. Nine. On the next number I count you're right there with that feeling. Number ten.

I'm counting quickly back. Stay with the feeling. As I count back you're going to an early childhood experience when you felt very sad. Ten, nine, eight, going back in time. Stay with your feelings. Seven, six, five, going back in time. Four, three, two. On the next number you're right there at this earlier experience. Number one. You're right there now. I'm going to ask you some questions. Are you inside or outside? Pick one.

PAT: (in a tiny, frightened voice) Inside.

RANDAL: Is it nighttime or daytime?

PAT: Daytime.

RANDAL: Are you alone or with others? (Pat is crying softly) Stay with your feelings. (Randal is softening his voice) Is there anybody else around?

PAT: My father.

RANDAL: Is there anybody else besides your father?
PAT: No.
RANDAL: Are you under four years old? Yes or no.
PAT: Yes.
RANDAL: Are you under two years old? Yes or no.
PAT: Yes.
RANDAL: Are you under one year old?
PAT: Yes.
RANDAL: Are you several months old?
PAT: Yes.
RANDAL: Okay, you're several months old. Feel your feelings. Stay with your feelings and tell me what's happening.
PAT: He's pinching me.
RANDAL: Where is he pinching you?
PAT: All over.
RANDAL: Is he pinching you for a particular reason? Did you do something to bother him or is he just doing it?
PAT: I don't know.
RANDAL: You don't even know. He's just pinching you all over. What room are you in?
PAT: The bedroom.
RANDAL: If I can come in, grab him and pull him away from you and you could never have to see him again, you could really tell him what you want to tell him and know that you're safe to do that. I'm putting unbreakable Plexiglas between you and your father and forcing him to listen to you. What is it that you want to tell him?
PAT: (sobbing) Stay away from me!
RANDAL: That's right. I want you to imagine now what your father is going to say. Suppose I'm insisting that he say something back. He's been pinching you all over and you're saying, "Stay away from me!" What would your father say in return?
PAT: She's a worthless little brat.
RANDAL: You heard him. What do you want to tell your father?
PAT: Go away!
RANDAL: Say it again.
PAT: Go away!
RANDAL: Good! Say it again!

PAT: Go away!

RANDAL: All right. Get in touch with your body. (whispering) You're doing great. Stay with it and get this out of your system forever. (speaking normally) Stay with the feelings in your body and describe what you feel.

PAT: My stomach hurts. I'm making my stomach hurt.

RANDAL: Yes, you're hurting your stomach. That's good to take responsibility for it. Do you notice anything else?

PAT: I'm having a hard time breathing.

RANDAL: How are you making it difficult for yourself to breathe? Is it in your throat or your stomach or your chest?

PAT: My chest.

RANDAL: So you're tensing your chest, is that right?

PAT: Uh huh.

RANDAL: And what are you doing to your stomach?

PAT: Tensing it.

RANDAL: Okay, we're going to do this process now. I want you to tense my arm. I want you to really feel all that tension inside and put all that tension into my arm. Really squeeze it. (Pat squeezes) Good. I want you to tell your father, "I hate you!"

PAT: I hate you!

RANDAL: Say it again.

PAT: (louder) I hate you!

RANDAL: Good! Again!

PAT: (voice breaking up) I hate you!

RANDAL: Squeeze now. Focus on your breathing. You're doing great. Breathe down into your stomach and tell me what you're feeling right now in your body.

PAT: I'm tensing my shoulders a little.

RANDAL: Uh huh. Do you notice anything else?

PAT: My stomach's better.

RANDAL: You're doing better with your stomach. Good. Check your chest out. How does your chest feel?

PAT: It feels okay.

RANDAL: Pat, your father is so mean, so cruel, and you went through terrible things no child should ever go through. (Pat is sobbing) I want you to bring the beautiful mother that is you here. I want you to hold this poor little girl. (Randal hands Pat a pillow and wraps her arms around it) You don't even have to say anything to her yet, just hold her. I want you to be the little girl now. Feel what it's like to have a good mommy that is there to protect you and hold you. Feel that comfort right now. (Pat cries softly) Be Pat, the mommy to this little girl. You've been comforting her and there is another thing you're going to do to comfort her. You'll say something to her father. Adult Pat, I want you to say whatever it is that you want to say to the father that was doing these terrible things over and over again to this poor little girl. What is it that you want to say to her father?

PAT: You're horrible. (sobbing) Oh, God.

RANDAL: I'm making him listen to you now so you can tell him exactly...

PAT: He doesn't listen to anybody!

RANDAL: Well, he's going to listen to you now, whatever it takes. We can strap him down, tie him down, but he's going to listen. He may try not to listen but you can get through to him what your feelings are. We may not be able to change him but we can keep him from ever coming around your little girl again. Things are going to be different now so what is it that you want to tell him? Tell him your feelings.

PAT: My feelings or her feelings?

RANDAL: I want you to tell him, as the mother to this little girl, how you feel about what he's been doing to her. Speak as yourself, the mother within you.

PAT: I just want to kill him.

RANDAL: Say, "I want to kill you."

PAT: (crying) I want to kill you.

RANDAL: Good. This is a safe place for you to have these feelings. Those terrible things that he did over and over again. If you could have a choice now, how would you like to kill him?

PAT: Just blast him apart so there is nothing left of him.

RANDAL: Uh huh. Get in touch with your body. What do you feel?

PAT: I feel okay.

RANDAL: How do you want to blast him?

PAT: I don't care. Just so there's nothing left of him.

RANDAL: Okay, what's the best way to make nothing left of him? Are you talking about a gun or a cannon or what? Make something up. Whatever you feel.

PAT: Sandy's dynamite. (an image from Sandy's session in class earlier that day)

RANDAL: Sandy's dynamite. That worked real well. Let's go to him now. You tied him to this chair. Where do you want to put the dynamite?

PAT: In his stomach, right in the middle.

RANDAL: Good. Stick it in his stomach. Get in there somehow and light the fuse with a long wick. All right. Send in a blast of air so it gets some oxygen. Here we go. Picture yourself lighting this dynamite now. Is the dynamite lit? (Pat nods) It's going to go off any second. Ready to watch him explode? (Pat begins sobbing) What's happening? What do you see over there where he was before? What's over there?

PAT: Nothing.

RANDAL: Good. He disintegrated into a million pieces. Millions of harmless, helpless pieces scattered throughout the universe. Talk to your little girl.

PAT: It's not your fault.

RANDAL: That's right.

PAT: You didn't do anything that a normal baby wouldn't do. It's his fault.

RANDAL: That's so true and she didn't know that. She was blaming herself so it's so good that you're telling her this. Tell her again. Make it really sink in.

PAT: It's not your fault. (sobbing)

RANDAL: Be the little girl. Be this beautiful little baby. If you could talk, what would you tell this woman who has just destroyed that terrible, mean man?

PAT: Where have you been?

RANDAL: Okay, switch and be Pat the mommy. Talk to your baby. She says "Where have you been?" What do you want to say to her?

PAT: I didn't know how to do anything.

RANDAL: Tell her you wanted to be there for her but you didn't know how until now.

PAT: I didn't think I could. I didn't know how.

RANDAL: Okay, switch and be the baby. She really has loved you all along and she really wanted to be there and she said she just didn't know how. But she's here for you now. What do you want to tell your mommy?

PAT: Don't leave me.
RANDAL: Switch and be Mommy.
PAT: I'll never leave you.
RANDAL: Switch and be the baby. She's holding you and she's telling you she'll never leave you.
PAT: I just want to go to sleep.
RANDAL: Okay, good. You've just been through a lot. That's a good sign that you're ready to sleep now. Doesn't it feel good to be in Mommy's arms? To be cuddled and held? (Pat is nodding) Mommy feels really good, doesn't she? Okay, be Mommy. Is there anything you want to say to baby before she drifts off to sleep?
PAT: I'm not going to let anything happen to you again.
RANDAL: Okay, be baby and take that in. Is there anything more you want to say to your mommy? Tell her something you appreciate about her.
PAT: You feel warm. You make me feel safe.
RANDAL: All right, be Mommy. Is there anything further you want to say to your little baby?
PAT: I love you.
RANDAL: Be the little baby. Is there any last thing you want to say to your mommy?
PAT: I love you, too.
RANDAL: (whispering) She's not going to leave you. She'll be here with you forever. As long as you live she'll be here with you. (speaking softly but not whispering) There will be times when you'll feel scared or sad or angry or upset in some way and your mommy will be here to comfort you inside and take good care of you. And one of the ways she takes good care of you is by taking good care of herself. Both parts of you. Pat, from this time forward you're going to take really good care of yourself. We talked about some of this last time and you came up with some good examples. Whether you repeat those same examples and let them sink in ten times deeper, or whether you come up with something new, I want you to talk about how from this time forward you're taking care of yourself.
PAT: I'm going to try not to feel guilty.
RANDAL: Let's make a stronger statement out of that.
PAT: I'm not going to feel guilty any more.
RANDAL: That's a very good one.
PAT: I'm going to accept that I make mistakes.

RANDAL: That's a very important one for you. It's okay to make mistakes. It's natural and human to make mistakes. "I accept that."

PAT: I accept it. And I'm not going to try and carry the world on my shoulders.

RANDAL: Good. Keep going.

PAT: I'm going to say what I want instead of going around the edges of it. Ask for what I need and what I want.

RANDAL: Give an example. Create a picture of you asking for something that you want in your life.

PAT: Well, I have two pictures. One picture was when I was asking to come and do this training and the way I approached it was really round about.

RANDAL: Do you mean asking us or talking to your husband about it?

PAT: Talking to my husband about it and justifying the reasons why it would be okay. The way I asked about going to level four was straight forward and it felt really good.

RANDAL: So you're starting to do that now. Great. Let's go on. Name some other ways you're taking care of yourself from now on.

PAT: I'm going to quit nagging everyone to do what they're supposed to do. That will lessen my tension a lot.

RANDAL: All right. What else?

PAT: Try to get away with Matthew more often.

RANDAL: Make a stronger statement.

PAT: We're going to go away more often.

RANDAL: Good. Trying is lying. Just do it.

PAT: (laughing) I like to leave my margin for failure in there.

RANDAL: Well, the world has changed now. You can allow for failure, only this is one of those ways you're not going to fail. You're going to do it. It's important for you to get away with Matthew. The two of you deserve it. You've been working hard and you're good parents with five kids. You deserve to get away and take care of yourselves. It's good for you and good for your kids. The kids will have a lot of fun while you're gone, too.

PAT: They love it when we leave.

RANDAL: Yeah, they get a different scene and more play time.

PAT: And my uncle gives them everything they want. They go to McDonald's for every meal.

RANDAL: That sounds like a form of paradise for your kids.

PAT: It is. They go to the one with the playground.

RANDAL: That's great. I'd like you to pick a date by a certain time or in a certain month in the near future when you two are going to get away.

PAT: Oh...October.

RANDAL: For how long?

PAT: Three days.

RANDAL: A long weekend, that kind of thing? So by October you get away with Matthew and you really have a good time and everybody will be so happy. Good. Give another example.

PAT: I'm going to stop agreeing with my mother just for everything to be okay. That one really hurts me internally. It hurts me when I agree with her viewpoint of the past.

RANDAL: You don't have to be the good girl who is just agreeable. You can say your feelings and be honest and not have to be approving of everything everybody does.

PAT: If she disowns me I have my own mother now.

RANDAL: And if she's worthy of being your friend then she'll honor your feelings about her stuff when she gets into that. Good example. You're coming up with many very good examples. This is re–creation.

PAT: I think I'm going to get a riding lawn mower.

RANDAL: Hey, it sounds like you're taking real good care of yourself now. Got a big lawn, huh?

PAT: An acre.

RANDAL: That's right, you live in the country. Of course if you get a riding lawn mower you might have to decide between you and the kids about who gets to use it.

PAT: They can use it, that's fine.

RANDAL: That's a good attitude. Sounds like fun. Say some more things about how you're going to do nurturing and fun things for yourself.

PAT: I was talking to Frank about getting some body work done on a regular basis and I think that would be really good for me. (Frank is a class member who is a massage practitioner)

RANDAL: That's a great idea. Have you done that before on a regular basis?

PAT: My sister, when she was living with us, did it. And I think I need to go to the book store once a week.

RANDAL: All right.

PAT: And I think I'd like to go fishing once a month. I love to fish.

RANDAL: Great! But you not only think you'd like to, let's say you'd like to fish once a month.

PAT: (laughing) I'd like to.

RANDAL: Do you want to commit to doing it once a month?

PAT: Yes.

RANDAL: Good. Would you do it by yourself or with your husband or with a friend?

PAT: Matthew has to be there to take the fish off the hook. I catch them, he cleans them.

RANDAL: Sounds like fun. You don't have to wait until October to go on a fishing trip. You can just go away for a day or two. Great. Come up with one more example. You've got the idea.

PAT: I want to get a Jacuzzi for my back. It really has helped me for the three weeks I've been using it while I've been up here for the class. I can go out and look at the moon while I soak.

RANDAL: That's a very good idea. You mentioned you hold stress in your back and especially when Matthew doesn't do his share around the house, how you take that on. I want to look at some other thing you can do for your back in addition to the Jacuzzi. How can you have a good back and still get Matthew to do his share?

PAT: Well, he promised me that he's going to take care of that.

RANDAL: Take care of what?

PAT: His behavior. That I don't have to.

RANDAL: So you don't have to throw your back out to get him to help.

PAT: That's what he says, so I'll hang onto my back until I see that what he says is what he does.

RANDAL: And?

PAT: And if he does what he says then I'll let it go.

RANDAL: And if he doesn't do what he says then what are you going to do?

PAT: Punch him in the nose.

RANDAL: Rather than punch your back out, right? There are other alternative things you can do. Punching him in the nose is one example. Give me another example.

PAT: Hit a pillow. Yell and scream.

RANDAL: Hit a pillow, yell and scream, get your anger out, rather than putting that burden onto your back. That's a way for you to take care of your back.

PAT: That's what I meant about not carrying the world on my shoulders because it always comes out in my lower back.

RANDAL: Okay, I'm going to take this pillow that is your inner child away. (Randal removes the pillow Pat has been holding) Of course you can have her back whenever you want. She's always there now. (Randal puts a different pillow in her hands) Now this is your lower back. I want you to talk to your lower back.

PAT: Okay. I don't feel like I can make a solid statement that I'm totally ready to give up the tension, so I'm going to approach it by saying I'm feeling it's a possibility. Giving up the back problem is a possibility.

RANDAL: Giving up hurting your back is a possibility.

PAT: Yes. (laughing) I'm getting there, Randal, don't push me too hard.

RANDAL: Rather than me pushing you, see this as me encouraging you to dialogue and make peace with yourself. You're doing fine. What I want you to do now is to become your lower back. Pat is saying that maybe she's getting ready to do something about not hurting you any more.

PAT: Well, I hope it's soon.

RANDAL: Switch and be Pat. What do you want to say to your lower back?

PAT: I'm working on it. I'm really working on it. And I've taken steps to start alleviating a lot of the pain with exercises. The pain is less than it was two months ago.

RANDAL: Good. I want you to know that what I'm doing is helping you to get clear about your feelings to your lower back. I know that it takes time to heal and I know that it takes time to change patterns and I accept that. I just want to make sure that you're being clear with your lower back, that you are working on it and that you do care.

PAT: I do.

RANDAL: Very good. After all, she's a part of you.

PAT: That's right.

RANDAL: All right, be your lower back and see how you're feeling now. Lower back, what do you want to say to Pat?

PAT: The exercises feel good and it feels good when Frank rubs my back. We can take him home with us! (laughing) And I felt less tension in the last three weeks which has felt good. The Jacuzzi has helped a lot.

RANDAL: You know, without even trying you'll find that you have a lot less tension. The burden you have just lifted from yourself you've also lifted from your back. You've stopped shouldering some tremendous burdens. You may even discover that you do fine without the Jacuzzi, but it'll be great to have anyway because it feels good. This is a healing process that is taking place. Your back is still sensitive and you're taking care of it. Your back is just going to take it all in and love it. Now be Pat. I want to wrap this up with your lower back by having you give your lower back some appreciation. What do you want to say to your lower back?

PAT: I appreciate your working even when I push you too hard and you tell me it doesn't work for you by giving me pain. You're still always there for me and I appreciate that.

RANDAL: Now be your lower back and talk to Pat about what you appreciate about her.

PAT: I appreciate your feeling the pain and slowing down. And putting the ice on me.

RANDAL: And the Jacuzzi.

PAT: And the Jacuzzi.

RANDAL: And the fact that you're working on all of this to heal. Be Pat and just relax. Go into your body and tell me what you feel.

PAT: I feel a little bit of tingling but my body feels good.

RANDAL: A little bit of tingling in various parts of your body?

PAT: Just all over.

RANDAL: That's a good feeling, an alive feeling. You're much more alive now.

PAT: A real aware feeling, I think.

RANDAL: Yes. You're free now. You feel like there's something that you were dragging around that's gone for good. You've separated yourself from that and in its place you're putting a beautiful, loving mother and a beautiful, healthy child that is going to continue to get nurtured by her. And there is one more thing that I want you to do. Visualize in your mind a perfect daddy for this beautiful little girl inside of you. What he would look like, how cuddly he would be and how gentle and kind and patient and all of that wonderful stuff. When you get an image of something about the way he looks and acts, go ahead and talk about it.

PAT: The only image that comes to mind is Matthew because he's such a great father. He's really good with the kids and he's really good with me.

RANDAL: That's great. He's a very good father. So picture Matthew within you as the daddy of your inner child and being his most loving and patient and joyful. Really having time for this little girl, which he does.

PAT: He does.

RANDAL: Good.

PAT: He always has, I just couldn't accept it.

RANDAL: Yes, and now you can accept it. As good as your relationship with Matthew has been all these years, it's about to take a quantum leap forward. You'll find a very special bonding and deepening love as you find yourself becoming so much more open to him and as he really appreciates that. It's going to be a beautiful upward spiral that continues to get better as you open up and become more loving and appreciative of him and he opens up and becomes more loving and appreciative of you. You two make sure each week to get personal time just with each other.

PAT: We do already. We do every day.

RANDAL: That's great. Neither of you have to go away on business trips, so you can be with each other every day.

PAT: And the kids really respect that.

RANDAL: That's wonderful. Is there anything further you would like to say or to ask before I bring you out of the hypnosis?

PAT: I want to say thank you.

RANDAL: You're welcome. And I want to thank you. You've done beautiful work. It took a lot of guts again to deal with these issues. I admire you so much for being a wonderful mother, for being healthy, for being an ethical, responsible person and for having survived. You have gone through so much. So much tragedy, so much trauma, so many things that no child should ever have to go through and yet you made it through and you survived. That says a lot for your character, for your integrity, for your being a very beautiful and special person. Most people who survived similar circumstances would be treating other people a lot worse than you do and/or treating themselves a lot worse than you have.

What you have been doing in many ways before now is being very hard on yourself. You'll now develop the habit of being good to yourself. You're going to be a great mother to yourself from this time forward. And you're not going to always be perfect. No one is ever perfect. Sometimes you may need to be selfish in relation to your kids or your husband. You may not feel like making dinner on a particular night, for example, and that's fine. But you're a good mother to your kids and you're also going to be good to yourself. You'll find a good balance there. There are many ways to nurture yourself and it's time you caught up on that and that's exactly what you're beginning to do. The process has already begun.

(Randal counts from one to five, giving suggestions as he brings Pat out of hypnosis) All the way back. (Pat blinks and opens her eyes and sits up) Before I have you say anything further, Pat, I'd like to see if anyone from the group would like to say anything to you right now.

JAN: I am just amazed at how you have come through all this with so little adverse affect.

PAT: I was determined to prove them wrong. That was always my determination. My mother, for as long as I can remember, told me how screwed up I was and what a problem I was. I left home at fifteen. I was determined and I never got in trouble. I never did drugs and I never was arrested or anything. I was determined that I was going to prove her wrong. And I'm real stubborn. It worked for me.

RANDAL: That stubborn streak has worked in so many ways for you and now you'll make sure it doesn't work against you.

SANDY: I just want to say I love you and I was glad to give you back that stick of dynamite.

SUSAN: I love you too, and I've learned so much about you since we've been here. Even more with these two sessions that you were uncomfortable with at first but you were trusting enough to go through it. I've learned so much from you and I appreciate it.

PAT: It felt like a matter of survival to do this.

RANDAL: Yes, I hear you. You talked about quitting smoking being like dying for you. You've been really dealing in so many ways with your survival. And you don't have to deal with that anymore. You can go on and not have this fear of dying in the back of your mind. Part of it was just repressing so much of yourself. You can express yourself now and that's going to manifest very creatively in your art work. I know you've already done great art work, and I'm really looking forward to seeing what you come up with in the weeks ahead.

NORM: As incredible as it may seem, no matter how negative the experiences one endures, there was a gift. You are now a full fledged therapist with the passion of understanding.

PAT: My biggest gift is that empty space. I don't even remember what my father looks like consciously. It's incredible.

RANDAL: This is a really big gift. And another one of them is your skill as a hypnotherapist.

MARLEEN: Could you say something about what it feels like that you did this for survival?

PAT: The way that I survived up to this point was not to really be vulnerable because if you were vulnerable you would fall apart and then you wouldn't be surviving. And to always be perfect and always be everything for everyone. If I got criticized I would just crumble. It was too much. I felt intuitively before I even did these sessions that this was an opportunity for me to really unload some of this crap and get rid of it. And as scared as I was to do it, I really trust Randal. I knew that he would push me just the right way to really get it out. I couldn't not do it. I was even feeling okay, up until this morning when I watched Sandy. I just wasn't in touch with my feelings and I was thinking today is the last day of this class. It was perfect the way that happened because even if I wasn't really feeling like I was into it, today was the last opportunity and I really want to get there. So that was just perfect. I now feel safe in life.

TAMMY: I told you you had it. I knew you had the strength.

PAT: You were right, Tammy. I can be wrong.

MARK: Thanks for your experience.

PAT: Oh, you're welcome. You have my number. If you need a therapist, just call me. (laughter)

MARY: Just an incredible story. I don't know if you know you have it, but I feel your strength.

RANDAL: (to Pat) Do you feel your strength?

PAT: Yes, I always have but I've always used it for other people.

CHAPTER 18

Lynette's Lack of Confidence

The Teenager Who Couldn't Stand Up For Herself

RANDAL: (choosing one of several volunteers from the audience at an International Hypnotherapy Conference) Lynette, do you want to come up here and take this seat? (Lynette comes forward from the audience and sits down next to Randal) Is it okay to mention your age?

LYNETTE: Yes.

RANDAL: (to the audience) Lynette is seventeen. Her mother is present and has given permission for her to do this. Would you say something about what you'd like to work on?

LYNETTE: Well, I'm not real self-confident. I kind of hide away when people look at me or I think people stare at me because they think I'm ugly or that I'm fat. I have a lot of trouble at school. I don't do my work because sometimes I feel it's not worth it. I'm not going to be able to amount to what I want to be. I don't want to go to school. I don't want to get up in the morning. I always want to ditch. I don't want to face my friends at school. I had a friend that I thought was a good friend but then she turned out not to be, so that kind of hurt.

Sometimes I feel like I don't have the support that I need. I don't like to look at myself a lot but I do because I want to make sure there is nothing out of place. I don't want anybody to say, "Oh, look at her. Something is wrong with her."

RANDAL: I want to read a little of what you wrote when I asked volunteers to write a summary about what they wanted to work on. (reading from a slip of paper) "Until recently I liked school and myself and I was doing good but now school work has gone downhill and I don't like the way I look." About a year ago you lost forty pounds and now you're gaining it back very fast. When you say you liked yourself and school until recently, was that until a year ago or six months ago or what?

LYNETTE: I really can't pinpoint the exact time. Probably about a year ago because I used to make straight A's without struggling at all and now it's a real struggle. It's really hard to make A's and B's and I've missed so much school. I just hate to go. I feel like I'm behind and other people are a lot smarter than me and it's not worth going because it's not going to work for me. Then I get scared because if I want to go to college I don't think I'm going to make it. I cry a lot. Sometimes I just sit there and it's like what's the matter? I don't know.

RANDAL: Does this seem to be a gradual development or was there a particular event you can pinpoint that was very difficult for you that happened last year or some other time?

LYNETTE: I really can't pinpoint anything. I know some things started happening. Well, my mom thinks it's my boyfriend. I don't, but she does. Also my friend back-stabbed me. That kind of hurt. I don't like to feel like I'm in competition so I try to get along with her but she thought we were in competition with everything that we did. And I always lost. And she always threw that up in my face.

RANDAL: Have you had this same boyfriend all along?

LYNETTE: Yes, I've had this same boyfriend since I was fourteen.

RANDAL: How do you feel about your relationship with your boyfriend?

LYNETTE: Well, at first I was kind of attached to him. I couldn't do anything without him. Then after awhile he went on vacation for about a month and I started doing things with my friends. It was good for me so I didn't want to be with him anymore. I thought that if I was with him I would miss out. I felt pretty good about myself and then I guess I kind of latched onto him because I felt like I'm never going to find anybody that is going to like me or love me as much as he does. I don't love him as much as he does me but I'd be scared that I'm not going to find anybody else to love me like he does. I feel like guys don't look at me. If I see someone cute I tell my mom I met this guy that was really cute but they don't ever want to talk to me. They always want to talk to my friends and I have a hard time there.

RANDAL: Was there anything particularly challenging for you when you were a child?

LYNETTE: Nothing that was challenging. The one bad thing that comes to mind is my sister. When I was little she used to beat me up a lot. Actually, she would beat me up real bad. My mom would be at work and we'd be at home together. I'd call my mom at work and tell her that my sister was beating me and she'd have to call the police or come home because sometimes my sister wouldn't let me out of the house.

RANDAL: How old were you when that was happening?

LYNETTE: I was six when it started and it happened all the way up until I was about thirteen.

RANDAL: How much older is your sister?

LYNETTE: My sister is six years older than me.

RANDAL: So when it started you were six and she was twelve.

LYNETTE: Yes, and it went on until she moved out when I was about thirteen. But it was really bad when I was younger. My sister has epilepsy and I always felt that if I hit her back she would have a seizure and it would be my fault so I never did.

RANDAL: I see. Have you ever gone into hypnosis?

LYNETTE: Yes.

RANDAL: If I were to suggest at some point that you go to a pleasant scene of some kind, what would be a good example of that? Do you have a particular favorite place?

LYNETTE: Not really. I like the beach. I don't like to get in the water though.

RANDAL: I talked earlier about ideomotor responses. Have you ever used finger signals for yes and no?

LYNETTE: No.

RANDAL: Is there anything else you'd like to say before we do the hypnosis?

LYNETTE: No.

RANDAL: All right, you can get comfortable on this cot here. (Lynette lies down and pulls a blanket across herself) Here's a pillow for you, too. You can rest your arms at your sides and we can both take off our glasses. (Randal puts Lynette's glasses on a chair along with his own) I'm near sighted so I can see fine close up. Are you ready?

LYNETTE: Yes.

RANDAL: I'd like you to look over here at my little finger (Randal holds his hand above Lynette's face) and take a nice deep breath and fill up your lungs. Now exhale slowly. I'm rotating my little finger as I'm moving it closer to your face. Relax now. Take a second deep breath and fill up your lungs. (pause) Now exhale, following my little finger. Relax now. And a third deep breath. (pause) Follow my little finger down until your eyelids close. (Randal moves his hand down and Lynette's eyes close) That's good.

I want you to turn your eyelids completely loose. Relax those tiny muscles around your eyes so much that they wouldn't work even if you wanted them to. Now imagine your eyelids are stuck tightly together. I'm going to count from three down to one and at the count of one you try to separate them but you'll find that they stick tightly together and the harder you try the deeper into hypnosis you go. Three, stuck tighter and tighter together. Two, sealing together. One, go ahead and try to open your eyelids but they're stuck together. (Lynette squints but her eyes remain closed) That's good. When I touch your shoulder relax, stop trying and go deeper. (Randal touches her shoulder)

Now I'm going to pick up your left hand by the wrist. Let your hand hang loosely and limply in mine. When I drop it and it lands beside you send a wave of relaxation all the way down your body and feel yourself go much deeper. (Randal drops her hand) I'm going to drop it a second time and this time you go deeper still. (Randal drops her hand again) That's good. I'm going to lift up your right hand and do the same thing. When I drop your right hand send another wave of relaxation down your body and feel yourself go much deeper. (Randal drops her hand) And a second time. When I drop your hand you're going to go much deeper. (Randal drops her hand) Much deeper. That's fine.

Just focus on your breathing. Let your breathing be slow and steady and deep and continuous. I'm going to push down on your shoulders as you exhale and you feel yourself go much deeper. Take a nice, deep breath and fill up your lungs. On the exhale send a wave of relaxation down your body and feel yourself go much deeper. (Randal pushes down as she exhales) Let's do that one more time. Take a nice, deep breath and on the exhale as I push down feel yourself go much deeper. (Randal pushes down) I'm going to gently rock your ankles and as I do let your whole body move gently and go deeper in relaxation. Relaxing just as you would if you were on a pleasant, beautiful beach. Resting on a beach towel in the sun or in the shade, however you would like to see and feel it.

Now please put your attention on your right hand. I'd like you to imagine the word "yes" in your mind's eye. There is a certain finger that will be your "yes" finger. I'd like you to keep seeing and hearing the word "yes" in your mind until one of the fingers on your right hand begins to lift and to rise. Just picture and hear and see the word "yes" until a certain finger begins to lift and to rise. (Lynette's index finger begins to quiver and Randal watches for several seconds before acknowledging it) That's good. I'm getting a definite quivering movement from the index finger on your right hand so that will be your "yes" finger. (Randal taps the finger)

Now imagine that there is a certain finger that is your "no" finger. It could be your thumb or your middle finger or your little finger. (Randal taps each finger as he names it) Hear and see the word "no" in your mind. There is a certain finger that will begin to lift and rise. Keep seeing and hearing the word "no" until a certain finger begins to move. (pause) A certain finger is your "no" finger. (Lynette's thumb quivers for several seconds) There we go. The thumb is your "no" finger.

Lynette, you've been describing your lack of confidence. I have a question for your subconscious mind. Is it safe and appropriate for you to recall any memories in your life that have to do with this feeling of putting yourself down or feeling negative about yourself or being afraid of what people will think of you? (Lynette's index finger rises) The answer is yes. We got a good, strong response with that. Another question: is it safe and appropriate for you to be open to your feelings and emotions as you recall these experiences? (Lynette's index finger moves) And the answer is yes.

I want you to know, Lynette, that I really admire you for being up here. It takes a lot of courage to do what you're doing. You're dealing with an issue of shyness and fear and lack of confidence, yet you have the guts to come up here amid all these strangers and do this. That kind of courage will help you over and over again to move forward and rise above difficulties in your life. You're going to do great. You may come up with some uncomfortable feelings now but that's okay. You'll be able to handle them. We'll be able to work them out together.

I'm going to count from one up to ten. With each number that I count you'll become more aware of a feeling. This feeling is being afraid that someone is going to criticize you or hurt you or put you down. (Lynette's body begins to shake) It's fine to let your body shake. You can let your body shake even more. That's your vital energy. You've got a tremendous amount of energy that you've been holding back. It's good to shake because this is a way to release that energy. You're doing fine.

Here we go. Number one, two, three. With each number that I count you're becoming more and more aware of that feeling. That feeling of being afraid that someone is going to hurt you or put you down or criticize you. Number four, five and six. You're afraid that someone is going to put you down. Seven, eight. Being aware of what that feels like now. Someone is putting you down and criticizing you or hurting you in some way. Number nine. On the next number that I count you're right there with that feeling. Number ten.

Now I'll count from ten down to one. You're going to go back to an earlier time in your life when you felt like someone was really hurting you in some way or putting you down. Number ten, nine, eight, going back in time. Seven, six, five, going back in time. Four, going back to an earlier time in your life. Three, stay with that feeling, two, going back to some time when you feel yourself being hurt or put down. Number one, you're right there with that feeling. I'm going to ask you some questions and you can respond with a quick answer. Lynette, this experience that you're becoming aware of now, are you inside or outside? Pick one.

LYNETTE: Inside.
RANDAL: Is it nighttime or daytime?
LYNETTE: Day.
RANDAL: Are you alone or with at least one other person?
LYNETTE: I'm with someone.
RANDAL: Who are you with?
LYNETTE: My sister.
RANDAL: Are you under ten years old?
LYNETTE: Yes.
RANDAL: Are you under seven years old?
LYNETTE: Yes.
RANDAL: Are you under five years old?
LYNETTE: No.
RANDAL: How old are you?

Lynette's Lack of Confidence

LYNETTE: Six.

RANDAL: Okay, you're six years old. You're with your sister. You're inside. Are you in your house or somewhere else?

LYNETTE: In our apartment.

RANDAL: What room are you in?

LYNETTE: The living room.

RANDAL: All right, that's the scene. You're there with your sister. What's happening?

LYNETTE: She's yelling at me.

RANDAL: Has she yelled at you before?

LYNETTE: Yes.

RANDAL: Does she do this often or does she only do this once and awhile?

LYNETTE: She does it a lot.

RANDAL: Is she yelling because she's upset at you or because she's upset at something else?

LYNETTE: She can't go outside because she has to watch me.

RANDAL: And how do you feel about that?

LYNETTE: I feel hurt because she says it's my fault she can't go anywhere.

RANDAL: She's blaming you because she can't go anywhere and she's also telling you that you have to stay inside, is that right?

LYNETTE: Yes.

RANDAL: Has she said this kind of thing to you before?

LYNETTE: Yes.

RANDAL: And what do you say in response to her?

LYNETTE: Nothing.

RANDAL: Do you want to speak up for yourself?

LYNETTE: No.

RANDAL: Why don't you want to do that?

LYNETTE: Because I don't want her to be mad at me.

RANDAL: You don't want her to be mad at you because she'll yell at you or what?

LYNETTE: She won't want to talk to me. (Lynette's body, especially her shoulders and chest, is shaking)

RANDAL: Let your body shake. You learned to hold back your energy then and now it's time for you to express that energy. (Lynette is shaking even more) That's good. It's time for you to stick up for yourself to your sister now. It's time for you to tell her how you feel. I can be here to help you. What would you like to say?

LYNETTE: Mom says you have to watch me but I can go outside by myself.

RANDAL: Okay, switch and be your sister. (Randal taps Lynette's shoulder each time he asks her to switch) What does your sister say in response to that?

LYNETTE: I don't care what mom says. You can't go outside. Not without me.

RANDAL: Switch and be Lynette. What do you want to say in response?

LYNETTE: Nothing.

RANDAL: I bet you can say something more than that. If you don't feel like you're going to be able to go outside you can at least tell her how you feel.

LYNETTE: I just want to go outside to the swings. You can watch me through the window. (to Randal) Mom said I could go outside but she won't let me go. (Lynette begins to cry) I don't want to say anything because she might hit me.

RANDAL: Let's deal with that. Has she hit you before?

LYNETTE: Yes.

RANDAL: This time we're going to create the situation a little bit differently, Lynette. She won't be able to hit you any more. We're going to put a barrier in front of her. Any time she tries to hit you she's going to hit this invisible Plexiglas barrier. She won't be able to get within a foot of you. Imagine that that's how it's going to be from now on, as if we could magically do that. What would you say to her if you could know that she can't hit you anymore?

LYNETTE: I wouldn't say anything because I would still feel bad. She would still be mad at me.

RANDAL: What's so bad about her being mad at you?

LYNETTE: I love her. I don't want her to be mad at me.

RANDAL: I believe that you really love her. I also want you to know that the opposite of love is not hate. The opposite of love is indifference. One thing you don't feel for your sister is indifference. You have a lot of love for her but she's really been tough on you. See how it feels to say, "I hate you." Try it out.

LYNETTE: (sobbing) I can't. I can't say that to her. I never say that to her. She says that to me.

RANDAL: Well, it's about time to get it out of your system and say it to her. That's not a very nice thing for her to do. You don't deserve for her to say such terrible things to you. She deserves to have it bounce off of you and go back to her. Say it back to her. Say, "I hate you." Just try it.

LYNETTE: (faltering) I hate...you. (begins to shake and sob)

RANDAL: Good for you. You're doing fine. Your body is starting to shake. Shake it even more. Go inside your body and tell me what you feel.

LYNETTE: I feel bad.

RANDAL: Where do you feel bad? Is it a particular part of your body or is it all over?

LYNETTE: It's all over.

RANDAL: What does "bad" mean? Do you feel tense or what?

LYNETTE: My feelings are hurt because I said that to her.

RANDAL: Your feelings are hurt or hers are?

LYNETTE: Mine. She doesn't care.

RANDAL: Well, if she doesn't care what does it matter? Maybe it's good for you to say that and get it out of your system. Breathe down into your belly and keep feeling your feelings. When somebody is telling you they hate you and yelling at you and hitting you and keeping you from doing things you should be able to do, it's not a time to be nice. If you weren't nice before maybe it would be even worse for you, but we're changing the rules now, Lynette. It's time for you to stand up for yourself.

LYNETTE: If I get her upset she might have a seizure. I hate it when she has those seizures. They're so ugly.

RANDAL: Has she ever had a seizure when she got upset at you?

LYNETTE: No.

RANDAL: Does she get seizures when she gets upset?

LYNETTE: Yes, when she gets real upset sometimes she has them.

RANDAL: Well, since we're all the way up to the present now and we're going back and recreating this experience for you, we can recreate it in a different way. I can understand how you learned to hold back your feelings because your sister had these problems. Even though she was mean to you, you were afraid of being mean back to her because you really love her. You didn't want her to get hurt because she has this physical condition. Now I would like you to imagine that your sister is saying and doing all those things but she doesn't get seizures anymore. What we're dealing with now is a different reality, and the rules have changed. It's a new day and you can express yourself with her. Imagine what that would be like if you don't have to worry at all about her having seizures. And I can also keep her from hitting you. Now I want you to tell her off. Tell her what's wrong with what she's been doing.

LYNETTE: (starting to breathe heavy) I can't stand you.

RANDAL: (loudly) Say that again!

LYNETTE: (sobbing, but louder) I can't stand you! You're always hitting me and I don't do anything wrong. You're such a bitch!

RANDAL: Good! That's telling her.

LYNETTE: Please just leave me alone. I don't want to talk to you.

RANDAL: I want you to use this pillow here. (Randal holds a pillow above Lynette's chest and guides her hands up to it) Take your hands and hit this pillow. Remember, this is a different sister. She's been a lot bigger than you but she's not going to be able to hit you back. You can hit her for all the times she hit you, and she can't get seizures any more. (Lynette punches the pillow moderately a couple of times) Say, "I hate you!"

LYNETTE: (crying and hitting harder) I hate you! I'm going to get even with you for once! (covers her face with her hands as she shakes and sobs)

RANDAL: Very good! Go inside your body. It's important for you to get this energy out of you. You don't have to hold it in anymore. You didn't deserve that. What do you feel inside your body right now?

LYNETTE: I feel calm.

RANDAL: Do you feel calm throughout your body?

LYNETTE: Yes.

RANDAL: Good. You weren't feeling very calm before. Do you notice how much better you're feeling?

LYNETTE: Yes.

RANDAL: Do you know why? You got that energy out of your system. She'd been hitting you all that time and now you hit back. You see, in therapy work we can get that energy out in such a way that you don't hurt anybody else. It's so good for you. You had been putting that negative energy into yourself, just holding back. Now you can express that energy. You're doing great. Notice how much more calm your body feels. You were really shaking before. Now take a look at your sister and remember that this is a special situation. She doesn't get those seizures anymore so you could hit her. She deserved it because she had been hitting you and you didn't deserve it at all. What would you like to say to her now?

LYNETTE: I forgive you.
RANDAL: Does that feel clear? Do you forgive her for all those things she did?
LYNETTE: Yes.
RANDAL: Let's see what your sister has to say. Switch and be your sister.
LYNETTE: Forgive me for what?
RANDAL: Be Lynette again and tell her what your response is to that.
LYNETTE: I forgive you for all the times you beat me and called me names and told me that you hated me. I love you. I know you love me. I know you didn't mean it.
RANDAL: Switch. What does your sister say?
LYNETTE: I don't beat you!
RANDAL: It looks like she hasn't gotten it. Switch and be Lynette.
LYNETTE: Then I forgive you for hitting me. You didn't beat me.
RANDAL: What's your sister's name?
LYNETTE: Laura.
RANDAL: Be Laura. Lynette has just said that for all those times you hit her and called her names and so forth, she's forgiving you. What do you say to that?
LYNETTE: Nothing. That's nice that she forgave me.
RANDAL: Say that to her. "That's nice that you forgave me."
LYNETTE: That's nice that you forgave me.
RANDAL: Good.
LYNETTE: She doesn't care.
RANDAL: What?
LYNETTE: My sister doesn't care.
RANDAL: Well, does that ring true or does that not ring true? Do you think she would say, "Well, that's nice that you forgave me?"
LYNETTE: Yes, but she'd be being sarcastic.
RANDAL: Oh, I see. She's being sarcastic. Lynette, you were just very kind and generous to your sister. Just like that, with a little bit of work on it, you became calm and you forgave her. That was very big of you. Now she's being sarcastic in response. How do you feel about that?
LYNETTE: I feel bad but at least I got it out. It doesn't matter to her but it matters to me. I don't need her to know that I forgave her because I do. If she wants to deny things then that's okay.

RANDAL: How do you feel about her denying it? Does it really feel okay with you? That's fine if it does, I'm just checking it out.

LYNETTE: Yes, it feels okay. She did it and I know she did. She may not realize what she did, but that's okay.

RANDAL: What do you feel in your body right now?

LYNETTE: I still feel a little scared.

RANDAL: Who or what do you feel afraid of?

LYNETTE: I'm still intimidated by my sister.

RANDAL: So it's unfinished. I want to say that you're doing very well. You're doing good work. If you're feeling intimidated by your sister it's time you pounded her down to your size, so we're going to do this again. (Randal holds the pillow above Lynette's chest) For all those times she hit you, I want you to hit her some more and say "I hate you!"

LYNETTE: (crying and hitting the pillow) I hate you! I hate you! I hate you! I hate you!

RANDAL: That's good. You had to hold back your feelings for all those years. That wasn't fair at all. You were treated very badly. It's good for you to get those feelings out now. You got so used to holding them in that you just got in the habit of it. It's important for you to stand up for yourself and express your feelings. Feel your power. Get bigger and make your sister and anyone else who has put you down smaller. You can stand up and be proud of yourself because you have a lot to be proud of. Go inside your body. What do you feel in your body now?

LYNETTE: I feel calm.

RANDAL: Now let's take a look at your sister. What do you want to say to her?

LYNETTE: I want to tell you that I love you and I still forgive you for everything.

RANDAL: What does your sister say in response now?

LYNETTE: I know that you forgive me and I love you, too.

RANDAL: She means it now, doesn't she?

LYNETTE: (crying) Yes.

RANDAL: She respects you a lot more now. You stood up for yourself and you knocked some sense into her. How does that feel?

LYNETTE: It feels good.

RANDAL: You got into all that negative energy that she had and worked things out and that's what is left. Love. (Lynette nods)

Good. You're beginning to get a sense of completion. Take a look at your sister over there and see yourself with her now. I'd like you to see her getting smaller and you getting bigger. You're beginning to recognize that when she did those terrible things it was as if there was this three year old part of her that was being a brat. Unfortunately she was a big brat and you were smaller than her physically. But now it's changed. You can see that she's gotten smaller and you've gotten bigger than her. Can you picture that?

LYNETTE: Yes.

RANDAL: Is there anything more you have to say to your sister? (Lynette shakes her head) Is there anything more she has to say to you? (Lynette shakes her head) Does it feel complete?

LYNETTE: Yes.

RANDAL: There is a shift taking place now inside of you, Lynette. You're feeling yourself becoming more expansive and strong and clear. And you're learning a great deal. Not only about what we've talked about, but there are all kinds of shifts taking place inside of you. You're finding yourself standing taller and feeling prouder and knowing that you can stand up for yourself. There was a time when you couldn't. There was a time when you had to hold back on your energy and you don't need to do that anymore. It's a different world. It's not like that anymore and it never will be again. We all have difficult times but you can stand up for yourself. And of course you can find many ways to do that without hitting, but with confidence and powerful communication.

Most of the time you don't even have to be concerned about standing up for yourself because you'll find that there is something different about the way people respond to you. People are liking you more. You recognize that you're feeling more confident, more self-assured, more attractive. It's a process. It doesn't happen overnight but it's a habit you're developing. You're noticing that sometimes boys do look at you in a positive way and you're noticing that people do like you and they like hearing what you have to say. You'll see. But first and foremost, you're finding yourself wanting to associate with people that you like and who like you.

Look back at six year old Lynette now. I would like mature seventeen year old Lynette to talk to six year old Lynette. You can be real proud of how this girl just stood up for herself. That was a difficult transition but she did it. What do you want to say to this six year old?

LYNETTE: You did real good and don't let anybody put you down. You should always speak your mind and stand up for yourself.

RANDAL: Now switch and be six year old Lynette. She really complimented you . How does that feel?

LYNETTE: It feels good.

RANDAL: I want to encourage you to do some visualization each day for the next few weeks. You can do it in hypnosis, if you want to go into self-hypnosis, or you can do it when you go to bed at night if you're not experienced in self-hypnosis. I'd like you to imagine that grown up you, with all of your experience and wisdom, is like an extra mother to this six year old. Visualize yourself being with this six year old and really nurturing her and taking good care of her. She was in a situation that was unfair and things were difficult, but now she's standing up for herself. I want you to be there to keep encouraging her that she's fine, that nothing like that has to happen anymore. You'll be there to protect her. Does that sound good? (Lynette nods)

And I'd like you to experience not only being the mother to the six year old within you, but also being that six year old and having adult you around to take care of her and protect her. You can also visualize someone else being with you, like your real mom or anyone else. You can imagine you have a perfect mom and a perfect dad that you can bring in there. Does anybody come to your mind?

LYNETTE: It's my mother.

RANDAL: So you can imagine being this six year old and having your mother there now even though she couldn't be there when it happened. She certainly wished she could have been there for you then and now she can be there within you. You can know that your mom is there and she loves you very much. She can be with you supporting six year old Lynette, and Lynette at all the different ages. Deep down in your subconscious mind you can have your mom there in spirit whenever you want her.

Now be yourself and look over at seventeen year old Lynette. I want you to recognize this very special young lady and I want you to compliment her. Tell her all the things you like about her and respect her for.

LYNETTE: There aren't any.

RANDAL: Keep looking.

LYNETTE: I always try to help people when they're in trouble or when they hurt. I'm a good friend.

RANDAL: Those are excellent examples. You have a very big heart. It may not be easy at first but you're going to get in the habit of seeing things you like about yourself. That's another thing you can do each night when you go to bed. You're going to find that practice makes perfect. It gets easier with time. It's like working muscles that are out of condition. You start getting them into condition by practicing. Find something else now that you like and respect about Lynette.

LYNETTE: When other people are down I try to make them laugh.

RANDAL: Once again I'm aware that you really care about people. You have a good heart. I think that's the most important thing in the world. A lot of people don't have that, but you do. You can be proud of yourself for that. If some people had the difficulties you had they might just feel sorry for themselves, whereas you're looking out for other people. You've been very generous and that's good. But just as you look out for other people, I want you to look out for yourself now. Imagine that you are somebody else looking at you as this young lady and you know how hard she's been on herself. What would you say to her?

LYNETTE: You shouldn't be so hard on yourself.

RANDAL: Stay with this detachment and see her as someone else. She's had a lot of unfair things happen and she's in the habit of feeling bad about herself. She needs to get some encouragement. Just as you'd like to make someone else feel better who's been hurting, what would you say to encourage her?

LYNETTE: You're strong and you don't give in to a lot of peer pressure.

RANDAL: That's very important, especially at your age. Peer pressure can be very challenging. Do you want to give an example of how she doesn't give in to peer pressure?

LYNETTE: All your friends smoke and you don't. You go to parties and everyone is drinking or doing drugs and you don't do it.

RANDAL: These are excellent examples. Others are doing that, but that young lady there, Lynette, she says no to that. That's very smart of her. And it's not easy at times. That shows fine character. Here is someone who has been feeling nervous about what people might think of her and yet she is not going to buckle under to peer pressure. Other kids don't have the strength that she does. You can feel proud of that young lady. She would be a good friend to have, wouldn't she?

LYNETTE: Yes.

RANDAL: Wouldn't you want to have a friend like that who wouldn't give in to peer pressure and who would really treat you well?

LYNETTE: I sure would.

RANDAL: Well, you can have a friend like that in yourself. You can treat yourself as a good friend. This is going to stay with you. You're starting to see what a special person you are. You deserve to have friends like yourself. You deserve to have a lot of good things coming your way. I'd like you to pick one more thing now. Take a look at her and say one more thing to her about what you like about her. (pause)

LYNETTE: I can't think of anything.

RANDAL: Well, you've just thought of some very important things. You were saying earlier that you used to get A's, is that right?

LYNETTE: Yes.

RANDAL: It seems to me that if you used to get A's when you were feeling good about yourself and now you're starting to feel good about yourself again, there's no reason why you can't turn that around and start getting A's again. I know you've missed a lot of classes and fell behind, but you can begin to turn yourself around. How do you feel about that?

LYNETTE: I feel like I can be a good friend but I don't like me. I don't like the way I look. I constantly think about it at school so I don't want to do my work. I just sit there and cry or put my head down and go to sleep.

RANDAL: I'm going to speak from some life experience now. Just hear me out. I've worked with a tremendous number of clients. You would be amazed at how subjectively people feel about their looks and how much of that has to do with confidence. The more you think positive things about yourself, the more attractive you look. I've worked with people over and over again who thought they weren't attractive, particularly as a teenagers, and then as they gained confidence they felt more attractive. I want you to allow for the possibility that first of all, you have a lot of attractive qualities physically as well as being a beautiful person inside. As you allow that beauty to come out more you begin to feel more beautiful. Don't close off to the fact that you might be surprised at how attractive you can be. Just keep an open mind about it.

Lynette's Lack of Confidence   335

I want you to know that I am very careful to never lie to somebody in hypnosis. You are attractive. I mean that deep down. You have so much going for you and I'm including physically. I'm sure a lot of boys will find you attractive as you continue to feel better about yourself. This is not an instant thing but it's something I encourage you to work on. Just trust. Notice somebody in the next few days or the next few weeks who is looking at you and smiling, seeming to be really interested in you, and just allow that possibility to start to happen.

I'm going to predict that you're going to look back some years from now and realize how attractive you feel, and you'll realize that all along you really were quite attractive. I don't expect you to believe me now one hundred percent, I just want you to hear me out because I'm telling you my experience. Can you just hear what I'm saying right now? (Lynette nods) Good. Go into your body. Do you feel good in your body right now? Do you feel clear?

LYNETTE: Yes.

RANDAL: Lynette, you have just done some very good work. You're beginning a process of turning things around. I can't emphasize too much how important it is for you to get into the habit of focusing on the positive. (this is Randal's only chance to work with Lynette, who lives in another state, so he is being especially thorough, including some creative repetition during the post-hypnotic suggestions and the encouragement for new habits) This is a very big process you've just done and I want you to think of it as a seed that's been planted. It's already begun to sprout, but it needs nurturing. I want you to be good to yourself. Think good thoughts about yourself. Appreciate the good things about yourself. If it's easier for you initially to appreciate what a good heart you have and what a good friend you would make, then work on that and just go from there.

When I was your age I had a lot of negative feelings about myself and a very low self-image. I felt very unattractive. I worked a lot on myself and expanded so much beyond that. For many years now I've felt very confident, attractive, strong and powerful. And you've got so many beautiful qualities, inside and out. It's just a matter of allowing that to happen for you. I've seen it happen for so many men and women.

You have just shown great heart and courage and determination. Here you are, having dealt with these terrible feelings about yourself in front of all these people here, because you care. Deep down you have a lot of desire and are really willing to reach out. I admire that in you tremendously. Many people would not have been able to do what you did. I'd say the vast majority of people your age, dealing with these issues, would not have had the courage to do this. You have great strength and that's going to help you so much. You can begin now to take really good care of yourself and become your own best friend. It's not an instant process but you work on it each day. Start looking for the good you can appreciate in your life and get in the habit of seeing the good side of things. Is there anything more you'd like to say or ask before I bring you out of the hypnosis?

LYNETTE: No.

RANDAL: Lynette, I want you to know that you're beautiful. I'll bet a lot of people in this room feel the same thing. (to the audience) Am I right?

CHORUS FROM THE AUDIENCE: Yes!

RANDAL: I'm going to begin counting from one to five and with each number that I count you become more and more alert, awake and aware. (Randal gives suggestions as he counts her out of hypnosis) You can open your eyes and take a deep breath. How are you doing?

LYNETTE: Fine.

RANDAL: You did an excellent job. You had never had an opportunity to speak back in that situation and it was very difficult for you at first, but you can see the kind of transformations that happen in doing that. Are you ready to sit up? (Lynette nods and Randal helps her up and guides her to the chair next to him) We'll just take a few more minutes here in the chair. Do you want to wear your glasses?

LYNETTE: Yes.

RANDAL: I'll wear mine, too. Look out there at everybody. (to the audience) First and foremost, let's show our appreciation to Lynette. (the audience applauds and Randal turns back to Lynette) Do you have any question or is there anything further you want to say about your experience?

LYNETTE: I just want to say it was a good experience. It's tough what happened between me and my sister. It hurt me a lot and I never had a chance to really get it out before now. I do feel a lot better.

RANDAL: That's great. Thank you.

CHAPTER 19

Craig's Lingering Resentment
The Absent Father

RANDAL: Craig, you wanted to work on something that you said goes back a long way. Would you like to do that now? (Craig comes up and sits next to Randal) What would you like to work on?

CRAIG: My parents divorced when I was around one and when I was fairly young, in the neighborhood of five or six, my natural father moved out of town. I lost contact with him, or he lost contact with me, for fifteen years or so. As a father now I'm wanting to go back and see how that affected me. For a long time in counseling I denied that it had any effect because my mother remarried and my stepfather was great, so I didn't feel like I really missed out. But I know that at some point I really need to go back and figure out that piece.

RANDAL: What do you mean by "figure out that piece"?

CRAIG: Even though I understand the events, I don't feel anything. It's a complete block, like a gap in the tape.

RANDAL: Does this stem from the time your parents divorced or when he moved away?

CRAIG: Before he moved away I saw him on occasional weekends and did things with him, so we had a relationship.

RANDAL: Do you remember some of that?

CRAIG: I remember some of it.

RANDAL: Are your memories generally positive?

CRAIG: Yes, when I was with him it was generally positive. He remarried and I have some not so positive, negative, I guess, is another word for it (laughter), memories of my stepmother. I do have a memory of waiting on a Saturday morning on the porch steps for him and him not showing up.

RANDAL: Approximately how old were you when that happened?

CRAIG: Four or five.

RANDAL: How did you feel when he moved away?

CRAIG: I don't remember when I was first aware that he had moved away. I don't remember if he told me or if my mom did. That's really where it becomes unclear.

RANDAL: After he moved away did you see him a few times or not at all for that long period of time?

CRAIG: I don't remember seeing him for a few years. I remember getting cards or a couple of phone calls. It might have been more than that but I don't remember it.

RANDAL: How would you describe this gap that you feel?

CRAIG: Most of my life I didn't think about it at all. I thought it was just fine and everything worked out for the best. Now I'm trying to do more self-awareness work in my life and I've realized it's a kind of protective gap, like denial.

RANDAL: Do you see your father occasionally now?

CRAIG: Yes.

RANDAL: Is your relationship with him positive?

CRAIG: Yes, it's generally positive. I've tried to make sure that nothing with me kept him from having a relationship with my son. I felt like that would rob my son of a grandparent and that didn't seem fair. Mostly he tries too hard out of guilt, which is annoying to me, so I can only take him in bits and pieces. We've never really talked about it.

RANDAL: Is there anything further you'd like to say that might be important in terms of your father or your early childhood?

CRAIG: I have a sense that between my mom not really liking my father and my stepmother wanting a new life, that neither of my parents encouraged our relationship. I also feel that he should have been man enough to put our relationship first. Well, not first, but at least give it a high priority.

RANDAL: Are you ready for some hypnosis?

CRAIG: Yes. (Craig switches to a reclining chair)

RANDAL: I'd like you to look out here in front of you and follow my fingers as they move toward your face. Follow my fingers. (Randal's hand moves toward Craig's face in a spiraling downward motion) Feel your eyelids getting heavier and heavier until they close down. (Craig's eyes close) Turn those eye muscles loose. I'm going to count from five down to one and at the count of one your eyelids lock tightly closed. At the count of one you try to open them and you find that the harder you try the tighter they seal and the deeper into hypnosis you go. Number five, four, stuck tightly together. Three, sealed as though they were glued. Two, on the next number the harder you try the tighter they lock and the deeper into hypnosis you go. Number one, go ahead and try but they're stuck together. (Craig's face muscles tense) When I touch your right shoulder relax, stop trying, and go deeper. (Randal touches his shoulder and Craig relaxes)

Focus on your breathing, breathing down into your stomach. Feel yourself going deeper with every easy breath that you take. I'm going to lift up your left hand and you can let it hang loosely and limply in mine. I'm going to drop it into my other hand and when I do send a wave of relaxation down your body. Take a nice, deep breath and fill up your lungs. On the exhale send a wave of relaxation down your body and go much deeper. (Randal drops Craig's hand as he exhales) I'm going to do the same thing with your right hand. Take another nice, deep breath and on the exhale send a wave of relaxation down your body. (Randal drops his hand)

I'm going to do the same thing with your right foot. Take a nice, deep breath and fill up your lungs. On the exhale you go twice as deep, way down. (Randal drops the foot as Craig exhales) That's very good. Now the left foot. Take a nice, comfortable deep breath. As I drop your foot send a wave of relaxation down your body and go twice as deep. (Randal drops his foot)

Continue going deeper and deeper relaxed as I put your finger and thumb together. Imagine that I've placed a powerful epoxy glue between your finger and thumb and that glue is hardening as I speak. I'm going to count from three down to one and at the count of one you will find your thumb and finger stuck together. At the count of one you can try to pull them apart but you'll find that the harder you try the tighter they squeeze together and the deeper into hypnosis you go. Number three, stuck tighter and tighter, sealing as though they were one metal band. Number two, stuck tightly. Number one, go ahead and try to pull them apart but they're stuck tightly together until I snap my fingers. (Craig attempts to pull them apart) When I snap my fingers the glue instantly dissolves and the fingers separate as you go much deeper. (Randal snaps and Craig's fingers separate) As I stroke your finger and thumb take away any sensation of the glue. You feel complete relaxation in your finger and thumb, as you do throughout your body.

I'm going to do some questioning with finger signals now, Craig, as you continue to go deeper with every easy breath. (Craig's ideomotor responses are established with his right index finger signaling for "yes," his thumb signaling for "no," and his little finger signaling for "I don't know," followed by successful practice questions)

We're going to be focusing on your feelings and your relationship with your father. I'd like to check with your subconscious mind about the appropriateness of where to go with that. My first question is, in issues regarding your natural father, is it safe and appropriate for you to be open to any and all memories having to do with your father? (Craig's little finger moves) The answer to the question is "I don't know." That answer came up fairly quickly and that might be a signal from the conscious mind. Generally an "I don't know" response takes some searching to get a completely subconscious response. I'm going to ask the question again and just think about the question without trying to let any finger respond at first. It might be the "I don't know" finger or it might be one of the other fingers that wants to respond. The question I'm going to ask will be similar to what I just asked. Is it safe and appropriate for you to be open to any and all memories having to do with your natural father as we go back in time? (after a pause Craig's little finger moves) Okay, we're getting the "I don't know" finger. That's fine.

My next question is, is it appropriate now for you to be open to your emotions and your feelings in communicating with your father? (Craig's index finger moves) The answer to the question is yes. Rather than take you back to a specific memory I'd like to take you back to your feelings with your father as a child and have you dialogue with him about that. Then if we do focus on any memories, I'm instructing your subconscious mind to only bring up safe and appropriate ones for you.

Craig, I'd like you to imagine that there is an old-fashioned grandfather clock in front of you. One of those real old ones that show the month, day and year. Imagine as I count down from twenty to one that you're going to go back to your childhood, back to your feelings, back to your sense of being a young boy. Going back to a young age, perhaps the age of four or five or six. Or your subconscious mind might choose to go to a different age, whatever is appropriate. On number twenty as I count down, nineteen, eighteen, you begin to see the date spin backwards. The day of the month, the month, and then the year. Seventeen, sixteen, the years are beginning to go backwards. Fifteen, fourteen, thirteen, as you get younger and younger. Twelve, eleven, I'm not counting ages, I'm just counting down. Ten, nine, you're going back in time. You're going back before puberty, almost as if your body is becoming smaller. Eight, seven, six, going back in time. Five, four, going back to being a young boy. As you go back you're going to be meeting with your father and you'll be able to talk with him. Three, two, back to being a young boy. Number one, being a young boy, whatever age that you are.

I'd like you to bring your father here. Even though you're a young boy you can feel that you're in a safe and secure environment and you can say whatever you'd like to say to your father. I'm going to count from five down to one and at the count of one you can say whatever pops into your mind. Five, four, three, two, one. Go ahead and say it aloud.

CRAIG: You're the greatest.

RANDAL: That's wonderful. How old are you imagining yourself to be as you talk with your father?

CRAIG: Four.

RANDAL: At the age of four what did you call him? Dad or Daddy or Father or what?

CRAIG: Dad

RANDAL: So what does Dad say when you tell him, "You're the greatest."

CRAIG: I think you're the greatest.

RANDAL: Very good. Is there anything else you'd like to say to Dad? Just be your four year old self.

CRAIG: You're so fun.

RANDAL: So you love your dad. Does your dad love you? (Craig nods his head) That's good. You can really enjoy being with your dad. Now if you were going to ask him something, something you'd like him to do or something you'd like him to do differently, what would you like to say?

CRAIG: Spend more time with me.

RANDAL: At the age of four are you called Craig?

CRAIG: Yes.

RANDAL: So imagine yourself actually being Dad. How do you respond to Craig when he says he'd like you to spend more time with him?

CRAIG: I will...but I get busy. I enjoy being with you. It doesn't always work out that we can be together.

RANDAL: When I touch you on the shoulder again you'll switch and this time you'll be four year old Craig. (Randal touches his shoulder) You heard what your dad said. What kind of response do you have for him?

CRAIG: You're a liar.

RANDAL: Uh huh. We're starting to see a pretty feisty kid here. Tell him how he's lying.

CRAIG: If you wanted to be with me you would.

RANDAL: It's good to tell the truth. It's good to tell what you feel. You're doing well. As I touch you on the shoulder switch and hear what your dad has to say to that. (Randal touches his shoulder)

CRAIG: I don't have anything to say.

RANDAL: Well, your son just called you a liar. He said, "If you want to be with me you would." You don't have any response to that?

CRAIG: He's right.

RANDAL: Say that to your son.

CRAIG: You're right.

RANDAL: Switch and be Craig. (Randal continues to touch Craig on the shoulder when he switches between young Craig and his father) What do you want to say to that?

CRAIG: I don't understand. We have fun when we're together. It doesn't make sense. It doesn't add up.

RANDAL: Now let's switch and be Dad.

CRAIG: There's nothing I can say. I'm a chicken shit. I can't say that but that's what I think.

RANDAL: Switch and be Craig.

CRAIG: I guess that's the way it is. I wish it weren't.

RANDAL: Go inside your body. What do you feel inside your body right now?

CRAIG: The whole situation seems unreal. It doesn't make sense. I can't grasp it.

RANDAL: How is it that it doesn't make sense? It seems vague or...

CRAIG: ...a different reality.

RANDAL: It's a different reality as a child than as an adult?
CRAIG: I don't have the ability to comprehend it.
RANDAL: Let me just say that your subconscious mind is zeroing in on what you're doing and is comprehending a lot right now. You don't have to consciously comprehend various aspects, just trust that you're doing fine. Your subconscious mind is doing some good work with this. What I'd like to do now is bring in adult Craig. Of course, adult Craig, you've been hearing this dialogue. Who would you like to talk to right now? Four year old Craig or Dad?
CRAIG: I don't know.
RANDAL: Go inside your body. Are you aware of anything physical inside or outside your body?
CRAIG: My hands are sweaty. My breathing is shallow.
RANDAL: Adult Craig, what would you like to say to Dad?
CRAIG: You're right, you were a chicken shit but that was then. You let me down but I guess you're human. Don't make me keep feeling pain by annoying me with your guilt.
RANDAL: Switch. What does dad have to say in response?
CRAIG: The hell I've created for myself is not being able to make up for lost time.
RANDAL: Be adult Craig.
CRAIG: Get over it.
RANDAL: Tell him what you want from him. You can tell him something you said before that he didn't respond to, or you can say something different.
CRAIG: To say "I'm sorry" and get over it.
RANDAL: Switch and be dad.
CRAIG: It doesn't seem that easy.
RANDAL: So what is it that you want from Craig?
CRAIG: I don't know. He's not the problem.
RANDAL: So what's your problem?
CRAIG: I always look back at lost time. Can't get it back.
RANDAL: How does that feel?
CRAIG: Guilt. Like I blew it for him and for myself.
RANDAL: Switch to adult Craig. Are you losing time yourself with your son?
CRAIG: No.
RANDAL: Do you have a good relationship with your son?
CRAIG: Great.

RANDAL: Good.

CRAIG: I'm never going to let what happened to me happen to him.

RANDAL: There's still some resentment there toward your father. Here is a chance for you to get it out, to say something to your father about all those times he wasn't there for you.

CRAIG: I can't put it into words.

RANDAL: I bet you can. Some kind of words.

CRAIG: Self-centered, inconsiderate asshole.

RANDAL: Your father's response?

CRAIG: You're right. You didn't do anything wrong. I'm sorry, but that doesn't cover it. I do better looking forward.

RANDAL: Be Craig.

CRAIG: I'll believe it as I see it.

RANDAL: Is there anything further you have to say to your father right now about your resentment?

CRAIG: Just don't fuck it up with my son.

RANDAL: Switch and be your father.

CRAIG: I won't let it happen again.

RANDAL: Switch and be Craig.

CRAIG: That's good.

RANDAL: What is it that's missing? Maybe you just spelled it out crystal clear and maybe there's some kind of a twist on it, but you were talking before the hypnosis about this gap. Is this gap from your father not being there or what?

CRAIG: Keep talking.

RANDAL: You're doing great. Talk to that missing part that made you want to do this session. What do you want to say to it?

CRAIG: It's just an underlying feeling that I always had to push down. I didn't understand it and it seemed too painful. There's no one to talk to about it anyway.

RANDAL: That can get pretty lonely, can't it?

CRAIG: Yes.

RANDAL: As a young boy did you sometimes feel very lonely?

CRAIG: Sometimes.

RANDAL: How does it feel to be very lonely and not have someone to talk to?

CRAIG: Scared.

RANDAL: What do you feel in your body when you feel scared and lonely?

CRAIG: Imagination.

RANDAL: Do you mean it's more in your imagination than your body?

CRAIG: Yes.

RANDAL: What do you feel in your body right now?

CRAIG: Tight.

RANDAL: Where do you feel tight?

CRAIG: Chest...stomach...legs...hands...shoulders.

RANDAL: (putting a pillow in Craig's hands) I'm going to give you this pillow and I want you to use your hands to put that tightness into this pillow. (Craig squeezes the pillow with one hand) Breathe down into your stomach. Be that young boy and say to your father, "I resent you."

CRAIG: (small voice) I resent you.

RANDAL: Now squeeze that pillow with both hands. (Craig squeezes) Say "I resent you!"

CRAIG: (a little louder) I resent you.

RANDAL: Squeeze it tightly and look into your father's eyes and say, "I resent you!"

CRAIG: I resent you. (squeezing tightly)

RANDAL: Squeezing tighter, that's good. (pause) Okay, let go now (Randal takes the pillow) and go inside your body. Is it more tight or less tight? What's going on?

CRAIG: There's tightness.

RANDAL: I thought so. Where do you feel it? The same places?

CRAIG: My whole body.

RANDAL: Do you feel it more now or about the same or less?

CRAIG: There's a little more.

RANDAL: All right, here is your father. (Randal puts the pillow in Craig's hands again) All the different parts of you - four year old Craig, adult Craig, all of the ages in-between, are saying that he's not spending time with you. He's even saying it to himself. He's not there for you. Give him a good squeeze and tell him what it feels like to be lonely.

CRAIG: (starting to cry) You just don't leave a little boy sitting on the steps waiting for you.

RANDAL: Say that again to him.

CRAIG: (still crying) You just don't leave a little boy sitting on the steps. It's not right.

RANDAL: Yes, it's not right.

CRAIG: Be a man. Take care...take care of the people you're supposed to take care of.

RANDAL: What does he say?

CRAIG: He can't say anything.

RANDAL: He won't say anything. I bet he could.

CRAIG: (whispers) Yes, he can. He knows.

RANDAL: (taking the pillow) All right, let go. Go into your body. What do you feel in your body? You're breathing more deeply now.

CRAIG: I feel exhausted...but I feel good.

RANDAL: Do you feel less tightness?

CRAIG: No tightness.

RANDAL: Good. The golden rule of Gestalt, as you've all heard me say before, is to do unto others as you do unto yourself. Rather than tensing and tightening yourself you get it out of your system, you communicate physically and/or verbally and release that tension out of your body. (pause) I want to talk to four year old Craig who got left on the porch there. How are you doing, four year old Craig?

CRAIG: Fine.

RANDAL: Are you still out there on the porch or have you gone in? What's going on?

CRAIG: I'm going to go play.

RANDAL: You say you're doing fine but you were feeling a lot of pain a little while ago, weren't you?

CRAIG: It's gone.

RANDAL: It's gone because you squeezed it out or you communicated about it or because you're done with it or what?

CRAIG: It's fine.

RANDAL: Go inside your body. Is your body feeling fine now?

CRAIG: Uh huh.

RANDAL: You just did some very good work communicating that. Sometimes we can really push ourselves down and hold ourselves back. It's so good to get that out. (getting a large pillow and giving it to Craig) I'd like you to bring four year old Craig here, who has been waiting on the porch all that time. I'd like you to talk to four year old Craig. You can tell him whatever you'd like to say.

CRAIG: It's going to be okay.

RANDAL: Do you want to hold him as you say that? (Randal puts Craig's arms around the pillow) Say some more to him.

CRAIG: If you look at the end of the story it looks okay.

RANDAL: Talking to four year old Craig, you have a nice father right here taking good care of you now, don't you?

CRAIG: Yes.

RANDAL: Four year old Craig, what would you like to say to adult Craig?

CRAIG: I'm glad to be with you.

RANDAL: Be four year old Craig and feel how good it feels. As Wavy Gravy said, it's never too late to have a happy childhood. Four year old Craig, in the here and now you have a real good dad with you. I'm talking about adult Craig. (Craig is nodding) You know that. You're getting a lot of good loving attention right now. Is there anything you'd like from him or is there anything else you'd like to say?

CRAIG: Let's hang out together more. Don't be so busy. I enjoy your company.

RANDAL: Adult Craig, do you think that would be good for both of you?

CRAIG: Yes. We can always do it more.

RANDAL: What would you like to do more of with your inner child?

CRAIG: It's a way of just being.

RANDAL: Now four year old Craig, is there anything you'd like to add? Is there anything you'd like to do more of together besides what adult Craig was just saying?

CRAIG: It's being one person instead of two people.

RANDAL: So you're both talking about the same thing then, adult Craig and four year old Craig? You're talking about a way of being integrated?

CRAIG: Yes.

RANDAL: And you both understand exactly what that means?

CRAIG: Yes.

RANDAL: So that's some good integration. You can commit to this way of being that honors your adult and also the child within, and allows them both to get attention and pay attention and to be present and alive. Talking to four year old Craig now, I'd like to check that out with your finger signals. Do you have a good understanding about this way of being? (Craig's index finger moves) The answer is yes. And is that something you will make a commitment to, that way of being present and alive and all the different aspects of that?

CRAIG: Yes, but it's not easy. It takes work.

RANDAL: It's not easy to do, it takes work, but yes. Adult Craig, do you understand what this is about, this way of being in the world with the child within and with your adult self?

CRAIG: I already started that but it takes time.

RANDAL: You're in the process of discovering that way of being, that sense of awareness, is that correct? (Craig's index finger moves) Yes. Knowing it takes work at times, it's challenging, but it's something you will commit to, is that correct? (Craig's index finger moves) Yes, good. Adult Craig, is there anything further you want to say to your dad before you say goodbye to him?

CRAIG: No, I just feel pretty tired.

RANDAL: Four year old Craig, is there any further feeling that you have toward your father as you say goodbye to him?

CRAIG: It just feels familiar.

RANDAL: You've done some good work. Go inside your body. What do you feel right now?

CRAIG: It feels more relaxed than it did but there is still some lingering tension.

RANDAL: Where do you feel that lingering tension?

CRAIG: The same places but not as much. It feels a lot better.

RANDAL: That lingering tension might be something residual from all the energy you put into squeezing that pillow and so forth. It may just gradually dissipate. There may be some ongoing letting go that happens in the hours and days ahead. Some of that may be surprisingly easy, even happening without any effort whatsoever.

CRAIG: Tell it to keep happening.

RANDAL: I am happy to encourage your subconscious mind although I feel it would keep happening to some extent anyway. Talking to your subconscious mind, there is a process of letting go and moving on and integrating that is happening. And there may be a process here that includes a pleasant surprise. The things that seemed like they were hard work before may become easier. Your subconscious mind is learning a great deal. It's learning about letting go and discovering deeper joy and wonder. Some degree of that got lost from that child and the child within is beginning to gain it back.

There is a feeling of liberation in letting go of the difficulties from the past that were holding you back. Time is healing and that healing is dramatically accelerating now because of certain realizations in your subconscious mind. Your communication with your father, your decision to let go and move on, is occurring on a much deeper level than it did before. You may even realize you gained as a child by using the challenges that came up around your father as a way to strengthen yourself, to transcend circumstances and deal with adversity. You have gained flexibility and creativity as a result of dealing with the difficulties that you had as a child. This has helped you to be a much more powerful and compassionate person.

You are an excellent father, which you're understanding on a deeper level now. It goes far beyond the things that you missed from your father not being there, to a true deep feeling of joy and love between yourself and your son. There are no two ways about it, you love the time you spend together. You're developing even better balance in your life, more good attention as a father to him and as a father to yourself.

Deep down inside, Craig, your subconscious mind is learning more completely that what happened back then wasn't your fault. You didn't do anything wrong. You knew that intellectually before and now you are understanding it down to the essence of your soul, that you are a good, deserving, lovable person. Your inner child at all ages, two year old Craig, four year old Craig, six year old Craig, knows that you deserve great abundance and love and attention. You are understanding more deeply than before, more thoroughly, that what happened then had to do with the problems and difficulties of someone else and it wasn't about you. Even though you naturally felt the difficulty of it, it wasn't your fault. You are a very good, lovable, loving boy.

I'd like to add something on a personal note. I truly find you, Craig, to be a very kind, enthusiastic, giving, wonderful person. I remember during Level One that you sent an email to the school about your enthusiasm for the course. I was so touched by your loving and positive energy. I've felt that throughout the course from you. You have a very supportive presence in the class. There are a lot of good things coming your way and you deserve them all.

It always inspires me when someone who has gone through something really painful turns that around rather than continuing that on as an adult. It's certainly easy to understand how people do that, so it always inspires me when individuals transcend that. Part of that for you is giving your children the loving attention that you didn't have much of from your father. Your father did love you, but he often wasn't there for you. Your family and the world is a better place as a result of who you are. You are a very compassionate and caring person and you can give that kind of loving compassion to yourself on a regular basis.

In a little while I'm going to begin to help you come back to your full conscious awareness. Is there anything you would like to say or to ask before I do that?

CRAIG: No.

RANDAL: Are you continuing to feel better? (Craig nods) In a moment I'll count from one to five and all aspects of you are back here in 1999. Bringing back adult Craig and child Craig and all the different parts of you that are all one. You're coming back to your full conscious awareness. Number one, gently and easily coming back. Number two, more and more alert, awake, and aware with each number that I count. Number three, hearing the sounds around you, feeling your body resting comfortably. Number four, getting ready to open your eyes. On the next number you open your eyes and you are then fully alert, awake, and aware. Coming back, number five. Open your eyes and take a deep breath.

CRAIG: (opening his eyes) It's bright.

RANDAL: We're going to take a break in a minute. You don't have to say anything right now, just feel your aliveness and your body. Feel yourself fully back. Are you doing okay? (Craig nods) I'd like to acknowledge Craig for doing a fine job and staying with it. Thank you.

RANDAL: (after the break) During regression there can be a kind of dance of, "Where are we going to go from here?" For example, early on I could have gone straight to a memory with or without an affect bridge, but because he signaled that he didn't know if it was appropriate to get in touch with his memories, I decided to go directly to a Gestalt dialogue at the onset of the regression. We did a process of some Gestalt dialogue between the father and the son as a young boy and as an adult, which eventually included some Transactional Analysis in working with the adult and the child. Is there anything you'd like to say, Craig?

CRAIG: It's a little hard to come back into the class.

RANDAL: Yes, now you have to start using your left brain.

CRAIG: It was great.

RANDAL: You did a good job. Does anyone have any questions?

ANNIE: When Craig went back to talk to his father as a child was that a memory of what he actually said?

RANDAL: I was encouraging him to make up a dialogue about his feelings. He could have remembered something but the kind of dialogue that is created between the child and the parent is typically something that the child would not have said, or would not have gone into much detail about. We're creating a safe place for the child to communicate things that in many cases would not or could not have been said.

ANNIE: To create an atmosphere?

RANDAL: Partly to create an atmosphere for working out the unfinished stuff that was talked about and also to work with anything else that might be relevant. For example, at one point I checked with Craig to see if there was a lost time issue with his own son, as there is in his relationship with his father, and he didn't feel that. I asked almost in a suggestive way to help him find a similarity if there was one.

PETER: I noticed that when you were talking to the child you said to say, "I resent you," and I just wondered if a child wouldn't say something more like "I'm mad at you." Do you want to try to talk to the child in a way that a child would talk?

RANDAL: Usually I try to encourage the use of vocabulary to fit the age and the circumstances. "I'm mad at you" may be more how a child would talk, although in this case "I resent you" seemed to me to be a bit more accurate to the situation at that moment.

Interview One Week Later

RANDAL: Do you have anything to report since our session?

CRAIG: It's been subtle and it hasn't fully capsulated yet. I was extremely tired Sunday night and all day Monday. It was about Tuesday morning before I felt back on my feet, so the emotional experience required a lot of energy.

RANDAL: You were dealing with important issues and intense underlying emotions that go way back for you with your father. You made huge progress, and there's still some apparent resentment you're working through. It's not surprising that you felt pretty exhausted afterwards.

CRAIG: There are a couple of things I want to remember to tell you. One feeling that I think I described at the beginning of our session is that counselors in the past have said, "Let's deal with this," and I always said there was nothing there. I really did have a sense, and I don't think I completely understand it yet, that there was almost a puzzle shaped piece that was added back in after our session. I'm still waiting for the result of that to unfold for me, but that in itself is a huge first step.

RANDAL: There is often a process or a shift that is sometimes subtle at first but it's a sense that something is different. You can accelerate this process with your self-hypnosis work. It may be valuable to do a follow-up session eventually.

CRAIG: I feel like it's one of those paradigms where not feeling the pain keeps the pain alive and by accepting the pain it kind of goes away. It's something I can understand intellectually, but I haven't worked on it enough.

RANDAL: Are you saying that you're feeling more of a sense of peace as you're working things through and coming to a place of acceptance?

CRAIG: Absolutely, but I feel I'm at the beginning of understanding that. It's not in a way that I can really describe or articulate.

RANDAL: One thing I'll say is that describing or articulating it is not nearly as important as feeling it. This is just one week later and the update already is very positive.

CRAIG: Two more things come to mind. I feel like I have a clearer feeling that I got a lot of it out and that there is still some left. But I feel that having gotten the biggest chunk of it out will make the rest an interesting and doable process. It doesn't seem like such a huge mountain now and the momentum can help carry through the rest of the work.

RANDAL: You made major progress in the work we did. We don't have to go from A to Z all at once. For now it may be a matter of letting things sort themselves out and allowing more puzzle pieces to fit in place and become more apparent. I would recommend self-hypnosis to nurture that inner child and help him continue to feel the loving father that is there with him. You're moving in the right direction, so we'll see where it goes and whether we'll do some more work together later.

CRAIG: Thank you.

Commentary: Although Craig still had some resentment toward his father at the end of the session, Randal used the power of suggestion and positive thinking to encourage as much progress as possible independent of any further sessions. In the dynamics of the therapist-client relationship, it's important to be aware of the tremendous power mental expectancy can play. It is also important for the reader to understand that these are class demonstrations and generally not part of a series of sessions. The thoroughness of the work and the suggestions reflect that intent as well as the fact that most students have already being doing a lot of hypnosis both with themselves and others and can continue to reinforce their own work with subsequent self-hypnosis.

Follow-up Session Two Months Later

RANDAL: (to class) In our previous session Craig worked on issues regarding his father. His parents divorced when he was one year old and his father moved away from the area when Craig was five or six. There were issues of abandonment and resentment, including regarding a time when he waited for his father on the porch and he never showed up. (to Craig) We left it that you would continue to work things through on your own and possibly do some more session work later, and here we are. Bringing it up to the present, what's happening now?

CRAIG: A lot. After the last session it felt like a missing puzzle piece got locked back in. I guess the whole issue has been more at the forefront ever since. This is probably the most conscious I've ever been about that period of time.

RANDAL: Our work really opened things up. You accomplished a lot with this long-term issue, and there's still some unfinished stuff.

CRAIG: One other relevant thing is that in the last couple of months I've been going through marriage counseling with a psychologist. I mentioned to her what we had done in class and her comment was that there is an underlying element of pain that I bring into my intimate relationships, and the issue with my father is the source of that developmentally.

RANDAL: So all your life this underlying issue you felt about your absent father has affected your relationships, including your marriage? (Craig nods) I know you expressed some concern two months ago about wanting to be a good father and your feelings were influenced by what happened with your father. It's not surprising that an issue that runs as deeply as this would affect your relationship with your wife in various ways as well.

CRAIG: I think the pain she referred to is not something I'm really conscious of even when she says that, because I tend to be a very outgoing, get a lot of things done kind of a person. It was almost surprising and it took awhile for me to accept that she was on target.

RANDAL: Just because something is said by me or someone else doesn't automatically mean that it's an insight. It might be a projection or it may be off a little. Do you feel that what she said fits for you?

CRAIG: I think part of it does.

RANDAL: Taking the part that fits and focusing right now on your father, how do you feel? Have your feelings changed in any noticeable way since our session?

CRAIG: I used to refer to him as an annoying man because in thirty seconds on the phone, certainly without trying to, it was just really hard to be around him. I feel like a lot of the struggle seems to have gone away. He doesn't bother me so much.

RANDAL: This is obviously a sign of your progress. My feeling is that if you didn't have those issues with him and/or if it was someone else, the phone calls wouldn't bother you. Is that correct?

CRAIG: Definitely.

RANDAL: So what do you want to get out of this session now? Is there something that stands out or some kind of pain you're feeling about your father or your life?

CRAIG: I don't really feel like I know what it is yet...self-discovery, I guess. The psychologist said that I bring an underlying pain into my relationships that I'm not aware of. I think that might be true and I'd like to figure out more about that so I can stop doing it.

RANDAL: Can you be more specific? Does something come up in your relationship, whether or not you can see it, that's tied in with your father?

CRAIG: One thing is that I think I try too hard.

RANDAL: Well, this certainly ties in with your father. You have been really annoyed about how your father tries too hard to be nice and you can tell that he must feel guilty. Can you say something about how you try too hard? Are you trying to be extra nice or to please or to go out of your way or sacrifice yourself, something like that?

CRAIG: All of that.

RANDAL: How is that a problem? I think there are a lot of people who would say, boy, I'd like to have that problem with my spouse or significant other trying too hard to please. (laughter)

CRAIG: I had a one on one session with the psychologist and she asked, "Do you think you're a good spouse?" And I said, "Yes, I think I'm a great spouse," and she said, "Then how do you reconcile that with the difficulty you're having in your marriage?" And I can't, other than on the one hand I try too hard and on the other hand I'm sensitive to rejection. I think that the trying hard is going to somehow...

RANDAL: Keep you from getting rejected?

CRAIG: Right. This is probably clearer to you than it is to me. (laughing)

RANDAL: Having a distance can help us to have more perspective than if we're in the middle of it. Is your sensitivity to rejection part of the difficulty that brought you to the marriage counselor?

CRAIG: Yes, that and...how did she put it...that different people have different styles of loving and behaving and I tend not to be open to other styles. I have an idea of how it's supposed to be and if it doesn't fall within that framework I take it as rejection rather than just accepting that different people have other ways of doing things.

RANDAL: So there is still an issue of rejection and that's not surprising. In spite of all the good work you did in the session, in the dialogue with your father it felt like there was still some unfinished resentment. Is there anything else that you think might be useful before we do the hypnosis?

CRAIG: One thing is that I didn't feel I was as deep in hypnosis in our last session as I sometimes go. I was down, but I don't know if I didn't go as deep because there was a room full of people or because of my adrenaline, or whatever.

RANDAL: I'll do a little more deepening than I usually do, which may or may not make a difference. I wouldn't worry about depth when we're doing this, but I'm glad you brought it up. (Randal directs Craig into the reclining chair and looks at his notes) Okay, the thumb on your right hand is your "no" finger, your index finger is your "yes" finger, and your little finger is your "I don't know" finger. (Craig nods)

I'd like you to look into my right eye and take a nice, deep breath. Fill up your lungs and exhale slowly. (pause) Now take a second deep breath and switch your focus to my little finger. Follow my little finger down until your eyelids close down. (Craig's eyes follow the finger and close) I want you to turn those eyelids loose, limp and relaxed. I'm going to count from three down to one and at the count of one your eyelids lock tightly closed. Three, stuck tightly together. Two, sealing together as if they were glued. Number one, go ahead and try to open them but they're stuck tightly closed. (Craig's muscles tense) That's good, now relax, stop trying and go deeper.

I'm going to lift your right hand and drop it into my other hand and when I do send a wave of relaxation down your body. (Randal picks up Craig's hand and drops it as he exhales) And again I'll drop it and you go much deeper. (Randal drops his hand) Now I'll shake your hand and I'd like you to take a nice, deep breath and fill up your lungs. On the exhale (Randal pulls Craig's arm suddenly and simultaneously shouts), sleep! When I use the word "sleep" in this context, I'm referring to hypnotic sleep, the sleep of the nervous system. Now I'll do the same thing with the left hand. I'm picking up this hand and dropping it into my hand. (Randal drops Craig's hand as he exhales) I'm dropping it again into my other hand and you go much deeper. (Randal drops his hand) Take a nice deep breath and fill up your lungs. (Randal takes Craig's hand in his) And on the exhale just relax and (pulling his arm and shouting) sleep! Deeper and deeper relaxed.

I'm going to push down on your shoulders. Take a nice deep breath and fill up your lungs. On the exhale send a wave of relaxation down your body (Randal pushes down on Craig's shoulders as he exhales) and feel yourself go much deeper. As I rub your shoulders feel yourself go much deeper, way down. That's good.

I'm going to squeeze your index finger and your middle finger together. I'd like you to imagine that it's as if they were one single unit, such as a block of wood. I'm going to take my fingers away and count from three to one. At the count of one you'll try to pull these two fingers apart but you'll find that the harder you try the tighter they squeeze together and the deeper into hypnosis you go. Number three, stuck tightly together. Two, sealing together as though they were glued. Number one, go ahead and try but they're stuck together until I snap my fingers. (Craig tries) When I snap my fingers it's as though that glue instantly dissolves and they become two separate fingers again. Three, two, one (snap, Craig's fingers separate), and now they separate, taking away any sensation of glue or being stuck. You can feel the fingers are two entirely separate fingers again.

Relaxing deeper and deeper, perhaps on a beautiful beach of some kind, a local beach or a tropical beach. Just as the bright light of the sun could be relaxing for you as you're resting on the beach, so the lights of the room can be relaxing. Your whole body is turning loose and limp like a rag doll. Relaxing as though you're soaking up the sunshine.

As you continue to go deeper with every easy breath that you take I'm going to do a couple of practice ideomotor questions with you. This is a question for your finger signals. Was last year known as the year of the new millennium? (Craig's thumb moves) The answer is no. Is next year considered to be the year of the new millennium? (Craig's index finger moves) The answer is yes. Good.

Craig, we've been talking about issues regarding your father, issues of rejection and issues of trying too hard. I'd like to check with your subconscious about this. (Craig's ideomotor responses establish that it is it safe and appropriate to be open to any and all memories and emotions having to do with his issues of rejection)

I want to encourage you to know that whatever comes up, you are here in a supportive environment. You can take that understanding deep within to all parts of yourself. I want you to understand that you are going to do well. It'll work out fine. For now though, I want you to become aware of a feeling that sometimes causes you discomfort. I'm going to count from one to ten. With each number that I count you'll become aware of a feeling that you sometimes get. A feeling of rejection. It's an old feeling for you, a feeling that goes way back.

Number one, I'm counting upward now. Number two, with each number that I count you're becoming more aware of a feeling of rejection. Number three, a feeling you know. Number four, a feeling of abandonment. Number five, a feeling that is growing stronger. Number six, perhaps feeling it in some part of your body. A feeling of rejection. Number seven, feeling that feeling more and more strongly now. A feeling of rejection, perhaps feeling hurt. Number eight, feeling it more and more intensely in your body. Number nine, on the next number you're right there with that feeling of rejection, that feeling of abandonment. Number ten.

I'll count quickly down as you go back to an earlier time in your life when you felt that same feeling of rejection. Number ten, nine, stay with your feelings as you go back. Eight, seven, you're going back in time now. Six, five, you're getting younger. Four, going back before puberty. Three, your arms and legs are shrinking, getting smaller. You're whole body is getting smaller as your go back. Two, on the next number I count you're back to a time long time ago when you were feeling rejected. Number one. Where are you now? Inside or outside?

CRAIG: Outside.
RANDAL: Is it nighttime or daytime?
CRAIG: Daytime.
RANDAL: Are you alone or are there others?
CRAIG: I'm alone.
RANDAL: Are you under ten years old? Yes or no.
CRAIG: Yes.
RANDAL: Are you under five years old?
CRAIG: Yes.
RANDAL: Are you under three years old?
CRAIG: No.
RANDAL: How old are you?
CRAIG: Four.
RANDAL: Where are you outside?
CRAIG: On the porch.
RANDAL: You're four years old, you're on the porch alone, and it's daytime. How are you feeling?
CRAIG: Everything seems so vast and empty. It stretches on forever.
RANDAL: When you say everything, do you mean looking out or is it emotions that you're feeling?
CRAIG: The world seems bigger and it seems empty.
RANDAL: What makes the world feel so empty?
CRAIG: It seems like there is no one in it.
RANDAL: Have you been on the porch for a long time or not?
CRAIG: I'm not sure.
RANDAL: Does it seem like a long time?
CRAIG: It seems like forever.

RANDAL: What are you doing on this porch? Are you there for a particular reason?

CRAIG: I'm walking on the grass.

RANDAL: Is this the same scene? You've been on the porch and now you're walking on the grass?

CRAIG: I'm not sure.

RANDAL: How do you feel as you're walking on the grass?

CRAIG: I keep looking.

RANDAL: What are you looking for?

CRAIG: Any people.

RANDAL: How old are you as you're walking on the grass and looking for people? Are you four or another age?

CRAIG: Four.

RANDAL: Are you walking on the grass near your porch or somewhere else?

CRAIG: My front yard.

RANDAL: Are you looking for anyone in particular?

CRAIG: Anybody.

RANDAL: How do you feel as you're walking on the grass looking for just anybody?

CRAIG: The world seems too big.

RANDAL: If the world seems too big how do you feel?

CRAIG: Small.

RANDAL: Is there some particular reason why you're out here like this or did you just go out here to look around?

CRAIG: (after a pause) I'm not sure.

RANDAL: I'd like to do finger signals now for your subconscious mind to give us some understanding. I know you're out on the grass but I want to ask about the porch for now. Does this have to do with the time that four year old Craig is waiting for his father and he doesn't show up? It may or may not have to do with this, I'm just asking your subconscious mind. (Craig's index finger moves) Okay, I see your "yes" finger. Does this feeling of the world seeming so big, does this have to do with this particular time that you waited for your father for a very long time and he never came? (Craig's index finger moves) The answer is yes. Does the image of you walking on the grass and looking around and the world seeming so big, not seeing anybody and feeling so alone, is that from this same experience when you're waiting for your father when you're four years old and he never comes? (Craig's index finger moves) The answer is yes, it's from the same experience. (taking Craig's hands and pulling his arms up in the air) I want you to reach out like this. You can hold your arms up (Randal lets go and Craig's arms stay outstretched) and say, "Dad, where are you?"

CRAIG: (in a little voice) Dad, where are you?
RANDAL: Do you hear him respond in some way?
CRAIG: No.
RANDAL: Ask him again.
CRAIG: Dad, where are you?
RANDAL: All right, rest your arms down and go inside your body. What do you feel right now? Do you notice anything in particular?
CRAIG: My heart is pounding...I can feel my pulse in my arms and my legs.
RANDAL: Is there anything else that you notice?
CRAIG: Kind of vibrating.
RANDAL: Where are you vibrating?
CRAIG: My arms and hands...
RANDAL: Are your legs vibrating?
CRAIG: I meant my legs and hands...excitability.
RANDAL: When you say excitability, do you mean that you feel excited?
CRAIG: Yes.
RANDAL: Okay, that's a good report. Keep breathing down into your stomach and feel your feelings. (pause) You're waiting and waiting for your father and looking around and the world seems so big and so empty. Use your finger signals. Is this feeling something that you've felt before? This feeling of the world seeming so big and you being so small and alone? (Craig's index finger moves) The answer is yes. Have you felt this painful feeling of aloneness at least as strongly as this before? (Craig's index finger moves) The answer is yes. This memory of being on the porch is a very important memory, but is there some memory that would also be important to go to that goes back even further? (Craig's index finger moves) The answer to the question is yes.

All right, get in touch with this feeling, Craig. The world seems so big and you feel so small and alone. You're feeling rejected, feeling sad. The world is empty and there is no one there for you. I'm going to count from five down to one and you're going to go back to an even earlier time when you felt similar kinds of feelings. Stay with the feeling of rejection. It's a big, empty world. There is nobody there for you. Five, four, going back even further in time. Three, two, going back in time. Number one, getting clear where you are now. You're feeling all alone. Feeling rejected. Are you inside or outside?

CRAIG: Inside.

RANDAL: Is it nighttime or daytime?

CRAIG: Daytime.

RANDAL: Are you under three years old, yes or no?

CRAIG: Yes.

RANDAL: Are you under two years old?

CRAIG: Yes.

RANDAL: Are you under one year old?

CRAIG: About one.

RANDAL: Where are you? Are you in your house or somewhere else?

CRAIG: My mom's apartment.

RANDAL: Do you know what room you're in?

CRAIG: Between the kitchen and the family room.

RANDAL: Are you on the floor or a bed or what? Do you know where you are?

CRAIG: On the carpet on the floor.

RANDAL: Is there anybody there with you in the room?

CRAIG: No.

RANDAL: Is there anybody there in the house with you?

CRAIG: No.

RANDAL: How do you feel as you're all alone there on the carpet?

CRAIG: Scared.

RANDAL: Are you expressing your fear in some way? Are you making any sound or are you crying?

CRAIG: Crying...looking around.

RANDAL: You're crying and looking around and nobody is there. Do you have any idea how long you've been alone here?

CRAIG: I was just coming out of a nap.

RANDAL: So feel this fear. You're only about one year old and you wake up from a nap and you're all alone. It's very frightening and you're crying. Is anybody coming?

CRAIG: Not for some time.

RANDAL: Eventually someone comes. Was it a long time to you?

CRAIG: Yes.

RANDAL: Eventually who is it that does come?

CRAIG: My mom.

RANDAL: She comes in and you've been all alone and crying. What happens?

CRAIG: She puts down her groceries and picks me up. It's fine.

RANDAL: You're feeling fine now?

CRAIG: Yes.

RANDAL: Does she seem to be concerned that you're alone and she's trying to take good care of you now?

CRAIG: She doesn't understand.

RANDAL: Your mom isn't aware of how terrified you were when you were all alone, which is a normal response for a baby. If you could talk, what would you say to her?

CRAIG: Just that I got scared.

RANDAL: You got very scared. If you could somehow communicate that to her, what does she say in response?

CRAIG: She explains that she just ran to go to the store and she thought I would be asleep.

RANDAL: Do you want to tell her how you feel?

CRAIG: You still don't understand how I felt.

RANDAL: Be your mother and respond to your baby who is trying to communicate with you about how very scared he was that you were gone.

CRAIG: Everything's fine.

RANDAL: Be Craig. How does that feel when she says that everything is fine?

CRAIG: I understand. Everything is fine.

RANDAL: And in the here and now everything has become fine. For awhile it wasn't fine and that's a feeling that happened to you at various times when you were very young. It happened at that point when you were only a year old and it happened when you were four years old.

CRAIG: That wasn't fine.

RANDAL: Let's go to the time when that wasn't fine. You've had this very frightening feeling before when you were very young and terrified of being alone. Now you're four years old, still very young, and you're having a similar feeling of being all alone and the world seems so big. You have a link with that earlier feeling that happened at least one time and may have happened more than once. It's a feeling that runs deep. You're four years old now and you've been waiting and waiting for your father and he still doesn't show up. If you could bring him here what would you say to him?

CRAIG: It feels like everyone was gone.

RANDAL: Switch and be your father. What does he say in response to that?

CRAIG: My mom and step-dad left the house and I was on the porch.

RANDAL: What is his response?

CRAIG: He didn't know that everyone would be gone.

RANDAL: Switch.

CRAIG: Be reliable.

RANDAL: What does your father say in response to that?

CRAIG: He looks confused.

RANDAL: Be four year old Craig and tell your father how you feel.

CRAIG: It seems too overwhelming.

RANDAL: What do you feel in your body right now?

CRAIG: Sweaty and cold at the same time.

RANDAL: Do you notice any other feelings in your body anywhere?

CRAIG: It feels like...excitability.

RANDAL: Where do you feel that excitability?

CRAIG: All over.

RANDAL: So feel that excitability. And you say it feels overwhelming to say how you feel. How would you act if you were feeling overwhelmed right now?

CRAIG: It seems like I'd explode.

RANDAL: What would you do if you exploded at your father?

CRAIG: It seems impossible to communicate how it felt.

RANDAL: (to the class) Is there a pillow in the room? (there is no pillow) That's interesting. That's never happened before. (someone hands Randal a folded jacket) Breathe down into your stomach. I want you to tell your father off. Criticize your father for leaving you alone.

CRAIG: I wish that I could take the pain and put it inside of him so that he could see how it feels.

RANDAL: Okay, here he is. (Randal hands Craig the folded jacket) I want you to find a way to put it inside of him. (Craig starts to squeeze the jacket) You want to squeeze it into him? Okay, squeeze it into him.

CRAIG: I'm imagining it into him.

RANDAL: Good, feel all that pain that you're taking through your body and out into your shoulders to your arms and your hands and put all of that pain into him there. Do you want to put it into some part of him or all over or what?

CRAIG: His head and his heart.

RANDAL: Okay, so here's his head. (tightening Craig's hands on the jacket) Put that pain into his head and say, "I hate you."

CRAIG: I hate you.

RANDAL: Good, now put that pain into his heart and say, "I hate you."

CRAIG: I hate you! (starting to push his hands forcefully into the jacket)

RANDAL: (loudly) Push it into him! That's good! Push it all into him! (pause, voice softening) Now breathe and relax. (taking the jacket away) What do you feel in your body now?

CRAIG: My heart beating in my head.

RANDAL: Where in your head is it beating?

CRAIG: The top and sides.

RANDAL: Do you notice anything else?

CRAIG: No, but I feel good.

RANDAL: How do you feel good?

CRAIG: Relaxed.

RANDAL: Are you feeling more relaxed than before?

CRAIG: And not excitable.

RANDAL: So you got the excitement out of your system. You were just feeling this pain in you and you put that pain that your father deserved into him. Is there anything further that you'd like to say to him?

CRAIG: He disappeared.

RANDAL: He seems pretty good at disappearing so let's bring him back. (pause) Is he back?

CRAIG: Yes.

RANDAL: So what does your father say in response to all this energy you just gave him? The pain and the anger and the hatred that you put into his head and his heart.

CRAIG: He's kind of blubbery.

RANDAL: Maybe he doesn't have anything particular to say. Maybe he just needs to cry right now. Be your father and feel what it feels like to have been in this position, to have abandoned your son and how upset your son is. Do you have anything to say?

CRAIG: It's current time.

RANDAL: By current time do you mean it's 1999?

CRAIG: Yes.

RANDAL: Where are you? Are you with your father in 1999 or is there something else going on now?

CRAIG: He's saying that he's trying to be better.

RANDAL: Respond.

CRAIG: I understand that you're trying. You can't erase the past but at least you're doing something about it right now.

RANDAL: Switch and be your father.

CRAIG: I am trying and I know that you won't let me in. It seems like no matter how hard I try you'll never let me in.

RANDAL: Switch and be Craig.

CRAIG: I like watching you try.

RANDAL: What it is that you like about watching him try?

CRAIG: Punishment.

RANDAL: So tell your father that. "I like watching you try because I feel like you're getting punished for what you've done."

CRAIG: I like watching you try sometimes. I like seeing you punished. Other times I just like to be away.

RANDAL: Switch and be your father.

CRAIG: I want to try but I get discouraged. I get really sad. You don't know how sad I am...and how sorry.

RANDAL: Switch and be Craig.

CRAIG: I do know.

RANDAL: Is there anything further you want to say about that?

CRAIG: Maybe someday I'll get tired of wanting to punish you but it hasn't happened. It should stop.

RANDAL: Gestalt founder Fritz Perls said that "should is shit." Don't tell yourself what you should do. What I'm concerned about is, who is getting hurt more by your continued anger toward your father? Is there some way that you punish yourself by doing that?

CRAIG: It avoids pain. And something else. I'm not sure what.

RANDAL: Is it worth it to hold on to your resentment toward your father?

CRAIG: It's not worth it. It's too much energy...too much pain in my chest. It's tight.

RANDAL: Feel that tightness in your chest, Craig. Tighten it more. I want you to really feel it so you know what you're talking about. (pause) Now I want you to put that tightness into your father. (putting the jacket into Craig's hands) Here's another chance. Go ahead. You've been holding onto a lot of stuff. Put that tightness into his chest. This is another chance to punish him. (Craig squeezes the jacket) That's good. Go ahead and get it out of your system. Say, "I hate you!"

CRAIG: (strong voice) I hate you!

RANDAL: That's good. Say it again!

CRAIG: I hate you!

RANDAL: Good. Getting it all out. Put it all in there. Go inside your body now. What do you feel?

CRAIG: My heart beating in my chest.

RANDAL: You're feeling that more. You weren't feeling that before, were you?

CRAIG: No.

RANDAL: How does your chest feel?

CRAIG: Fine.

RANDAL: You were feeling some tightness before and now you don't have it, is that right?

CRAIG: It felt like a wad of black.

RANDAL: How does your chest feel now?

CRAIG: It feels strong.

RANDAL: Okay, look at your father. What do you want to say to your father?

CRAIG: He disappeared. Can't picture him. It just seems like he disappeared.

RANDAL: That's fine.

CRAIG: He's back.

RANDAL: What do you say?

CRAIG: I'd like to feel glad when I hear your voice on the phone.

RANDAL: What does your father say?

CRAIG: I'd like that, too. I'd like it if you were glad...I'd like it if he would stop trying so hard.

RANDAL: Who is that talking?

CRAIG: Craig.

RANDAL: Tell that directly to him. "I'd like you to stop trying so hard."

CRAIG: It would help if you would let go and stop trying so hard.

RANDAL: Switch and be your father.
CRAIG: It's hard to let go but I want to.
RANDAL: What would you like from Craig?
CRAIG: Keep giving me a chance so that we can have a normal relationship, whatever that is.
RANDAL: Switch and be Craig.
CRAIG: I'd like to do that. I'm not sure where the balance point is but I'd like to be honest and let you know when I find that balance.
RANDAL: Be your father. How do you feel about what Craig just said?
CRAIG: I feel all right.
RANDAL: Is there anything further you'd like to say to Craig?
CRAIG: I'd like a fresh start...as much as possible.
RANDAL: Switch and be Craig. How do you respond to that?
CRAIG: Even normal parents are wrong sometimes.
RANDAL: So you're reminding him of that.
CRAIG: Even the best parents are wrong sometimes.
RANDAL: You're reminding yourself of that, too. Dealing with reality.
CRAIG: (laughing) All of us are well aware of that.
RANDAL: Switch and be your father.
CRAIG: I wish that it could be more but I'll have to live with it.
RANDAL: Be Craig. Is there anything you want to say in response to him?
CRAIG: No.
RANDAL: Is there any final statement to your father?
CRAIG: It's all been said.
RANDAL: Look at your father and tell him how you feel about him right now.
CRAIG: You're actually a pretty nice guy.
RANDAL: Be your father. Is there any last statement you'd like to say to Craig?
CRAIG: I wish I could do more during your hard times. It doesn't matter to me whether you do good or bad.
RANDAL: Be Craig. Any response to that?
CRAIG: No. Just a statement to myself.
RANDAL: And that is?
CRAIG: Just for the realization of trying too hard, trying to be good.
RANDAL: Can you say goodbye to your father for now?

CRAIG: 'Bye.

RANDAL: Father, can you say goodbye to Craig now?

CRAIG: 'Bye and thank you.

RANDAL: Do you want to thank your father?

CRAIG: (laughing) Yeah, thanks.

RANDAL: Very good. You've come a long way with this process. Can you feel ways in your life that you can identify deeper realizations about letting go and not trying so hard?

CRAIG: Yes.

RANDAL: You've been working through some resentment still left after the first session and getting improvement in your relationship with your father. You've come a lot further. I want to encourage you to have a lightness of being, an expansiveness in your chest and in your heart. You are understanding more deeply that the more you can let go and move on, Craig, the more you're doing for yourself and the more you stop punishing yourself. It's a real irony about life that when we hang onto feeling vengeful or hurtful or wanting to punish someone else, we often hurt ourselves at least as much as the other person. I want you to recognize deep down that you really do love yourself. You can be good to yourself and let go of those feelings toward your father and forgive him. A lot of people in a situation like his might have acted a lot worse or not cared enough to try to make up for it.

By forgiving him you are most importantly forgiving yourself. When a child feels abandoned the feeling inside is, to some degree, a feeling of not being deserving. "This happened because something about me is not okay." I want you to know that you are okay. You deserve love and affection and approval. You've got a wonderful life and you're a wonderful husband and father. As you understand that deep down in your heart it helps you to take in even more, Craig, all the love that is there for you.

There is a tremendous amount of acceptance and appreciation around you. The more you accept that and open up, the more you feel deeply fulfilled and satisfied within. You don't have to try hard. Just be yourself. You are a lovable person just being who you are. If you want to do something for someone you do it just because you want to, not because you're nervous about being rejected, whether it be with your wife or your child or anyone else.

And sometimes you do really good things for yourself, just taking care of yourself. You have an abundance of many things, including people who are there for you. You can trust them and you can be there for yourself, too. Deep down inside that child is recognizing that he deserves to have plenty of attention. He can't always have attention, that's life. But you are giving that child within you plenty of attention. Is there anything you would like to say or to ask before coming out of the hypnosis?

CRAIG: Self-soothing. Inviting myself to be soothing to myself, rather than others.

RANDAL: Yes, you recognize that you sometimes need to be able to put yourself first. You're a good father and you're a good person but you need balance in life. Sometimes you put yourself first and take care of yourself. You recognize that other people sometimes need to do that for themselves too. It's part of the ebb and flow of balance in life and relationships. Is there anything else that you want to say?

CRAIG: No.

RANDAL: (Randal gives suggestions to help Craig gradually come out of hypnosis and Craig opens his eyes) How are you doing?

CRAIG: Fine.

RANDAL: Is there anything you'd like to say about any aspect of the session?

CRAIG: It seems like there was more revelation this time. More going on inside. I wish I had all the thoughts and images on videotape, too.

RANDAL: (laughing) Yes, I really felt that there was some shifting going on as things were developing. It felt like the times when you put that energy into your father you were really releasing a lot from yourself. The irony is that by getting all of that negativity out of the way you can feel what's beneath that. Among other things, your father is a pretty nice guy after all. We'll take a break now and then come back.

RANDAL: (after a break) How was your depth of hypnosis this time? Was it the same or different?

CRAIG: It was much deeper. And our conversation before the hypnosis tonight was like priming the pump. Revelations and understandings were pouring in during the hypnosis. It was almost overwhelming how much revelation I got.

RANDAL: Do you want to describe any of that?

CRAIG: There were pieces that were totally new this time. I knew I had been on the porch waiting for my father but I hadn't remembered any details, like being on the grass. All of a sudden the front lawn and the street went all the way to the horizon. It was like a movie, not like reality.

RANDAL: You did some really good work here. Does anyone have any questions for Craig?

BARBARA: Do you think the next time you have a conversation with your father it might be different?

CRAIG: It doesn't seem like it'll be one hundred percent different but it seems like it might be better.

RANDAL: Of course you have memories and habits, which you will continue to work with, but I think you may be surprised at two things. First, I feel that you made a real shift deep down and you might be surprised at some differences there. (Craig laughs and Randal laughs with him) In spite of yourself. And secondly, I think this process will continue to develop.

CRAIG: It feels like a beginning.

RANDAL: Definitely. Anybody else?

SUSAN: I'm curious that your mom would leave you alone as a one year old and then that your mother and step-father would leave you alone at four. I would think there would be some issues with your mother as well. Randal, could you say something about why you didn't explore that direction further?

RANDAL: I had him dialogue with his mother and he quickly worked through that. I'm not looking for or trying to make a judgment about who did what to Craig when he was a child. The great irony about the value of regression is that it's all about what the person is bringing into the here and now. Craig made a telling comment after his terrifying experience as a one year old being left all alone. He said he was fine now with his mother but not with his father. What happened with his father being gone was not okay but with his mother, she made a mistake and he can accept it. That's something I'm not here to judge.

SUSAN: It just seemed that the abandonment issues with his mother may be carrying through into the here and now.

RANDAL: Well, let's check it out. (to Craig) Do you have any response to that?

CRAIG: It seems clear that when she was single, it was just her and me, it was a frantic situation of, "I forgot something at the store." It didn't seem that bad.

RANDAL: The abandonment issues had been carrying through to the here and now, but the blame was toward the father.

SUSAN: What about when you were four and your mom left you there alone before your dad didn't show up?

CRAIG: Well, at that time it seemed like everyone had abandoned me. I was kind of mad that I couldn't go back inside the house even and I wasn't sure I wanted to because I might miss my dad. But I was also looking across the street to where my friends lived and no one was outside. There wasn't a car on the road. I felt like the whole world abandoned me, not just my dad.

RANDAL: You made that very clear and I continued focusing on your dad because that was the one that was continuing to the present.

NANCY: Do you usually focus on just one of the parents?

RANDAL: I don't necessarily focus on just one. In this particular case the feeling of abandonment was coming from all over. It wasn't just the mother and the step-father, but the kids across the street and the whole world that were gone. No one was there or even driving by. But the big feeling was dealing with his father who he already had an issue with at that point.

KAREN: In relation to the mother and father issue, Craig's mom never did actually leave. She went to the store but Craig was with his mom all the time and his dad had literally left.

RANDAL: Yes, his mother was consistently with him when he was growing up and this one time she left for a little while because she thought she could get away with it. She made a mistake, but she came right back. Thank you, Craig.

Interview One Year Later

RANDAL: I've been reviewing the transcripts of our sessions. To summarize, the issue was your father's absence, not being there for you, highlighted by an experience at age four of you waiting for him on the porch for a very long time but he never showed up. In the first session you made some good progress and in the second session we did further work with that, including the discovery of a major earlier similar experience. You re-experienced a vast, fearful emptiness as a baby when you woke up from a nap and your mom wasn't there. You had been terrified for what seemed like a long time until she returned. You quickly worked through that scene with your mom and we returned to the ongoing issue with your dad.

It was important, I feel, to have gone to and worked through the initial sensitizing event, as well as the secondary reinforcing event with your father. At the end of that second session you talked about getting a lot more realizations as well as the much more detailed recall. Can you give us an update?

CRAIG: First of all, I've been in counseling at various points in my life, including marriage counseling, and a family history would always be taken. I'd say my parents were divorced when I was one and my dad left the area when I was five and the therapist would say that's a crucial issue, we can work on that more. Then I would say, "No, that's not an issue." (laughing) Clearly it's an issue, but to me it was a non-issue until recently. I really believed then that that would be a waste of time and energy. Now the pendulum has swung from denial to acknowledgment. I talk about it and if someone brings up a similar kind of thing I don't mind throwing my experience out on the table. I've told my son about it, not in a big, overly dramatic way, but he knows. Now it's part of my experience.

RANDAL: How old is your son?

CRAIG: He's twelve. Since our sessions I moved away from the Bay Area but I really worked hard to keep that connection with my son and spent a lot of time on the road going back and forth to keep that alive. I've since moved back to spend more time with him. Another big piece of that is that my father came back into my life when I was in my twenties and I think I referred to him as annoying then.

RANDAL: (laughing) You certainly did. Partly because he would try too hard. Then lo and behold, that was an issue for you also, about trying too hard in relationships. In our second session you brought up that you were in counseling, trying to deal with the relationship with your wife and maybe your son as well.

CRAIG: Another part of it is that I'm not trying so hard anymore. Things seem to work much better by keeping more balance and letting people like me sometimes and not like me at other times, and that's just fine.

RANDAL: That's terrific. Seeing how far you've come, it's clear that certain difficulties you've had in relationships in your life have to do with this unfinished pain that went back to your father. You weren't recognizing it but it was apparent to your counselor and perhaps to others in your relationships.

CRAIG: Everyone in the room that day got it. As I was telling the story I was watching people going, "Oh, brother." I was the last one in the room to figure it out. Another thing, too, that is a result of this, is that I've spent the majority of my life either in a relationship, or to use an archaic term, chasing skirts. I was always looking for a relationship and in pursuit all the time.

RANDAL: Yes, not feeling like you could own it. Even when you had attained it, maybe you still felt like you weren't there. For those who have unresolved abandonment issues, even when they have attained everything, there can be this feeling of being afraid that they're going to lose it. In your case that was the part of you that was trying too hard, just like your father was doing, to try to make things work out.

CRAIG: Right, and I don't feel that anymore.

RANDAL: That's great.

CRAIG: That's really great!

RANDAL: (to the class) Are there any questions for Craig?

NANCY: When you said you were chasing women, was that related to abandonment by your mother? You were going to keep chasing after women because she abandoned you?

CRAIG: No, not really. It was more like Randal said. There was a missing piece and I wasn't dealing with that missing piece. I was out doing things to keep busy and keeping my emotions busy. I was doing things in relationships on a superhuman level, going overboard, which is what I hated about my dad. I was acting that out.

RANDAL: Fine job, Craig. Thank you.

CHAPTER 20

Gerrie's Fear of Abandonment

A Year in a Drawer

The important issue of abandonment has been a significant factor in several of the cases in this book, and was the primary issue for Craig in the previous chapter. This session regards a more severe abandonment history than Craig's, but with a client who, in spite of her residual fears, had already progressed a long way in overcoming many of the effects of this trauma.

RANDAL: (calls on Gerrie, who has raised her hand to volunteer for a session in class) Come up and have a seat, Gerrie. You wrote me a letter saying you wanted to do some therapy with me. Is this going to be about the issues you discuss in the letter?
GERRIE: Yes.
RANDAL: Go ahead and tell us what you'd like to work on.
GERRIE: Well, it all happened when you worked with Liz and she went into an age regression. As she started to go back in time I started to panic. I didn't understand what was going on with me. I was so uncomfortable that I wanted to leave the room. I thought, well, that's crazy. I better stay and see what's going on. (to Liz) Some of the insights came to me while you were talking to your mother in the session. Then more insights came after I talked to my husband and later during that night.
I've worked a lot on healing because I was abandoned when I was five weeks old. My mother and father both left their homes when they were young and met in Denver. They got married but didn't tell either of their families. Then they had me and the

depression hit. My mother took me to a neighbor's house when I was five weeks old and then she had a truck come and pick up all the furniture, which she sold to get enough money to go to Chicago. When my father came home that night a very angry neighbor handed him a little crying baby and he didn't know what to do. He told me later on there was only a dresser left in the apartment and our clothes.

My father kept me until I was nearly a year old. Then he swallowed his pride and went to his great aunt who lived in Denver and asked her if she would take me and raise me and she said yes. She hadn't seen him since he was a young boy and didn't even know I existed until that day. The reason he took me to her is that I was dying. My great aunt brought me to the doctor and the doctor confirmed this, saying I would be dead in a week. So here I am. (applause) Well, I've had to do a lot of healing up to the time my great aunt took me. I've also done some healing work to forgive my mother, but it dawned on me that I don't know what happened to me within that length of time.

RANDAL: Which length of time? From the time your mother left until you were taken to your aunt?

GERRIE: Yes. I had such feelings during Liz's session of danger and foreboding and wanting to leave the room and all, that I think I've not thoroughly examined that period. I'm not sure I want to.

RANDAL: Well, you've done a lot of work on yourself. Do you know why the doctor said you only had a week to live? Was there some kind of diagnosis?

GERRIE: What they call it now is failure to thrive. I couldn't lift my head. My whole buttock area was raw because diapers hadn't been changed, things like that. I was too weak to lift my head until I was much older. I didn't walk until I was a year and a half. I hadn't gained much weight and I was still very tiny.

RANDAL: So you weren't eating properly and so forth?

GERRIE: Well, my dad says that he kept me in the bottom drawer for a long time and went to work for ten hours a day. That was back when people worked ten hours a day instead of eight. And for the first couple of weeks he didn't know what to do so he got a can of condensed milk and an eye dropper and was feeding me that. By the time my great aunt took me I couldn't tolerate milk at all so I was raised on vegetable juice.

RANDAL: As I'm getting a sense about your terrible experiences, to have to survive such abandonment and such a difficult infancy, I want to say that people don't have to necessarily recall major traumas in therapy. The purpose would be if there is still a problem that is affecting you in your life now. The fact that Liz's regression to early childhood triggered your feelings of foreboding and danger is an apparent sign that this hasn't been completely resolved for you. Besides this example, are there other times when you feel excessively or inappropriately in danger or when you feel not really fully alive?

GERRIE: I feel the danger just before I do something big in my life and I've been able to overcome that pretty well, but I've often wondered why it's there. Why is the danger so bad that I want to run and escape, and why do I have to work so terribly hard on doing some of the good things I want to do? Things that are accomplishments. In some of my other work on healing of memories I've often thought it was because my great aunt, who I call Mom, would always say, "Oh no, you can't do that." She was so afraid something would happen to me and my dad would blame her.

RANDAL: So she was over protective?

GERRIE: Yes, but now I don't think it's that so much. I think it's maybe some of this danger I feel that's coming up. I mean I really felt that.

RANDAL: You've already come a long way in your life. I feel this is residual stuff, which is miraculous, considering your early experiences. Who you are, what you've done and how comfortable you are in life and with yourself, it's obvious that you've done tremendously well considering the terrible traumas you went through. But there is this matter of getting rid of that feeling of danger and of feeling that much more alive. We can explore this and get a sense from your subconscious mind about whether to further expunge this in order to help you release it, or if the part you're still in touch with could possibly be beneficial to you. Does that sound good?

GERRIE: Yes.

RANDAL: Tell me again the feeling you got in touch with when Liz was going back in regression. You referred to a feeling of foreboding and danger.

GERRIE: Yes. I've had those feelings before but this time when she was going back I wanted to scream. I could hear the scream in my head and that frightened me.

RANDAL: There's definitely some unfinished stuff here. We'll check it out with your subconscious mind and see if this is a good time to work further on it. Do you use your right hand or your left hand for ideomotor?

GERRIE: My right.

RANDAL: (Randal motions to the mat and helps Gerrie to lie down) Are you ready?

GERRIE: I'm ready.

RANDAL: (leads Gerrie into hypnosis with rapid induction methods) I'd like you to put your attention on your right hand, Gerrie. (Gerrie's ideomotor signals designate her index finger as "yes," her thumb as "no," and her little finger as "I don't know")

Now if your subconscious mind doesn't know how to properly answer a question or didn't hear the question or for some reason refuses to answer, then you can signal with your middle finger. (Randal taps her middle finger) You'll find that your subconscious mind has great knowledge and in many cases it can answer with a "yes" or a "no" response.

All right, Gerrie, I want to call your attention to the feelings that were coming up for you when I was working with Liz last Sunday on her regression. You had certain feelings of danger and foreboding, of wanting to scream. The question I'm going to ask your subconscious mind is whether it is safe and appropriate for you to deal with those feelings that were coming up when you were watching Liz work. Is that safe and appropriate for you to work on at this time? (Gerrie's right index finger lifts) Okay, I'm getting a "yes" response to that.

Is it safe and appropriate for you to consciously remember any and all memories that have to do with those feelings of danger and foreboding and wanting to scream? (Several fingers twitch and move on Gerrie's right hand) I saw a twitch of your "yes" finger, a twitch of your middle finger and then a more major movement of your "I don't know" finger, so I'm sensing that your subconscious mind is not sure.

I'm going to ask your subconscious a question that is a little different now. Would it be safe and appropriate for Gerrie to remember some of the memories that have to do with the feelings of danger and foreboding and wanting to scream that she felt when she was watching Liz work? (Gerrie's index finger rises) The answer is yes. Now talking to the subconscious mind, would you be willing to commit to only bringing up any memories to Gerrie's conscious mind that are safe and appropriate for her to become aware of and work on at this time? (Gerrie's index finger rises) The answer to the question is yes. Good.

Another question. As you bring up certain memories for Gerrie to work on that have to do with these feelings of danger and foreboding and wanting to scream, is it safe and appropriate for Gerrie to be open to her emotions as she recalls those selected memories? (Gerrie's index finger rises) The answer to the question is yes.

Gerrie, I want you to know that you are here in a very supportive environment with me and the class and with God. (Gerrie is a church deacon) You are surrounded by love. What you are going to get in touch with is something you went through that was very difficult for you at the time. You have all of your resources now and all of this support to help you get to the other side, in which you can feel a great sense of letting go of something that you've been holding onto until now. I want you to know as you get in touch with these feelings that I'm here for you one hundred percent, Les (Gerrie's husband) is here for you one hundred percent, the class is here for you one hundred percent, and you're going to do great.

I want to say that I really admire and respect you for the tremendous growth you have made in your life. For having come so far after having such great and difficult circumstances in very early childhood. You have shown tremendous courage, integrity, love, commitment, determination, strength and endurance, and a very strong motivation to live and thrive and grow to be the good, kind, loving, generous, healthy person that you are. We can all admire you greatly for the journey you've taken and continue to take as you move forward. This is another step on that journey as you intuitively recognize that it's time for you to move on. Speaking of the hero's journey (referred to in class earlier that day), here we go.

(Randal begins to increase his voice tempo) I'm going to count from one to ten. With each number that I count you're going to become more and more aware of that feeling of foreboding you felt when Liz was going into regression on Sunday. That feeling of danger and foreboding and wanting to scream. On number one and with each number I count, becoming more and more aware of that feeling. As I count you stay in hypnosis but you get more in touch with that feeling. On number two, getting more in touch with that feeling. Number three and four, more in touch with that feeling of danger. Number five, that feeling of foreboding. Number six and seven, that feeling of wanting to scream. Number eight, like the flood gates of a dam, feeling it throughout your body. Number nine, on the next number I count you're right there with that feeling. Stay with that feeling now. Number ten. You're right there with that feeling.

I'm going to take you back to an earlier time in your life when you felt that same feeling. Stay with that feeling. Number ten, nine, eight. Going back in time, going back to a much earlier time in your life. Seven, six, five. Going back in time. Four. Going back to that feeling of danger, back to that feeling of wanting to scream. Three, two. On the next number I count you're right there with that feeling. Number one. You're right there. (Randal taps Gerrie's forehead) All right, you can easily stay in hypnosis as you speak now. Are you inside or outside? Pick one.

GERRIE: Inside.
RANDAL: Is it nighttime or daytime?
GERRIE: It's nighttime.
RANDAL: Are you alone or with others?
GERRIE: I'm alone. (Gerrie starts to cry)
RANDAL: (slowing down and softening his voice) Okay, stay with your feelings. It's okay to cry. How old are you? Are you under three years old, yes or no?
GERRIE: Yes.
RANDAL: Are you under one year old, yes or no?
GERRIE: Yes.
RANDAL: Are you an infant?
GERRIE: Yes. (begins to cry like an infant)
RANDAL: Stay with your feelings. It's okay to cry. What are you feeling? Are you feeling sad or scared or what?
GERRIE: Scared.
RANDAL: Where are you right now? Are you aware of where you are?
GERRIE: Inside.
RANDAL: Inside. Is it completely dark? (Gerrie nods) You said it's nighttime. Are you all alone in the room or do you just feel all alone?
GERRIE: All alone.
RANDAL: Being alone and feeling scared, have you felt this often?

GERRIE: Yes.
RANDAL: You've felt this feeling over and over again?
GERRIE: Yes.
RANDAL: Stay with the feeling. You're scared and you're all alone. Who do you want to call out for? Mommy or daddy or who?
GERRIE: I don't know.
RANDAL: I'm going to check something out here. I'm going to have you lift up your arms and say "Mommy!" Just start calling out for Mommy. (Randal takes Gerrie's arms and holds them out in front of her) I want you to raise your hands and arms upward. Reach up and call out and say, "Mommy, where are you?"
GERRIE: (crying, then very softly) Mommy, where are you?
RANDAL: "Mommy, please come. Mommy, please come."
GERRIE: (very soft whisper) Please come.
RANDAL: It's okay to cry. You can rest your arms back down. (Randal helps her move her arms down) It's okay to cry. Does Mommy say anything? Is she there? (Gerrie shakes her head) So Mommy's not there. You're still all alone. How do you feel about that?
GERRIE: (whispers) I want to die.
RANDAL: I understand how you want to die in such a terrible circumstance, because this has happened over and over again and for so long, for such grueling long periods, hasn't it?
GERRIE: Yes.
RANDAL: Okay, reach out for Daddy now. (Randal takes Gerrie's arms again and stretches them out in front of her) Say, "Daddy, please come."
GERRIE: (barely a whisper) Daddy, please come.
RANDAL: Does Daddy come? (Gerrie is whimpering and her face is all scrunched up) Does he sometimes come?
GERRIE: Sometimes.
RANDAL: Let's bring Daddy here. (Randal puts Gerrie's hands together and they fall to her stomach) Tell him how you feel.
GERRIE: I don't think he cares.
RANDAL: Tell him that. Say, "Daddy, I don't think you care."
GERRIE: I don't think you care.
RANDAL: "I don't feel like you care."
GERRIE: He's afraid of me.
RANDAL: Is that what he says? Be Daddy. What does he say?
GERRIE: Cries out. He says he hates me.

RANDAL: It's okay to cry. What do you feel? Go inside your body and feel what you feel. (pause) Check from your head to your toes. Do you notice any part of your body?

GERRIE: I feel sad.

RANDAL: Where do you feel your sadness? Do you feel it anywhere in particular or all over or what?

GERRIE: All over.

RANDAL: Breathe down into your stomach and feel that sadness. What do you want to say to Daddy about him saying he hates you? You can say anything you want. I'm here. I can protect you. You can be safe and say anything you want to Daddy.

GERRIE: I don't know what I did to have you hate me.

RANDAL: Look over there at him instead of becoming him. (Randal chooses some detachment from the traditional Gestalt dialogue because of the combination of her extremely traumatic infancy and her father's very negative response) Just get a sense about what he says in response now. "I'm talking to you, Daddy. What did I do to make you hate me?" What does Daddy say in response to that? (pause) Listen to him. I'm going to count from three to one. At the count of one you can hear him. Three, two, one. (Randal taps Gerrie on the forehead) What does he say?

GERRIE: If you weren't here she would still be with me.

RANDAL: When I touch your shoulder switch and be Gerrie. Be his little baby. Your father is blaming you for your mommy having left him. What would you say to him about that if you could speak?

GERRIE: I'm sorry. (crying) I'm sorry.

RANDAL: I'm going to help you out here, Gerrie. I want you to say, "It's not my fault." See how that feels. Just say "This isn't my fault."

GERRIE: This isn't my fault.

RANDAL: What does Daddy say in response to that?

GERRIE: He's crying.

RANDAL: See him crying. Become Daddy who's crying right now. Gerrie just said, "It's not my fault." What do you want to say to her?

GERRIE: I don't know what to do. I can't take care of you.

RANDAL: Thank you, Daddy. Now be Gerrie. What do you want to say to him?

GERRIE: I don't know.

RANDAL: Okay, I'd like you to imagine you can bring your mother here. She's here now. You can say anything you want to your mother about how you feel toward her.

GERRIE: What did I do to make you leave?

RANDAL: When I touch your shoulder I want you to hear your mother's response. (Randal touches her shoulder) What does your mother say in response?

GERRIE: Nothing.

RANDAL: She's here but she has no response?

GERRIE: No. She's saying that I didn't do anything.

RANDAL: I'd like you to hear her out further. Mommy, give Gerrie a sense of what made you go. You can hear your mommy's response now. What does she say? (Randal touches Gerrie's shoulder)

GERRIE: I had to leave.

RANDAL: Finish this. "I had to leave because..." What does your mommy say?

GERRIE: I wanted to do my own thing.

RANDAL: Now be Gerrie. How do you feel about her saying that? It wasn't you, I just wanted to leave because I wanted to do my own thing.

GERRIE: I am your thing.

RANDAL: (Randal claps) Yes, you are. I'm glad that you're sticking up for yourself here. What does your mother say?

GERRIE: (sadly) I wish I didn't go away.

RANDAL: Okay, feel that sadness. And elaborate.

GERRIE: I just wasn't ready for you.

RANDAL: Is there anything else you want to say or is that all for now?

GERRIE: Just that.

RANDAL: Switch and be Gerrie. (Randal touches Gerrie on the shoulder) She's sorry she went away and she felt that she wasn't ready for you. Respond.

GERRIE: We would have had great fun together.

RANDAL: Switch and be your mother. (Randal touches Gerrie on the shoulder)

GERRIE: It wasn't you that I ran away from.

RANDAL: Do you want to say something about what you ran away from? (pause) Tell Gerrie something about what you ran away from.

GERRIE: The marriage.

RANDAL: Switch and be Gerrie. (Randal touches Gerrie on the shoulder) What do you want to say in response? (pause) How do you feel toward your mother right now as she's explaining to you that it wasn't you she was running away from, it was her marriage?

GERRIE: Bewildered.

RANDAL: I don't know if she fully comprehends what she did. I think it's time for you to tell her. You've got her here finally. Tell her what you've been going through.

GERRIE: I think she was wrong.

RANDAL: Say, "You were wrong."

GERRIE: You were wrong.

RANDAL: Yes. And tell her about that now, Gerrie. You can tell her off.

GERRIE: How could you leave a little baby?

RANDAL: Good for you. Tell her, "That's a terrible thing that you did to me."

GERRIE: That's a terrible thing that you did to me. (Crying)

RANDAL: That's right. Feel the feelings in your body as you're saying that. What do you feel in your body right now? Do you notice anything in particular?

GERRIE: I don't feel so sad. I feel mad.

RANDAL: Uh huh! You're feeling mad. I think there's a lot for you to be feeling mad about right now. Say, "I hate you!"

GERRIE: No, I don't hate you. I hate what you did.

RANDAL: Good! Say, "I hate what you did."

GERRIE: I hate what you did.

RANDAL: Keep breathing down into your stomach and feel your body now. Do you feel anything in your mouth and your jaw and your neck? Get in touch with that area.

GERRIE: Less tension.

RANDAL: You're getting some stuff out that you've been holding onto for a long time. This is good. Listen to your mother now. What does she say in response?

GERRIE: It was something I felt I had to do.

RANDAL: Is there anything else?

GERRIE: No.

RANDAL: Switch and be Gerrie. (Randal touches Gerrie's shoulder) How do you feel about what your mother just said? Is that good enough?

GERRIE: Yes.

RANDAL: How are you feeling towards your mother right now?

GERRIE: I'm glad she said it wasn't my fault.

RANDAL: You know that's true. You've come a long way with this process already. It feels very good to know deep down in your subconscious that it's not your fault. As a baby, you felt it was your fault. It's good to hear that from your mother. Now look at your mother. I want to get a sense of whether or not there are any more feelings that need to be expressed. It's not for me to say whether you've done that or not, it's for you to tap into. What do you feel toward your mother right now?

GERRIE: I just want to hold her and have her hold me.

RANDAL: (Knowing Gerrie and being aware of the current clarity of her voice and body language, Randal trusts that this unusually rapid completion of her anger toward her mother's abandonment is a sign of how far Gerrie's development has come, and not a sign of denial.) What does Mother say in response to that?

GERRIE: Yes!

RANDAL: Very good. Okay, here's Mommy. (Randal places a pillow on Gerrie's chest and Gerrie hugs it) Feel Mommy holding onto you. (Gerrie sobs) It's been a long time coming. Mommy, what do you want to say to your little girl?

GERRIE: I love you.

RANDAL: Good. Say that again.

GERRIE: I love you.

RANDAL: Now be Gerrie and take it in. Your mommy loves you. She made a terrible mistake, but she really does love you and it wasn't your fault. Just feel your mommy's love for you. There's a void that's gradually getting filled now. All that emptiness that was there before is starting to get filled by the love that is coming into you. That love that you always deserved. You didn't know that you deserved it at the time because you felt responsible for your mother leaving. But you did deserve it. You always were a good girl. You didn't do anything wrong. You're a good girl just the way you are, and your mommy loves you. Does it feel good to hold her after all this time?

GERRIE: Yes.

RANDAL: Do you love your mommy?

GERRIE: Yes.

RANDAL: Keep breathing down into your stomach and feel that love. Is there anything else you want to say to your mommy? You don't have to say anything else, I'm just wondering.

GERRIE: No.

RANDAL: Okay, you can just be there and enjoy holding each other and feeling that love. Is that what you'd like to do? (Gerrie's "yes" finger rises twice) Good. Your "yes" finger moved. Okay, Mommy, is there anything further you want to say to Gerrie right now?

GERRIE: No.

RANDAL: Just take your time and feel the love that's there as you hold each other. Besides taking it in and enjoying it, your subconscious mind is learning a lot right now. It's learning more about how you developed certain ideas about yourself and about the world. It's learning about things you thought about your mother, having to do with blame and abandonment. You're learning some very important truths right now. They're sinking deep down into your subconscious mind.

In fact right now, even as you're feeling love for your mommy and from your mommy, you can use your adult reasoning mind to recognize what decisions were made by this little girl who had such difficult experiences at a young and tender age. There were certain decisions that you had transcended to varying degrees and in some ways to a large degree, but there were still some things deep down that were having a certain hold on you until now. What decisions were made by this girl that had still been affecting you until now? When you're ready to talk about that you can signal with your "yes" finger. (Gerrie signals with her "yes" finger) Okay, what do you want to say about that?

GERRIE: I thought things were my fault but I didn't know that I did.

RANDAL: What happened is crystal clear to you now, isn't it? You blamed yourself for your mother having left you. That's what any infant in your position would have done. Now you recognize that there was nothing that you did, nothing about the way you were that caused her to go. Do you understand now that it's not your fault, that you don't ever need to have these feelings again?

GERRIE: Yes.

RANDAL: Good. Say, "I'm a good person."

GERRIE: I'm a good person.
RANDAL: "I'm a lovable person."
GERRIE: I'm a lovable person.
RANDAL: "I deserve love."
GERRIE: I deserve love.
RANDAL: "I deserve acceptance."
GERRIE: I deserve acceptance.
RANDAL: "I deserve approval."
GERRIE: I deserve approval.
RANDAL: "I deserve love for who I am, not just for what I do."
GERRIE: I deserve love for who I am, not just for what I do.

RANDAL: People can also love you for what you do but they love you for who you are, Gerrie. You are lovable just the way you are. That's the key. It goes way deep down there. There are all kinds of cords that are being cut now. There are all kinds of new experiences that are wide open for you in the world. Deep down you used to have a feeling that was automatic, a knee jerk response. You felt guilty. You felt that some things that happened were your fault. Feelings like that came up because of the abandonment by your mother. But you're not feeling that abandonment anymore. Your mother made a terrible mistake. It was from her own shortcomings, not from you.

Deep down you recognize that you've always deserved love. And now that you are a full grown adult and you have all the capabilities that you have, you can give yourself that love and that approval and that support that you couldn't get before. And you can always love that beautiful baby girl within you that deserves all that love. You treat her very well. You're very accepting and proud of her. What do you want to say to that little girl of yours? Be adult Gerrie and talk to little baby Gerrie.

GERRIE: You're very brave.
RANDAL: Yes! Tell her other ways you're proud of her.
GERRIE: You're not bad. And you're not ugly.
RANDAL: Let's turn both of those around and say, "You're good and you're beautiful."
GERRIE: You're good and you're beautiful.
RANDAL: Good, here she is (Randal rocks Gerrie's hands on the pillow she's still holding), and you're telling her these things right now. Switch and be little baby Gerrie. (Randal touches Gerrie on the shoulder) Feel your mommy that you have from now on.

Your inner mommy who loves you very much and that you can have whenever you want her. Hear what she said. You're brave and you're beautiful and you're good. How does that feel?

GERRIE: Wonderful.

RANDAL: Do you love your mommy?

GERRIE: Yes.

RANDAL: Tell adult Gerrie something you appreciate about her.

GERRIE: We made it through.

RANDAL: You made it through! That's right, because it was a close call for her. It was something of a miracle that she made it through. Tell your inner mommy what qualities she not only had but used very actively to make it through and be the beautiful woman she is now. Tell big Gerrie about those qualities.

GERRIE: You wanted to be good.

RANDAL: Is wanting to be good part of what helped Gerrie to get through? Wanting to give her love and herself?

GERRIE: Yes. And loving life.

RANDAL: And the part of Gerrie that in spite of all those terrible experiences, still loved life.

GERRIE: I'm glad I lived.

RANDAL: Switch and be adult Gerrie now. (Randal touches Gerrie's hand) Feel how far you've come. Talk about life affirming, being so near death and having gone through hell so often, and yet you still loved life! And if you still loved life then, think how much you can love life now with how much more you have. You've come so far and now you can go even further.

GERRIE: When things go wrong I won't blame myself anymore.

RANDAL: Yes, you recognize it's not your fault. You're great just the way you are. That's such a deep experience that you are getting. (to the class) Does anybody have anything to say to Gerrie? You might say your name first and then say whatever you'd like to say to her.

ELIZABETH: This is Elizabeth. I love you, Gerrie.

RANDAL: Take it in, Gerrie.

KRISTA: This is Krista. I love you just the way you are.

A CHORUS OF VOICES: You're a beautiful person.

STEPHANIE: Gerrie, this is Stephanie. You're so courageous and brave. I really admire you.

LINDA: This is Linda. I'm glad that you lived and I'm glad that you're here today and that you shared this. I just love you so much.

Gerrie's Fear of Abandonment 389

JOANIE: This is Joanie. I love you, Gerrie. You're really special.

NORM: This is Norm. Your soul has to be huge for you to survive so much and you give to the world the knowledge that anyone can survive whatever they have to. You are a great gift.

WENDY: This is Wendy. You are an amazing inspiration, Gerrie. Certainly to me and I think to everyone here. I love you.

LES: Gerrie, this is Les. I want to thank you for being my wife and for being present for me for the past 45 years. For bringing into our lives the freedom and joy and love that is you. I thank you for that. For being a helpmate and for helping me to learn how to live life. Thank you so much. I love you. (Randal motions, inviting Les to come forward and he kneels down to embrace and kiss Gerrie)

RANDAL: (holding Gerrie's hand) There are a lot of tears in this room. You're an inspiration to all of us. We really love you and admire you. You've come through so much and that shows in all the love that you have within you. And you don't have to do anything, you can just be yourself because it's there naturally. Your light is shining and it's blessing everyone. You are healing this planet so much just by being yourself and being alive.

You're beginning to feel such an uplifting feeling of freedom and joy and aliveness. You're going to see so much color in the world and so much beauty in the days ahead. You'll feel more alive than you've ever felt as all of this sinks in more and more, and as you feel yourself living your life so fully. Feeling the love you feel for Les, for your family, for your extended family, for your friends, for your classmates and for the people you work with. Especially feeling the love for yourself, for the wonderful inspiring woman that you are. Now is there anything more you would like to say or to ask before I bring you out of hypnosis?

GERRIE: I love my mom and dad.

RANDAL: Okay, let's bring your father here. What would you like to say to your father?

GERRIE: Thanks for bringing me to your aunt. We made it through.

RANDAL: Good. Be your dad. What does he say to Gerrie?

GERRIE: Thank you. (crying)

RANDAL: Do you love your little daughter?

GERRIE: Yes.

RANDAL: So tell her that.

GERRIE: (whispering) I love you, Gerrie.

RANDAL: You've already said that you love your daddy. Would you like to bring him here and hold him now?

GERRIE: Yes.

RANDAL: Good. And Daddy, is there anything further you have to say to Gerrie? You don't need to, I'm just checking to see if there's anything more. (Gerrie shakes her head) You can just hold her and show her you love her. (Gerrie cries) That's good. (pause) You're finding many shifts in the days ahead, Gerrie, including a lot of things just becoming so much easier. And feeling your heart being so very open to the good and the beauty and the love that's around you. You're discovering that there's even more than you knew there for you. It's just natural, it just there.

Now I'm going to count from one to five. You're returning to a whole new state of feeling like you've just been born. Feeling so good. Number one, gently and slowly beginning to return to your fully alert, fully aware state. Number two, more and more alert, awake and aware. Number three, more and more alert, awake and aware with each number. Number four, getting ready to open your eyes. On the next number you are fully alert, awake and aware. Coming back, number five. Open your eyes, wide awake, fully alert. All the way back. (Gerrie opens her eyes) Take your time and just relax. You don't have to get up.

GERRIE: (whispering) What a trip! (Gerrie and Randal share a long hug as Gerrie whispers in his ear)

RANDAL: God, I love this work. We'll talk more about this after a fifteen minute break.

RANDAL: (after the break) Gerrie, will you come back up here? (Gerrie sits opposite Randal and her face is glowing) How are you doing?

GERRIE: Well, I'm fine.

RANDAL: Is there anything else you'd like to say right now?

GERRIE: When you mentioned the tension in my neck and shoulders, it was like a steel bar was just taken off. It was a very physical feeling.

RANDAL: That's great.

GERRIE: And I had an insight during the session. Whenever I get a friend I feel I have to give presents. I'm always giving presents. And Les has said, "Why do you have to do that?" And I say,

"Well, I don't know." It dawned on me that I was doing that to try to buy love. And I don't have to do that any more. Whew!

RANDAL: You never had to and now you know deep down that you don't have to buy love. There is plenty of it there for you.

GERRIE: My grandkids even say, "Grandma, you didn't have to do that."

RANDAL: Another part of your growth process is developing new habits. There may be some times when you start to think about a present to give and then realize, "The best present in the world is myself. I'll be myself and we'll visit and we'll have a great time." It will be good practice for you to get used to the fact that you can just be yourself.

GERRIE: That's a wonderful gift, to know that.

RANDAL: During the break I reviewed the five page letter you wrote to me. You were discussing some of the issues in detail. You told the dramatic story of how your mother abandoned you and the neighbor didn't have any food for you all day and so forth. And how your father really did do his best out of what little he knew about what to do, but he was going through his own struggles and the depression. He was a very young man and he lost his job and had gone from place to place. And how wonderful it was that you were able to find a loving family with your aunt. You described different feelings you've had in your life. Great waves of apprehension and dread and at times feeling that something was holding you back. And you said, "I thought I had completely forgiven my natural mother but maybe not." Now you don't have to be held back anymore at all.

GERRIE: No!

RANDAL: I look forward to checking in with you in class next week and getting an update. Are there any questions for Gerrie or me?

CALVIN: I'm curious to find out what happened with the father. At the beginning he seemed to disappear and then he came back at the very end.

RANDAL: We got to a point in the process where her father was starting to cry. It felt like he was reaching out and had stopped blaming her. After making some progress with the father, I felt she was ready to focus on the mother, which was particularly urgent and important. I knew I could come back to him, so I went on with her.

As usual when I'm doing Gestalt with someone, I periodically had Gerrie go inside to get in touch with what she was feeling. Often that will lead to what needs to be done next. When Gerrie was feeling all that tension I had her communicate about it. Had she described more vividly feeling the tension in a particular way, I may have had her act it out with her arms or with a pillow or whatever.

I'll mention that I was surprised at how quickly Gerrie was able to go through her feelings toward her mother. It's not for us to speculate that a person should have more anger or more grief or spend more time telling her mother off, unless there is more going on inside that is unfinished. When she talked about the burden being lifted, well, what else do you have to say? That felt genuine. If she was saying (in a strained voice, clenching his fists) "I want to hold you, mother," and there was that obvious tension, that would be a sign that she was unfinished. In that case I could have encouraged her to go inside and gone on from there. When everything has been dealt with what is left, if the person is ready to go that far in the session, may be to spontaneously say, "I love you."

STEPHANIE: I noticed that at one time when she wasn't expressing her anger you worked with her. You said something like, "Let me help you. Let me encourage you to say..."

RANDAL: Yes, I came in when she was specifically blaming herself. Her father was saying, "Look what you put me through. It was because of you that your mother left." She was just a little baby and starting to say, "Oh, I'm sorry." I wanted her to turn that around. In Gestalt, we recognize that underneath guilt is resentment and I can't think of a more perfect example of someone feeling guilty who had every right to feel resentful. Gerrie was basically saying, "I feel guilty for what I did. I made Mommy leave you. I'm bad. Maybe if I keep acting good enough people will be willing to accept me and start loving me." I wanted her to stand up for herself, and it worked. Her father immediately took responsibility and felt his grief.

Incidentally, another thing Gerrie mentioned in her letter is that her mother had a problem with drinking. She drank heavily every day, including during pregnancy. And it was a terrible childbirth situation. (reading from letter) "When it came time for my birth they had no money for drugs or a nurse to help the doctor deliver so my dad had to hold her down. It was a gruesome story..." So we can begin to imagine the affect that was having on a very sensitive baby, way back through the pregnancy and birth.

HOPE: Obviously Gerrie is a very strong person who has done a lot of growing. If you were working with someone who was not like that, would you divide it into more than one session or would you still have gone as far as you did?

RANDAL: Well, this was quite a ways to go in one session and it was because she had done a lot of work.

GERRIE: About twenty years.

RANDAL: With someone who had not come so far already I might divide it into any number of sessions to get as far as we did. We often progress dramatically and quickly with hypnosis, especially in regression work, so it might only be several sessions. Sometimes even early on in therapy you can move surprisingly quickly, but keep in mind that you also want to help the person integrate the experience into their lives and to start creating new habit patterns and so forth. In my practice, my regression work is usually part of a fairly brief series of sessions that tends to emphasize the post-hypnotic suggestions for integration.

This is something that Gerrie, with her background and experience, can do with herself in self-hypnosis. We could have another session privately or later in class that would be useful, but this session feels like a completion in itself. (to Gerrie) Gerrie, be sure to keep on track with your new ways of being, feeling great just the way you are and giving yourself some self-hypnosis regularly for the next several weeks for reinforcement. If something else comes up we can talk about it and see if we want to do any more sessions.

BRUCE: (to Randal) I'd like to ask you what your emotional level was when you finished with Gerrie. I know you've done this process a million times. As a therapist, how did you feel?

RANDAL: I had been crying during the process and I felt a tremendous amount of love and admiration for Gerrie. I felt a wonderful joy to be a part of her growth and the great honor of that. I knew that I would need a time during the break to be by myself, to just sit for a few minutes. I talked to several people afterwards and then I was able to be alone for a few minutes and go inward. I can be affected very strongly by a session and still not feel like I need to go off and be by myself but this time I needed to have a break. I feel exhilarated and I don't know if I would call it tired, but I've expended a lot of energy. It's not really being tired but more of a sense of relief and a deep sense of satisfaction and joy.

Interview One Week Later

RANDAL: We're going to do a little follow up with Gerrie. Do you want to come up? (Randal and Gerrie hug and sit down) Do you have any thoughts or realizations since we did the session?

GERRIE: Well, it was a beautiful session and I felt very good about it. Yesterday in class I went into group hypnosis with the holotropic work and my mother came to me. She was about twenty five years old and dressed in a beautiful chiffon dress, wearing shoes to dance in. They had taps on them. She put out her arms to me and I was dressed the same way and was about the same age and we had a wonderful dance together. I truly love her, which is very powerful.

RANDAL: All right. (applause) In spite of all the work Gerrie had obviously done before that session, it was impressive how quickly she was willing to move through understanding and forgiveness toward her mother. This is a big part of what we hope to ultimately accomplish. It can certainly take a lot of work, especially in cases of such extreme trauma, but if you can achieve forgiveness that is often the final stage in healing.

GERRIE: There were many sessions. Not officially hypnotherapy. Healing of memories and so forth. Spiritual things.

RANDAL: In fact you thought you might have reached the point of forgiveness before but it turned out that there was still some deep residual stuff.

GERRIE: Thank you for helping me through all that. I have a wonderful relationship with my mother now. There is no bitterness or anything there. It's just a marvelous feeling.

RANDAL: Great! Are there any questions for either me or Gerrie?

DEBBIE: What a wonderful lady you are, Gerrie. Congratulations.

GERRIE: Thank you.

ELIZABETH: I second that.

RANDAL: All right, the motion has been seconded. All those in favor say "aye". (loud applause and unanimous "aye's") None opposed. Motion stands. (Randal and Gerrie hug)

CHAPTER 21

Hypnotic Dreamwork as Regression

The Integration of Gestalt Dreamwork and Hypnotherapy

Working with the subconscious mind gives us the potential for deep transformation, and one of the vitally important functions of the subconscious mind is dreaming. Dreams are direct existential messages from the subconscious. To enter the dream and work with it directly is an opportunity for profound subconscious shifts.

The last two chapters of this book are about Hypnotic Dreamwork™, which I originated by integrating hypnotherapeutic modalities with Gestalt dreamwork. My book, *Become the Dream: The Transforming Power of Hypnotic Dreamwork*, focuses deeply on this powerful form of regression, including work with a tremendous variety of dreams. While several hypnotherapy books had a brief section on dream analysis or mentioned post-hypnotic suggestions regarding dreaming, *Become the Dream* was the first book about the integration of hypnosis and any form of dreamwork.

A dream can be considered a form of reality while it is happening. Since hypnotic regression is a revivification of recent or distant memories, and vividly recalling dreams (as done in Gestalt and Hypnotic Dreamwork) tends to induce hypnosis, these kinds of dreamwork are actually forms of hypnotic regression.

Dreams can be fleeting and disappear from conscious memory quickly. But whether or not we ever consciously remember our dreams, we all go through cycles of dreaming during a full night of sleep. Dreaming is a natural and necessary function for our mental health and well-being. For those who never or rarely remember their dreams, there are many ways to develop dream retention, and various hypnotic methods provide some of the most effective ways to do this. In addition, hypnotherapists can use both guided and elicited hypnodreams, as described in *Become the Dream*.

It has not been generally recognized that the methods of Gestalt dreamwork tend to initiate or deepen a hypnotic state. This is a major reason why Gestalt methods are so effective. By further utilizing this spontaneous entrance to the subconscious, we can add even greater value to the techniques of Gestalt.

The Gestalt Perspective on Dreamwork

The vast majority of methods to discover the meaning of dreams are interpretive. The role of the therapist is to analyze the dream or, in some cases, to help the patient or client analyze it. The overwhelming number of books about dreamwork attempt to help the reader understand how to interpret dreams.

Gestalt methods, on the other hand, do not analyze or interpret. Rather than understanding intellectually, the purpose is to experience the dream and feel significant aspects of it at a core level. Rather than analyze, the dreamer becomes the dream and all of its different parts. The deeper meaning of the dream is found with Gestalt methods through your heart, your gut, your senses and your feelings.

Most people have had the experience of waking up from a particularly intense or frightening dream with a pounding heart or gasping for breath. In spite of being asleep, the body experiences the processes of the dream. Dream images can produce the same physiological effects as the actual event would in reality. When a dream is taking place it is absolutely real to the dreamer. In its own way, it is reality while it is happening.

Our dreams are metaphors for our existence. They are even more than that. Our dreams are direct messages that express our subconscious experience of ourselves and the world. The Gestalt perspective of dreams is that every part of a dream is a part of the dreamer. This not only refers to the different persons in the dream, but all places, animals, objects, clothing, body parts, moods, weather and so forth. These parts have been fragmented or projected onto the world. By becoming the part we are taking back the power of that part. Gestalt therapy founder Fritz Perls, who was so fascinated by dreamwork that his work focused primarily on that in the years before his death in 1970, said, "You are greater than your wildest dreams."

Gestalt helps us to own all the different parts of ourselves. Anything we dream about has certain qualities and potentials that we are not fully accepting. We may not be in touch with our eyes, our ears, our center, our sexuality, our spontaneity, and so forth. Anything that a dreamer becomes aware of in a dream, even atmospheric conditions or time, is a different part of the person that has been projected to one degree or another onto the world. Even a character in the dream which is apparently immoral or repugnant has something of value which the dreamer can incorporate.

By becoming the parts and dialoguing between different parts, we take on a certain power that each character has and become so much more than we are when we project those parts externally onto people or things. Some Native Americans have traditionally identified with different animals or birds and felt the power inherent in that symbol. There are certain advantages or strengths in any character, whether it be survival, cleverness, creativity, playfulness, ability to hide, etc.

Gestalt is an existential therapy predicated on awareness. Using our heads takes us away from the here and now, which we experience externally through our senses and internally through body awareness and emotions. Understandings can and do occur during Gestalt, but are a result of the direct experience of becoming dream characters, interacting with other dream characters, and experiencing our spontaneous physical and emotional processes.

Many who are considered dream experts have stated that there is still so much that we don't understand about the meanings of dreams. But in fact your own creative subconscious mind, which formulated your dreams, knows exactly what they are about, and Gestalt dreamwork is a powerful tool in getting to the answers.

Dreams hold the answers without trying to intellectually figure them out. A formal interpretation could be wrong, or not as important as other aspects of what the dream is about. Unlike different methods of dream interpretation that say a particular object or activity always means the same thing for all people of all ages in all cultures, in Gestalt dreamwork, dreamers are led to experience what it means for them. The most important meaning is the truth of one's experience. As the therapist, if you feel your client might be missing something obvious you can encourage him or her to stay with the feeling and notice if there is also something else. But again, that is turning it over to and trusting the dreamer's subjective experience, rather than giving (or requesting) analysis.

Many individuals have gotten value from various methods of dream interpretation, and my statements regarding interpretation are in the context of Gestalt dreamwork strategies. These methods provide us with non-analytic tools which steer completely away from interpretation and are consistently effective in giving us deep understandings of our dreams and solutions to the issues the dreams address. When used properly, Gestalt dreamwork methods produce meaningful revelations time and time again. And they keep the client tending toward hypnotic states as opposed to analysis, which tends to bring the client out of hypnosis. Avoiding interpretation keeps us focused on direct access to the wisdom of the greatest ally and potential therapist of all, our own subconscious minds, and also allows the potential for deep healing by way of the increased suggestibility inherent to hypnotic states.

Accessing the Subconscious with Gestalt Dreamwork Methods

The first step for the therapist is to have the client describe the dream in present tense while vividly imagining it. Encouragement may be given to close the eyes and make gestures and movements to experience the dream more intensely. Very significantly, this revivification of the dream brings the person's full attention right into the subconscious, the part of the mind that created the dream. The key to profound, deep therapy is to work with and effect the subconscious mind. By definition, any method that gives us direct access to our inner minds while awake is hypnotic. In other words, this first step in Gestalt dreamwork is a hypnotic induction. (Through many traditional hypnotic inductions, a person initially opens to the subconscious mind by becoming very relaxed and passive. Gestalt dreamwork is one of the many alternative forms of hypnotic inductions.)

Next, the therapist typically has the dreamer describe him or herself as being one of the characters of the dream, emphasizing to stay in touch with his or her feelings. If the description is brief, some elaboration may be encouraged. The therapist will usually then have the dreamer become at least one more additional character. This increased identification with specific parts of the dream frequently further deepens the hypnosis.

A very common Gestalt dreamwork procedure is to have different characters dialogue. This is communicated directly in the first and second person, rather than talking to the therapist about the other character. When you dialogue between the different parts, switching and becoming first one part and then the other, this gives the opportunity to work through struggles between conflicting parts (and/or increase communication and appreciation between complementary, harmonious parts), integrating characteristics of each part into a more balanced whole. Questions between the characters are to be avoided or turned into statements. A question is considered a form of manipulation, a way of not taking responsibility. It also is usually a request for an intellectual explanation, which tends to diminish the hypnotic state. The Gestalt dialogue is traditionally done while sitting in a chair and facing an empty chair. It usually works well to have the dreamer get up and switch chairs when moving from one character to another.

Another Gestalt practice is to periodically have the dreamer describe what is happening internally. This is especially good when a person has begun to tap into an emotion, whether or not there appears to be resistance to that emotion. Going inward will tend to take a person deeper into hypnosis and deeper into the experience. As the person describes his or her inner feelings you might turn to an inner dialogue to further develop that experience. For example, if a person has begun to make physical movements, you can encourage him or her to exaggerate those movements or become the body part that is doing that, in the same way the person would become a direct character in the dream.

Keep working with dialogue between characters until you complete the communication or get a natural coming together of some of the characters. It is important that the therapist not take sides. What usually happens as you stay with a person in dreamwork is a gradual appreciation and integration of the different sides. The appreciation is automatic with wish fulfillment dreams, but in frustration dreams you initially emphasize the clashing parts and work with those, letting them have total space to be themselves. You encourage each part to express and be itself, whether the part is upset at the other, or afraid, or whatever the feeling is. If the dreamer becomes ready to complete this process, a mutual respect and acceptance often develops between characters at the conclusion of the dialogue.

Most dreams for most of us are frustration dreams or have significant elements of frustration. Both frustration and wish fulfillment dreams are valuable and have their advantages. Working with a wish fulfillment dream, for instance, can be very healing when the subconscious mind finds a discovery or solution, or immerses itself in the joy of its power and sense of accomplishment, or success, freedom, peace or whatever the relevant feelings are. A dream segment can be so brief that it may not be clear at first if there will be something frustrating or challenging to work with. You simply find out by having the person do the dreamwork process.

Combining Additional Hypnotic Processes with Gestalt Dreamwork

Most people are able to do Gestalt dreamwork in the traditional posture, making movements and switching chairs as they switch characters, and so forth. Some may find this distracting and become more responsive after receiving a hypnotic induction. Also, the dream may be experienced more deeply and emotionally by some after an initial hypnotic induction, which is one possibility for bypassing resistance or to help someone who is using Gestalt dreamwork methods but having difficulty identifying with the parts of the dream. The subconscious connections of this deeper state can bring the dream more to the surface.

If I do dreamwork after a hypnotic relaxation induction I don't have the person get up and switch chairs because that would be difficult and distracting. Instead of switching chairs, I can tap a person on the shoulder or hand to encourage a switch to a different part, or just announce to make a switch.

With the integration of hypnosis, we can take traditional Gestalt work further. For example, Hypnotic Dreamwork can include further integration with direct and/or indirect suggestions. Traditional Gestalt therapy focuses just on the person's process, but there is so much you can suggest for further integration of the process while the subconscious mind is open to suggestion. Actually, the subtle support throughout of the person's process, including encouragement of full expression of each character, is a form of indirect suggestion.

Typically, I avoid direct post-hypnotic suggestions during the process of the Gestalt dreamwork, to not interfere in that way with the person's internal process. Once we are at or near the conclusion, I often give various kinds of suggestions for appreciation, reinforcement and further integration. For example, encouragement may be given that integration continues to take place in the days and the weeks ahead, and in further dreams. Depending on circumstances, the hypnotic support can take place at different times during the process, not just at the conclusion. Positive suggestions laced throughout the dreamwork may fit well once it is clear it is a wish fulfillment dream.

Sometimes before doing direct hypnotic suggestions, I will begin that process with a few brief hypnotic deepening techniques. The deepening can intensify the suggestibility, and it is also a signal for the client to become more passive and receptive. Additionally, hypnotic deepening can be used to increase the effectiveness of the process at any stage of the dreamwork.

As previously stated, Hypnotic Dreamwork is actually a form of hypnotic regression. But what follows refers to non-dream regression. During Hypnotic Dreamwork a dream can be transformed directly into regression when appropriate. Regression work is often valuable when a person is working on a particular issue or recurring pattern because on a subconscious level, the person hasn't let go of something that is still affecting the way he or she sees and experiences the world. Perls said that a person's experiences are retrieved "not in his memory but in his behavior. He repeats it, without, of course, knowing that he is repeating it."

Traditional Gestalt dreamwork stays with just the dream and the dreamer's here and now experience. But with the understanding we have of hypnosis and regression, we can also return to an earlier similar experience. For example, using the affect bridge, a person can tap into a strong emotion that the dreamwork has brought up and regress to specific significant experiences that happened out of the dream state at an earlier time.

When dreamwork turns into another form of regression, various regression modalities can be integrated into the work. For example, while dream analysis is not associated with Gestalt dreamwork, encouraging the client to do his or her own brief hypno-analysis at the conclusion of a regression can be important and appropriate. When I lead such an analysis it is usually regarding the understanding and release of misconceptions that the client had continued to be stuck with in the here-and-now experience of himself and the world. I am usually able to help keep this self-analysis very brief so that it normally does not interfere with the hypnotic state.

Any additional form of hypnotherapy can be integrated when appropriate. For example, there are various ways ideomotor questions can be used to request information or get feedback from the subconscious. Other hypnotic tools that can be selectively used include grounding and centering techniques, indirect suggestion, hypnotic metaphor, time distortion, bibliotherapy and inner child processes.

Since hypnotic deepening techniques are typically a part of Hypnotic Dreamwork, a brief period of suggestions for returning to full conscious awareness is usually applicable to ensure best results, including avoidance of a possible lingering lethargy.

Common Steps in Hypnotic Dreamwork

1. The dreamer describes the dream in present tense while vividly imagining it, often with the eyes closed. Sometimes it may help to describe the dream again more expressively, including making gestures and movements to experience the dream more intensely.

2. The dreamer describes him or herself as being one of the characters of the dream, endeavoring to stay in touch with his or her feelings. Then the dreamer becomes at least one more dream character.

3. Have some of the characters dialogue directly to each other.

4. Periodically have the dreamer describe physical awareness. Sometimes a dialogue may develop from this, that is a similar process to the dialogue of the dream characters.

5. Keep working with steps two through four with selected characters until there is understanding and acceptance, or a completion of the communication that each side needs to make.

6. Any additional form of hypnotherapy, such as ideomotor questions or regression methods, can be integrated when appropriate.

7. Brief further hypnotic deepening techniques may sometimes be used to increase identification of the dream or therapy process, or to initiate a detailed hypnotic suggestion period.

8. Post-hypnotic suggestions for further integration and acceptance.

9. Suggestions for returning to normal awareness followed by a posthypnotic interview.

CHAPTER 22

Marilyn's Dream
The Crumbling Mountain

RANDAL: Marilyn, come on up and we'll work on your dream. (Marilyn walks up and sits beside Randal) As we discussed, shall we mention to the group the experience you had when the class first started? (Marilyn nods) About a month and a half ago, during a break, Marilyn shared with me that she had been reading my book, *Become the Dream*, and she was very excited about a particular part. After the break I was demonstrating the Elman rapid induction method and Marilyn was the volunteer. While she was in hypnosis I threw out a few brief suggestions and some spontaneous appreciation for her earlier comments. Can you tell the class what you experienced the next day?

MARILYN: I had been waking up every night for the past year, since my husband died, with a palpitating heart and feelings of anxiety. I couldn't overcome it and then after this event it was suddenly gone. It went away completely.

RANDAL: And the event was simply those few words of appreciation. Never underestimate the potential of hypnosis. Even a brief heartfelt acknowledgment can be so powerful. In this case it stopped a year of heart palpitations.

MARILYN: That's right.

RANDAL: That's wonderful. Now you recently said you would like to work on a dream. When did you have it?

MARILYN: I had it just after the class started in June and it was very powerful and exciting. I don't usually remember my dreams so this one really made an impression on me.

RANDAL: Go ahead and tell it now in the present tense. You can do it with your eyes open or closed. Just describe it as though it's happening now.

MARILYN: Okay. (Marilyn closes her eyes) I'm an observer and I'm standing watching something going on at this enormous mountain. At the base of the mountain there is a large black truck with a long truck bed. It's being filled up with huge boulders and then the truck drives away. Just as the truck gets out of the way an avalanche of boulders begins falling down where the truck had been. I'm out of the way observing from a distance. I'm in a safe place.

Then when that bunch of rocks falls down it loosens up the next layer and they begin tumbling down in a big avalanche. I was really impressed. I thought, "Wow, this is really something." I could hear the noise and the thundering and everything. Then that caused the next layer above, the whole top of the mountain...

RANDAL: (reminding Marilyn to return to present tense) "This causes the next layer..."

MARILYN: This causes the next layer, the final layer of rocks, to come tumbling down. The whole top of the mountain is coming all the way down. Millions of rocks and dust and debris. I decide to go up the base of the mountain after it's all over because I'm fascinated and because it looks different. A voice within me says, "Aren't you afraid that more stuff is going to come down?" And I say, "No, I'm not going to be hurt. Nothing else is going to come down."

I feel very confident to go up to the base of the mountain and I'm looking at it. All of the top soil and everything has been shorn away and it's kind of creamy white with a tiny bit of sand on it. I'm stroking the side of the mountain there and it's rather like a glacier had gone by and stripped it. The mountain, the base of it, is stripped of everything from these rocks coming down. And I don't understand the dream.

RANDAL: The point is not to understand the dream, but to become the dream. You'll understand at a deeper level by avoiding trying to understand.

MARILYN: I did figure out that I think I have rocks in my head. (laughter)

RANDAL: Of course we can stop here because you already have the answer. Next? (more laughter) All right. So the last thing you remember in the dream is standing there and feeling that white, creamy surface and looking around. Are there rocks around where the mountain was and is that where you're standing?

MARILYN: The side of the mountain is left at the bottom and somehow I've climbed around the debris that has fallen and gone over to inspect the base of the mountain.

RANDAL: So what was a mountain is now much lower and you've found your way up to the flat area.

MARILYN: It's still the side of the mountain.

RANDAL: Let's get right into that active scene where the rock slide is occurring. Describe yourself as one of these rocks.

MARILYN: Well, I'm the first rock in the truck. I'm really big and powerful and I'm out of here. I'm gone and I'm not going to get hurt. I'm the foundation and it's going to be a big mess because the whole thing is going to come down.

RANDAL: So you know that.

MARILYN: I know that because I've been holding it all up.

RANDAL: So you're being taken away. How do you feel about that?

MARILYN: I guess I feel fine. I hadn't thought about that. I know I'm safe because I'm out of the way.

RANDAL: You're in the here and now and you're being taken away and that feels good. You feel safe.

MARILYN: Yes.

RANDAL: Now we'll move on. You can be one of the rocks coming down or you can be a whole avalanche of rocks coming down.

MARILYN: The next whole layer.

RANDAL: Okay. Be this next whole layer and describe yourself.

MARILYN: I'm the next layer of big boulders. The foundation has come out from under us and there is nothing more to hold us up. The weight on top of us is tremendous and we can't hold it anymore without the ones beneath. I, or we, have to let go...

RANDAL: Let's say "I" for now. I know you're also talking about "we" with all these different rocks, but you are also this layer, this mass. I'm hearing you say that "my foundation is being taken away."

MARILYN: My foundation has been taken away and I'm crumbling under the weight of everything. It's crumbling and I've got to move. I can't stay here any longer. There is nothing underneath me.

I just have to let go and give way and it's going to cause a lot of trouble, a lot of havoc, but I've got to come down.

RANDAL: How does that feel? You can't hold on any longer and you've got to give way and come down.

MARILYN: I'm feeling very uncomfortable about it, that I'm not doing the job I'm supposed to do, holding up this mountain. I feel worthless if I'm just falling down. My whole life purpose is gone. It's all been pulled out from under me. Those people took my foundation away. It's gone. It's ruined. Not only do I have no foundation but this whole mountain has no foundation now. It's havoc.

RANDAL: I'd like you to talk to those people now. Face your chair toward this empty chair and in the empty chair we're putting the people who took your foundation and all those rocks away. Talk to those people and tell them how you feel.

MARILYN: (eyes open now) I don't know who you are. Somebody was driving the truck. Somebody put me in the truck and took me away. But you really ought to be more careful about what you do and have more consideration for mountains, because if you're going to undermine things then everything is going to break down. You should be more responsible and not cause all this destruction.

RANDAL: Now I'd like you to personalize it more and say, "I want you to be more careful about undermining me." You're the rocks that are about ready to fall now. Talk about how these people are affecting you.

MARILYN: Your actions have really devastated me. I feel I don't have my purpose in life anymore. I no longer have my job of holding up this mountain and of being the foundation. You've taken away my foundation and it's ruining everything for all of us here on this mountain. This whole big mountain that I am. You had no permission to do that. You're so stupid to take away the foundation. It's really a stupid, idiotic thing to do and you ought to have more sense.

RANDAL: That's good. (Randal motions to the empty chair) Now I'd like you to switch and be these people who took away your foundation and respond. (Marilyn switches chairs, which she will continue to do throughout this and subsequent dialogues)

MARILYN: I don't know who you think you are, lady, talking to us like that. We have a job to do. Don't bother us. We're busy and that's just too bad about the mountain. That's life. We have to take these foundation stones somewhere else and that's why we have this big truck. We need these big foundation stones to do a big job.

RANDAL: What do you want to say in response?

MARILYN: I don't feel like saying anything but I know how I feel and I feel really frustrated and helpless and without any power. And that even though I'm a big, strong, enormous rock I have no power or control over what happens to me.

RANDAL: "...over what you are doing to me."

MARILYN: Over what you are doing to me.

RANDAL: Go inside your body and notice what you feel right now.

MARILYN: I feel very frustrated because in spite of the fact that I'm a powerful rock, I don't have any power at all if something comes along that wants to do something different.

RANDAL: Do you notice any specific feelings in your body? Any sensations anywhere from your head to your toes?

MARILYN: Yes, it's a kicked in the gut feeling. A helpless kind of frustration that I have no control over outside events. It hurts.

RANDAL: All right. (to the class) Would someone get a pillow that is not being used right now? (someone hands Randal a pillow) Thank you. (to Marilyn) This person over here kicked you in the gut and I want you to do that back. Let's take it literally. I'd like you to lie down and I'll hold the pillow here. (Marilyn lies down with her feet in front of the pillow) This is the person. Start kicking him and say, "I'm kicking you."

MARILYN: (Marilyn starts kicking the pillow) I'm kicking you and I'm so frustrated because you're bigger and stronger than I am and you think you know it all. You just ought to know what it feels like to be treated this way, even though I'm a rock and you do it anyway. I despise you. You should be ashamed of yourself. This is terrible to do to people or to rocks or to anything or anybody. You ought to see how horrible it feels to be kicked right in the gut.

RANDAL: Good. Relax. Stay right where you are and go inside your body. Do you feel the same or different?

MARILYN: I feel better.

RANDAL: (laughing) Isn't that interesting? Come on back up here. (Marilyn sits in the chair) Now I want you to become this person you just kicked in the gut because you felt he was kicking you. Respond to the rock that just kicked you back. What do you have to say to that?

MARILYN: Lady, you're pretty tough. (laughing) I didn't think you had it in you. You're a very tough lady. A tough rock.

RANDAL: A pretty tough lady rock.

MARILYN: I didn't know rocks could kick like that. I'm a pretty big man and you really did me in. I'm a very powerful man and I work at this quarry and nobody pushes me around. But you sure socked it to me, lady. You're a very strong rock. I don't know how you managed to get me down like that but you sure trounced me.

RANDAL: Good. Now switch and be the rock again.

MARILYN: Well, I'm really not finished with you. (laughter)

RANDAL: (laughing) Okay, go for it.

MARILYN: You're just lucky you got away because you deserve to have this entire mountain of rocks pour down on you. And more than kicking you in the guts, I'd like to just stand on you and stomp your guts out for ruining my mountain.

RANDAL: Go ahead and do that. (Randal puts the pillow down away from the chair) Go ahead and stomp. That's the guy who did that to you. Really get into it. (Marilyn stomps on the pillow) Good.

MARILYN: (continues stomping) This is what I'd love to do to your guts because that's how you made me feel. I'd love to just stomp on you and stomp on you or send this whole mountain of rocks on you and just let you splat. That's what you deserve. With all your power and everything, you're a terrible person. Shame on you.

RANDAL: All right.

MARILYN: That's me, isn't it? Is that me? (laughing)

RANDAL: Well, right now this is you. (Randal points to the empty chair and Marilyn moves into it) Now you are this man. What do you want to say to the rock that just stomped you?

MARILYN: Lady, it would have been better if the whole mountain had come down on me because then I wouldn't have had to live through it like this. I feel terrible. My stomach really hurts. I'd rather be dead than have what you just did to me.

RANDAL: Can you describe the hurt in your stomach?

MARILYN: She stomped on my guts and they're hanging out all over the place. Blood and everything. I feel really awful.

RANDAL: Tell lady rock what you want from her.

MARILYN: I got your message and I get your point. I'm sorry I ruined your mountain and I won't do it again.

RANDAL: Now switch. Come over here. You're doing great. What do you want to say in response to him now? (Marilyn is silent for a couple of minutes) Take your time.

MARILYN: (with a big sigh) I was really in a deep place but I couldn't talk.

RANDAL: That's okay. I could tell. Go ahead now.

MARILYN: It didn't solve the problem. The destruction is done and it can never be repaired or put back together again.

RANDAL: Say, "I can never be..."

MARILYN: I can never be put back together again. I am totally destroyed down to my very bones. It's just one of those things.

RANDAL: What is it that you want from him?

MARILYN: I just hope you know never to go out and destroy anything again in nature without thinking ahead of time what your acts cause.

RANDAL: Let's switch and check that out.

MARILYN: I'm really sorry, lady. I understand how you feel. I feel the same way. I won't do that anymore. And thank you for helping me to understand that.

RANDAL: Switch and let the rock respond.

MARILYN: I don't have anything more to say to this creature.

RANDAL: Okay, you got what you were asking for. You're still in the terrible situation you were in, but do you feel finished with him?

MARILYN: I am finished with him.

RANDAL: "I'm finished with you."

MARILYN: I'm finished with you now. Thank you for listening to me. Goodbye.

RANDAL: Before we go on I want to point out for you and the group that it's good to get this integration when it occurs, in whatever way the client chooses. But it's not something to force. Notice that I didn't in any way try to make them work things out with each other. I just asked each side to share itself and say whatever it needed to get out. An aspect of this tragedy came to a conclusion with what needed to be communicated between the two parts. Both parts spontaneously thanked the other part, which is great.

What I want to do at this point, Marilyn, is have you go inside yourself and be aware of this sense of destruction. You have collapsed and you are a jumble of rocks. You are no longer a mountain. Describe yourself as being a jumble of rocks. How do you feel?

MARILYN: I no longer feel like a solid, strong unit. I no longer go up to a peak. I don't have a pinnacle. All the top part of me is down, the middle part of me is down, and I'm really destroyed down to bedrock. I'm laying in pieces all over the place and there is no possible way ever again to put me back together to be that tall mountain that I was.

RANDAL: How does that feel?

MARILYN: I feel I'm many parts and I know the many parts of myself are going to be dispersed all over the place from this quarry area. It is rather like a quarry at the base of this mountain although I haven't been a deeply dug down mountain. I was mostly being quarried from the base of the mountain. So I know the trucks are going to come back and take all of my parts and send them all over the place. I don't know where. (Marilyn's voice is getting shaky) And I'm sad about that. I've lost the unity and strength that I had. I only know that all these separate parts of myself will be gone, except that underneath part that held all those little rocks is still there and it's smooth.

RANDAL: So describe this underneath part. Despite the fact that you've lost so much and so many parts are being dispersed to other places, describe the base of you that you still have.

MARILYN: Everything is shorn away from me. There is nothing that can cling to me any longer and I'm smooth. Just a tiny bit of sand comes off. But when people come up to me to touch me, as I did in my dream, when I touched myself, there is nothing to fear about anything coming down because I'm very safe. I'm safe for people to come up and inspect. I won't hurt anybody. I won't tumble down on anybody because all those additional parts of myself are no longer there to come loose. They're all gone and will be taken away. So it'll take me many centuries to grow back my crest again. Nothing will grow on me now. It's so smooth.

RANDAL: "I'm so smooth."

MARILYN: I'm so smooth. There will be no more rocks on me or trees or plants. Or anything.

RANDAL: How does that feel?

MARILYN: Barren. (tears are trickling down Marilyn's face)

RANDAL: Be this barren base of a mountain.

MARILYN: (whispers) I feel like crying.

RANDAL: It's okay to cry.

MARILYN: (sobbing quietly) I feel like I have lost so much and it's all going to be carted away. But what I am is so powerful and strong under there. But I don't know what it's for. I don't know what I'm for. I'm just like a thing coming out of the earth. Big. I don't know what my purpose is.

RANDAL: Stay with that feeling. (Marilyn sobs) It's good to cry. There is a tremendous loss here.

MARILYN: Yes. I've lost all my parts. All the parts of myself that were a part of all I am. They're gone.

RANDAL: Let's talk to those parts now. They're over here in this chair. What do you want to say to the parts you have lost?

MARILYN: I don't know what I'll do without you because you're such a part of my being. I'm going to miss you. I guess you'll be put to good use. I don't know whether it's something that was part of this foundation that I am. I don't know where you came from. You look sort of forlorn sitting here in this pile of rubble but somewhere you will become useful in time. (sobbing and speaking haltingly) And you will always be a part of me. So wherever you go I go. All over. (crying) It's a weird dream.

RANDAL: Stay with your experience. I'd like you to switch and be the rocks and talk back.

MARILYN: Even though we're little and not very big and powerful, we'll always remember you and remember that we were a part of you. We were way up there in the sky. We will always take the memory of you with us because we rocks know what it is to have memory. We remember everything. We'll try to do our best to uphold your tradition of being strong rocks and to serve whatever purpose there is in life to the best of our ability, however we are used. And I'll miss you. All my selves will miss this mother rock. I'm feeling like a mother who has lost all her children.

RANDAL: Let's switch and say that over here. (Marilyn switches chairs) Say that now.

MARILYN: That's the feeling I get. A mother who's suddenly lost all her children. They've all fallen away.

RANDAL: Talk to your children some more over here. What else do you want to say to them? You're the mother, the base of the mountain.

MARILYN: You're all my children, all of you, and I give you my strength and my purpose and my love and it will always be with you wherever you go. You will never be without me. I am within you, I am a part of you, I radiate from within you. Wherever you go, little rocks, my blessings will go in you and through you and radiate out from you even as I do to you now. Everyone who touches one of you will be touching me. You are all my children and you have learned a lot from sitting on me. So maybe in the long run the men who undermined me did the right thing because now you'll be more useful than you were just sitting on me. Now you all have a job before you. Everywhere you go, you'll go forth and radiate the energy that I gave you in whatever job you're doing.

RANDAL: Switch and be the little rocks.

MARILYN: Okay, mother. Thank you for giving us this talk because now we know our purpose and we know what we're supposed to do. We will honor you by going out and reminding people that we are a part of you, that we are a part of this planet. No matter where we are, when people look at us and touch us, they will know that we were a part of the planet and a part of you, mother. We will be good kids and do our job.

RANDAL: Very good. Let's switch again. Does that feel complete or is there anything further you'd like to say?

MARILYN: I feel kind of bad that I tromped on that man for pulling the rug out from under me.

RANDAL: Do you feel finished with your children now?

MARILYN: Yes. I need to see the man again.

RANDAL: Good. Bring the man back here and talk to him.

MARILYN: I want to apologize for kicking you in the gut and stomping on you because I didn't realize you were a part of the plan. You had a purpose in undermining me and causing me to fall apart. We can't just sit here with all our children clinging to us and decorating us and being proud of our children hanging on us. Sometimes we have to have the rug pulled out from under us in order to release all these good parts of ourselves that have to go out and do a job. So I apologize to you for wrecking things. I got a bit emotional about that for a rock. I didn't see the purpose of it. I know now that you were an instrument for that purpose. No matter how terrible something is I have to look at it as all part of integration, of the relationships between humans and rocks and nature. There are no mistakes. Everything really is part of a great plan, no matter how onerous it seems or how painful it was for me.

RANDAL: Now switch and be him.

MARILYN: Well, lady, thank you for your apology. I really didn't know that I was part of a plan. I feel hurt but I think they can put me back together. I don't know whether I want to stay in this business or not. It can be dangerous. (laughter) I didn't know rocks could act up like that. So thank you for your apology and while I mend my guts I'll think about all I've learned from this experience.

RANDAL: Okay, switch. Is there anything else or does that feel finished?

MARILYN: Well, I want to say you're quite a man. You've got a lot of guts, too. (laughter)

RANDAL: All right. Close your eyes and focus on your breathing. (Randal gets up and stands behind Marilyn) Take a deep breath and as I push down on your shoulders send a wave of relaxation down your body. As I rub your shoulders feel yourself going deeper. Focus on your breathing. (since the dreamwork has already put Marilyn into a hypnotic state, this deepening process is very brief) Feel your center and feel how powerful you are and how far you've come. All the way through this process, Marilyn, you've come so far. From a feeling of having lost everything, to a recognition of how you've transformed and gone on to the next stages. You've seen the big plan and you're a part of that.

You're recognizing some great spiritual truths. You've transformed a tremendous loss into an appreciation that while it has been a great loss, you have experienced a transformation as well. All these different parts of yourself are going further into the world to have many different purposes. These different parts of you now transform into your children. They're good kids, all going out in the world, able to go much further and do much more and be of much more value.

You are all of this, Marilyn. You have been something very special for millions of years as this big, powerful mountain and you still have that as well, even though you are no longer the same. You are the essence of this high, beautiful mountain that is you. You are all of that and much more. You are the base of this mountain that is still firm and strong and solid, and now you can also be so much more by going out and having influence throughout the world, laying foundations and being part of more structures, helping so many people to have security and protection and shelter and transportation. There are so many different things that you can be part of.

The base of you knows that you have all of these different purposes in which you are providing much value and can receive much appreciation. That tall, big, beautiful, proud mountain is you. Just as you have been giving life for many years, you have had many trees, many plants, many animals, you continue to be that which gives life and which is a part of life. There are many good things you do in being this beautiful mountain with many strong, powerful rocks. There are various ways that you can inspire and help people to live in greater harmony with themselves and the earth as we evolve.

You've come so very far, Marilyn, from your initial feeling of devastation to your feeling of transformation and rebirth. You just made a more thorough integration and a beautiful completion with that man and with you as that man, giving appreciation to each other. His awareness and growth is a part of you, too. It was very admirable that he developed that respect to the rocks and to the mountain and that you can understand and appreciate the tremendous sadness that occurred and move on now. That beautiful forgiveness, of taking responsibility. Recognizing that you are healing and you will heal.

You can take all of that knowledge and move on and do whatever you're going to do from here with a greater awareness and appreciation and connection with the whole scheme of things. "I am a part of all that I have met, yet all experience is an arch where through glows that untraveled world whose margin fades forever and forever as I move." That's from James Joyce's *Ulysses*. (tears are running down Marilyn's face and Randal continues in a whisper) Marilyn, you are the truth. Take your time. Whenever you're ready you can come back and open your eyes. Fully alert, rested, refreshed and feeling good. (Marilyn takes a deep breath and then opens her eyes slowly and giggles) Take your time. That's fine. Mountains tend to move slowly. (more giggling from Marilyn)

MARILYN: You said some incredibly beautiful things for me to live up to.

RANDAL: You're already living up to them. (Randal and Marilyn hug)

MARILYN: I appreciate it very much. I had no idea what that dream was all about. I just thought I had rocks in my head. (laughter)

RANDAL: It's quite a bit more profound than that, isn't it? And you are a lot more profound than that. You say there is a lot to live up to, but just be yourself. You don't have to try to do anything. All of this is you.

MARILYN: I really feel so much stronger. It's amazing. (laughing) I really do.

RANDAL: You've done a tremendous amount of integration.

MARILYN: Thank you. That was wonderful.

RANDAL: You look radiant. Those eyes are so bright.

MARILYN: I'm kind of embarrassed now.

RANDAL: What is there to be embarrassed about?

MARILYN: You said all those nice things. (laughing)

RANDAL: Well, I guess you just have to put up with that embarrassment. (laughter) Let's show our appreciation for Marilyn. (applause) I want you to know that you deserve all of those things. Now take a look around and make connections with all these people.

MARILYN: I'm going to cry. (Marilyn pauses for a moment to cry) You've all been such good friends. It's so nice to see your faces and I feel so one with you. I send you lots of love and I radiate love to you all. I wish I could give you all a little rock filled with love. (laughter)

RANDAL: You've done it already.

MARILYN: I'll bring some rocks to class tomorrow from my garden and give you all a rock to remember me by, okay? And it will be filled with love.

RANDAL: That's beautiful.

MARILYN: I feel wonderful. It's so nice to know you all. It's like being in a family and it feels really good. (crying) It's a safe place because I've been alone for a long time and it's really nice to have all of these friendships. I've only had one close friendship for fifteen years and that was my husband. As I was explaining to some of you, I haven't been socializing for about fifteen years so I'm really enjoying meeting all of you and having these relationships and your friendship and your love. Thank you very, very much. I really appreciate it.

RANDAL: I know I can speak for the group when I say that we really appreciate you and your willingness to deal with the incredibly painful feelings that were coming up. You stayed very much in the present, dealing with one challenging thing after another. All these things that you were feeling and struggling with, kicking and being kicked, that led to these transformations. It takes guts to do that, and your willingness to do it in front of the group adds to everyone's experience and to the bonding of the class. Thank you very much.

It's now time for me to come out as a psychic. I can sense that you're going to be getting some hugs pretty soon. I just sense these things. (laughter) I'd like to make some comments about this beautiful dreamwork that Marilyn did but I don't want us to get in our heads right now. I want us to stay in our hearts and our senses and our feelings, so we'll take a break. When we come back I'll say a few things and we'll take some questions.

RANDAL: (after the break) Gestalt dialogue is an integral part of the depth of this work. Traditional Gestalt dreamwork processes include becoming various parts of the dream and dialoguing between some of the parts. Also going within and becoming a part of your body that is reacting to the dreamwork, and sometimes that can develop into a dialogue. But what is not part of traditional Gestalt is the post hypnotic suggestions I gave Marilyn at the end. I want to emphasize that until those suggestions I did not attempt to influence anything beyond supporting whatever part was expressing itself. Gestalt is about full self expression of any part without judgment of those parts. A basic element of Gestalt is that you don't take sides. I might say that you take all sides. I'm supportive of each part in actualizing itself, rather than being strictly neutral. I'm encouraging each side to say what it has to say, but I'm not giving interpretation or advice about additional ideas to express.

Besides avoiding taking sides, another thing to avoid in Gestalt is analysis. Don't try to figure out the meaning, and instead have a person come to his or her experience. I was encouraging Marilyn, and you can see the power Marilyn has. She had all the resources within. I just gave her guidance in becoming and switching between parts and in getting in touch with herself.

In doing dreamwork I don't try to hurry up a process or make two parts come to full integration. It's great when integration happens, but it doesn't always happen or it may be partial. Marilyn eventually came spontaneously to appreciation and gradually developed major completions and integration.

We went beyond traditional Gestalt to bring in hypnotic processes with the use of Hypnotic Dreamwork™. Since the person is usually already in at least a light hypnotic state you can add a few hypnotic deepening techniques and then give post hypnotic suggestions, as I did with Marilyn. Or sometimes dreamwork can spontaneously develop into a regression in the more traditional sense, or it can involve the use of ideomotor methods. You can integrate any hypnotic form into dreamwork if the timing is appropriate.

It's exciting that we have the wonderful tools of hypnosis to integrate into this great work. Gestalt dreamwork is so effective, and then to add additional hypnotic modalities takes a system that is already powerful and adds a whole new dimension. Are there any questions?

DOUG: It seemed obvious that this dream had to do with the loss of her husband of fourteen years and her personal support. I want to ask Marilyn what her experience was. Did this have to do with your husband?

MARILYN: Yes, Doug, it quite possibly had something to do with the death of my husband and the support being taken out from under me. It even crossed my mind that maybe it was part of a divine plan, that he was taken from me partly because I had a big work to do, and as long as I was spending my time in devotion to him I wouldn't be out doing what I was supposed to do. Since he died I'm doing all the things I needed to do for fifteen years but didn't.

DOUG: You seemed very positive about the way things progressed and as you worked your way through you progressively got very strong.

MARILYN: Yes, although I feel as though I've just had an operation. Physically I feel kind of drawn and strained. Everything outside is bright and seems different. I feel like I've just been born or had a baby or something like that. I feel very different but I also have an inner strength that I didn't know I had. And what I was experiencing toward the end was so profound and deep that I was too shy to really share it, so I hope you can all read between the lines. I was a little embarrassed to say how profound it really was, what I was getting about the children and the mother. It had nothing to do with me, Marilyn. I would say it was the higher self. It was definitely a transcendent experience.

RANDAL: That's what it felt like. I think many of us can read between the lines and feel, in a spiritual sense, that you were dealing with some very deep things .

MARILYN: Exactly. I have never before felt so in touch with the earth as I was. I had never really perceived this thing of gaia or the consciousness of being one with the earth. Also, when I said, "You are all my children," it was coming from the higher self and referring not only to everyone in the room, but everyone everywhere. It's like it was a higher voice speaking through me rather than me.

RANDAL: It was really profound.

MARILYN: I think that having had this experience confirmed for me something very powerful and deep that I only thought was perhaps in my imagination. Working with you, Randal, accelerated it for me. It's given me confirmation, and a greater strength and sense of reality about my invisible being that I needed to get in touch with. And it's an acceleration process.

RANDAL: That's well put. You've been progressing well all along and now this was an acceleration process.

Interview One Week Later

RANDAL: (Marilyn comes up and sits next to Randal) Hello there. You look great!

MARILYN: (laughing) Thank you.

RANDAL: How have you been doing these past few days? Have you had any insights or feelings since our session that you'd like to share?

MARILYN: One major feeling I got from our session was that this was a metaphor, a gift given to me to be able to share the idea that our inner strength is like a rock. There are always parts of ourselves that get disseminated and given out but nothing is lost or wasted.

RANDAL: I feel like you really went to the depths of despair with your dream and your feeling of, I don't know, hopelessness? That's just a word that comes to mind. I don't know if it fits.

MARILYN: Yes, hopelessness.

RANDAL: A feeling of having lost everything, of incredible destruction and despair. There was nothing that could be done about that. Then out of those ashes the Phoenix rose with what you created from that, and the rebirth was a wonder to behold. That's a confirmation of what you just said.

MARILYN: Yes. It really surprised me and I'm very happy to have had the opportunity to go into the dream in depth. It has had a lot of meaning for me as a core lesson and as a really powerful metaphor. I'm happy I was able to share it with everybody.

RANDAL: Also you said there were things that were hard to verbalize, which you partly touched upon, about the depth of realization you had gotten. I could sense the power of that for you. (to the class) Let's give Marilyn our thanks. (applause)

Commentary

The coincidental story that was told prior to the dreamwork regarding the tremendous impact of the death of Marilyn's husband on her, helped us have a greater understanding of some aspects of the meaning of this dream. But the value and purpose of Hypnotic Dreamwork is not about understanding our clients' dreams, nor is it even necessarily about helping our clients develop a conscious understanding of the meaning of the dream. Marilyn's realizations about the association of the dream and dreamwork to life events and difficulties were valuable, and may have become so obvious as to be inevitable in this case. But any realization of the association of the dream to her struggles with her husband's death, or any other struggles in her life, did not necessarily have to occur for her to get profound impact from the Hypnotic Dreamwork.

References

Chapter One: Regression Hypnotherapy and Its Profound Potential

Isen, Hal, (June 20, 2001) Photographic evidence of how we shape reality. *Core Wisdom On-Line: The Electonic Newsletter of Hal Isen & Associates, Inc.* Volume 1, Number 6.

Jourard, Sidney M., (1971) *The Transparent Self*, Van Nostrand Reinhold.

Chapter Four: Accessing Gestalt for Emotional Clearing

Boyne, Gil, (1989) *Transforming Therapy, A New Approach to Hypnotherapy*, Glendale, CA: Westwood Publishing Co.

Perls, Frederick S., (1992) *Gestalt Therapy Verbatim*. New York: Gestalt Journal Press

Perls, Frederick S., (1973) *The Gestalt Approach & Eye Witness to Therapy*, Palo Alto, CA: Science and Behavior Books, Inc.

Yontef, Gary, (1993) *Awareness, Dialogue and Process: Essays on Gestalt Therapy*. New York: Gestalt Journal Press.

Chapter Six: Direct vs Indirect Suggestion

Barber, J. (1977) Rapid induction analgesia: A Clinical Report. *American Journal of Clinical Hypnosis*, 19, 138-147.

Erickson, M., Hershman, S., & Sector, I. (1961) *Practical Application of Medical and Dental Hypnosis*. Brunner/Mazel: New York.

Erickson, M., Rossi, E., & Rossi, S. (1976) *Hypnotic Realities: The Induction of Clinical Hypnosis and Forms of Indirect Suggestion*. New York: Irvington Publishers.

Hammond, D. C. (1984) Myths about Erickson and Ericksonian hypnosis. *American Journal of Clinical Hypnosis*, 26, 236-245.

Hammond, D. C. (1990) *Handbook of Hypnotic Suggestions and Metaphors*. New York: W.W. Norton & Company.

Harrington, Pat. (1990) Choosing a hypnotherapist. *Recovering Magazine*.

Lankton, S., & Lankton, C. (1983) *The Answer Within: A Clinical Framework of Ericksonian Hypnotherapy*. New York: Brunner/Mazel.

Matthews, W. J., Bennett, H., Bean, W., & Gallagher, M. (1985) Indirect versus direct hypnotic suggestions - An initial investigation: A brief communication. *International Journal of Clinical and Experimental Hypnosis*, 33, 219-223.

Meyer, Robert G. (1992) *Practical Clinical Hypnosis: Techniques and Application*. New York: Lexington Books.

Yapko, M. (1986) In B. Zilbergeld, G. Edelstein, & D. Araoz (Eds.) *Hypnosis: Questions and Answers*. (223-231) New York: Norton.

Yapko, M. (1990) *Trancework: An Introduction to the Practice of Clinical Hypnosis*. New York: Brunner/Mazel

Chapter Fourteen: Recovered Memories

Brown, Daniel, Scheflin, Alan W., Hammond, D. Corydon, (1998) *Memory, Trauma Treatment, and the Law.* New York: W. W. Norton & Company.
Butler, Katy, (June 26, 1994) A House Divided. *Los Angeles Times Magazine,* 12.
Butler, Katy, (July 24, 1994) Memory on Trial. *San Francisco Chronicle, This World.*
Cheek, David B., M.D. (1994) *Hypnosis: The Application of Ideomotor Techniques.* Boston: Allyn and Bacon.
Churchill, Randal, (not yet published) *Ideomotor Magic: The Hypnotherapy Training Guide.* CA: Transforming Press
Courtois, Christine A., (1999) *Recollections of Sexual Abuse: Treatment Principles and Guidelines.* New York: W. W. Norton & Company
Cousins, Norman, (October 1, 1977) The Mysterious Placebo: How Mind Helps Medicine Work. *Saturday Review,* 9-17.
False Memory Syndrome Foundation (December 5, 1992) *Newsletter* 1.
Hovdestad, W.E., & Kristiansen, C.E., (1996) A field study of "false memory syndrome": Construct validity and incidence. *Journal of Psychiatry and Law,* 24, 299-338.
Joseph, Rawn, (September 25, 1997) The Reality of Repressed Memories: A Neuroscientist Explains How Victims Can Forget, Then Remember, Horrible Trauma. *San Francisco Chronicle.*
Kalichman, Seth C., (1993) *Mandated reporting of suspected child abuse: Ethics, law & policy.* Washington, D.C. American Psychological Association.
Kanovitz, J., (1992) Hypnotic memories and civil sexual abuse trials. *Vanderbilt Law Review,* 45, 1185-1262.
Loftus, Dr. Elizabeth, and Ketcham, Katherine, (1994) *The Myth of Repressed Memory: False Memories and Allegations of Sexual Abuse.* New York: St. Martin's Griffin
Lowenstein, R.J. (December, 1992) President's message. *International Society for the Study of Dissociation News,* page 4.
Nalder, Eric (November 5, 1995) False Memories. *The Seattle Times.*
Ofshe, R., & Singer, M.T. (1994) Recovered-memory therapy and robust repression: Influence of pseudomemories. *International Journal of Clinical and Experimental Hypnosis,* 42, 391-410.
Ofshe, R., & Waters, E. (1996) *Making Monsters: False Memories, Psychotherapy, and Sexual Hysteria.* Berkeley, CA: University of California Press
Terr, Lenore, (1995) *Unchained Memories: True Stories of Traumatic Memories, Lost and Found.* New York: Basic Books.
Yapko, Michael,Ph.D., (1994) *Suggestions of Abuse: True and False Memories of Childhood Sexual Trauma.* New York: Simon & Schuster.

Annotated Bibliography

Here is recommended reading that is relevant to major themes of this volume.

Hypnotherapy

Canfield, Cheryl, *Steps Toward Profound Healing, Healing Ourselves, Healing the World*. Transforming Press, 2002. Born out of the author's own experience with advanced cancer, this book uses practical and inspiring steps to explore the connection between mind and body, and our intrinsic potential to tap into our subconscious resources for profound healing. A priceless guide for therapists and clients.

Hammond, D. Corydon, Editor, *Handbook of Hypnotic Suggestions and Metaphors*. W.W. Norton and Company, 1990. This practical desktop reference is the largest collection of hypnotic suggestions and metaphors ever compiled, with contributions from over 100 experts in the field.

Hunter, Marlene E., *Creative Scripts for Hypnotherapy*, Brunner/Mazel, 1994. A wide variety of scripts for hypnotherapists, with a wealth of elaborate metaphorical imagery.

Isen, Hal, and Kline, Peter, *The Genesis Principle: A Journey into the Source of Creativity and Leadership*, Great Ocean Publishers, 1999. Hypnotherapist Hal Isen has led transformational programs for 100,000 persons over four decades. Based on the Kabbalah's Tree of Life, this guide to self-transformation and greater creativity provides deep wisdom for therapists and clients.

Jacobs, Donald T., *Patient Communication for First Responders,* Prentice Hall, 1991. This is an excellent book for developing communication and suggestion skills during hypnosis, including the hypnotic states often resulting from emergencies.

Kroger, William S., *Clinical and Experimental Hypnosis*, J.B. Lippencott, 2nd edition, 1977. This major text covers an exceptionally wide range of material and makes a very effective reference book.

Tebbetts, Charles, *Self-Hypnosis and Other Mind-Expanding Techniques,* Westwood Publishing, 1987. A good introduction for the hypnotherapist to help teach self-hypnosis to clients. In addition, the rules outlined in this bestselling book for structuring autosuggestions are relevant for proper use of direct suggestion during hetero-hypnosis.

Zimmerman, Katherine, *Hypnotherapy Scripts, Volume I and II,* TranceTime™ Publishing, 1996. Many of the scripts are infused with good ideas for regression explorations that can be used in group or individual sessions.

Regression

Many books in other sections of this bibliography are very relevant to the subject of regression, including all of the books in the section which focuses on recovered memories.

Barnett, E. A., *Analytical Hypnotherapy: Principles and Practice,* Westwood Publishing, 1989. This well-researched book includes many transcripts of hypnotic regressions, with considerable use of Transactional Analysis and ideomotor methods.

Boyne, Gil, *Transforming Therapy: A New Approach to Hypnotherapy,* Westwood Publishing, 1989. The first book to combine Gestalt and hypnotherapy, by the therapist who integrated these two fields. Emphasizes a collection of transcripts in which transformational hypnotic regression modalities are integral to the process.

Churchill, Randal, *Catharsis in Regression Hypnotherapy: Transcripts of Transformation, Volume II,* Transforming Press, 2004. This is the companion volume to *Regression Hypnotherapy,* exploring powerful therapeutic directions in conjunction with the abreactions that frequently develop with the use of the affect bridge and Gestalt in hypnosis.

Elman, Dave, *Hypnotherapy,* Westwood Publishing, 1964. This classic, originally entitled *Findings in Hypnosis,* is the summation of Elman's theories and techniques. Among his major contributions to the field, he was a pioneer in the development of regression and hypnoanalysis strategies.

Recovered Memories

Brown, Daniel; Scheflin, Alan W.; & Hammond, D. Corydon, *Memory, Trauma Treatment, and the Law: An Essential Reference on Memory for Clinicians, Researchers, Attorneys, and Judges.* W.W. Norton & Company, Inc., 1998. Exceptionally comprehensive and balanced, this massive book is the definitive work on the subject of recovered memories and the law.

Courtois, Christine A., *Recollections of Sexual Abuse: Treatment Principles and Guidelines*. W.W. Norton & Company, Inc., 1999. This well balanced, exhaustively researched book provides clinicians with information about the controversy of delayed memories of sexual abuse and sound guidelines for working with these issues.

Terr, Lenore, *Unchained Memories: True Stories of Traumatic Memories, Lost and Found*, Basic Books, 1995. Child psychiatrist Lenore Terr, an expert in trauma and repressed memory, has been a powerful expert witness in high-profile court cases.

Yapko, Michael D., *Suggestions of Abuse: True and False Memories of Childhood Sexual Trauma*. Simon & Schuster, 1994. Yapko explores the interrelated subjects of memory, repression and suggestibility. He reveals the alarming ignorance of many mental health professionals and provides guidance for working with memories in therapy.

Ideomotor Methods

Cheek, David B. and LeCron, Leslie M., *Clinical Hypnotherapy*, Harcourt Brace, 1968. This out-of-print classic introduces the subject of ideomotor methods and gives an excellent overview of hypnotherapy.

Cheek, David B., *Hypnosis: The Application of Ideomotor Techniques*, Paramount Publishing, 1994. An interesting many-faceted study of the field of hypnotherapy with insights from 50 years of clinical practice, including extensive utilization of ideomotor methods.

Churchill, Randal, *Ideomotor Magic: The Hypnotherapy Training Manual*, Transforming Press. This teaching text, to be published in 2006, explores strategies accessing the awareness, knowledge and wisdom of the subconscious mind that, combined with regression modalities, can yield profound results.

Mutke, Peter H. C., *Hypnosis: The Mind-Body Connection*, Westwood Publishing, 1987. Emphasizes teaching the finger-signal form of ideomotor methods within self-hypnosis. An in-depth guide to recommend to our clients to augment the learning of this skill, there is much information of value to therapists as well.

Rossi, Ernest L., and Cheek, David B., *Mind-body Therapy: Methods of Ideodynamic Healing in Hypnosis*, W.W. Norton & Company, Inc., 1988. The term ideodynamic is a synonym for ideomotor. This 519 page text includes hundreds of engaging case reports from Cheek's clinical work, complemented by Rossi's chapters linking this often intuitive work to the latest research in psychobiology.

Gestalt Therapy

An additional resource is The Gestalt Therapy Page, http://gestalt.org, a joint project sponsored by The Gestalt Journal and the International Gestalt Therapy Association. This resource-rich website includes many good links and a massive bibliography of books relevant to Gestalt therapy.

Churchill, Randal, *Become the Dream: The Transforming Power of Hypnotic Dreamwork.* Transforming Press, 1997. The first book about the integration of hypnosis and any form of dreamwork, by the originator of Hypnotic Dreamwork™. Gestalt dreamwork is synergistically augmented by powerful hypnotic modalities, including regression strategies where appropriate.

Kelzer, Kenneth, *Deep Journeys: Experimental Psychotherapy with Dreams, Personal Archetypal Tales and Trance States.* North Atlantic Books, 1999. This beautifully written book describes and demonstrates the unique synthesis of methodologies, including hypnotherapy and Gestalt, that make up the author's Deep Journey method for effective, long term transformation.

Downing, Jack, *Dreams and Nightmares,* Gestalt Journal Press Edition, 1997. This is the only book of Gestalt dreamwork transcriptions that includes inserted ongoing detailed commentary by the therapist.

Perls, Frederick, *Gestalt Therapy Verbatim,* Gestalt Journal Press Edition, 1992. Gestalt therapy's colorful primary founder helped put his work at Esalen on the map with this classic. Includes a superb theoretical overview of Gestalt and a large collection of dreamwork transcripts.

Perls, Frederick, *The Gestalt Approach & Eye Witness to Therapy,* Science and Behavior books, Inc., 1973. Perl's last and most comprehensive work, can be read as one entity or as two separate works. He was working on both books at the time of his death.

Yontef, Gary, *Awareness, Dialogue and Process: Essays on Gestalt Therapy,* Gestalt Journal Press, 1993. Called "the most significant addition to the body of Gestalt therapy literature in almost two decades," this 570 page collection of Yontef's writings includes the definitive overview of the theory and practice of Gestalt. Highly recommended as a training text and as a resource for graduate students and scholars.

Become the Dream
The Transforming Power of Hypnotic Dreamwork

*Randal Churchill, the originator of Hypnotic Dreamwork™,
writes the book that transcends interpretation*

The "unique and revolutionary" *Become the Dream,* the first book about combining dreams and hypnotherapy, is winner of the 1999 Founders Award for Excellence in Professional Literature. Integrating a wealth of hypnotherapy modalities with Gestalt dreamwork, Randal Churchill demonstrates Hypnotic Dreamwork, based on original work he began developing in 1970.

• The vast majority of dreamwork methods rely on analysis and interpretation. By contrast, Gestalt dreamwork brings the dreamer into a deeper experience of the dream itself and allows the individual to find the unique relationship of the dream to his or her own existential experience. The addition of a wealth of hypnotic techniques takes the dreamer much further, with a variety of effective options such as hypnotic deepening, ideomotor methods, regression and positive suggestions for further insight and integration.

• The first two chapters of the book provide a foundation for understanding the potential value of hypnotherapy, Gestalt dreamwork, and the integration of these forms of therapy. The third chapter gives insights for developing dream recall and lucid dream skills. A later chapter emphasizes the author's signature processes of elicited and guided hypnodreams. The rest of the book focuses primarily on transcripts and commentary of a wide range of fascinating dreamwork sessions, which draw the reader into an intimate look at therapy from the inside. With sensitivity and skill, the author demonstrates the remarkable potential of this unique work to tap into the receptivity and wisdom inherent in the subconscious mind and the potential for profound change.

• *Become the Dream* is a powerful and practical teaching tool for professionals in any of the health and counseling fields, and an inspiring and provocative book for anyone seeking self-knowledge and actualization.

"This fascinating book is unique and revolutionary... an important addition to the fields of dream therapy, hypnotism, Gestalt therapy and psychology. *Become the Dream* is a major breakthrough, a text of university and universal level, worthy of worldwide acclaim."
 - From the foreword by Ormond McGill, *The Dean of American Hypnotists*

280 pages, hardbound, with a beautiful dust cover. Price: $29.95.

Visit the website, **www. transformingpress.com**, for much more information, including the Table of Contents, foreword, reviews, a sample chapter, and an order form to get an autographed copy.

Transforming Press, www.transformingpress.com
phone & fax: 209/962-6403 • email: info@transformingpress.com

Praise for *Become the Dream* from the Fields of Psychology, Gestalt Therapy, Hypnotherapy & Dreamwork

"Randal Churchill is one of the best hypnotherapists working today, and a superb teacher of this powerful transformative art. He has poured his heart, his soul, and over 25 years of hands-on experience into his new book, which is filled with information on the best methods and techniques for working with dreams, hypnosis, regression and the subconscious mind. ...Essential reading for counselors and therapists."

- Dr. Jim Dreaver, author of *The Ultimate Cure*

"*Become the Dream* is a very welcome addition to the literature of Gestalt Therapy. Gestalt dream work, when practiced skillfully, is more art form than therapy, and I'm happy to see that Randal Churchill understands truly the art of working with dreams."

- Robert K. Hall, M.D., Psychiatrist, Lomi School Founder

"*Become the Dream* promises an awareness that goes beyond the bounds of our five senses. Combining hypnosis and dreamwork as Churchill has done confirms the ancient aboriginal understanding that dreaming is an intangible world that is an intimate and indispensable aspect of the tangible one. Avoiding the typical conscious interpretations of dreams, Churchill shows how transformation is more likely when dreams are experienced via the hidden power of hypnosis."

- Dr. Donald Trent Jacobs, author of *Patient Communication for First Responders*

"Randal Churchill's caring style and humor provide an added dimension to this inspiring and pioneering work. Become the *Dream* illuminates the personal and existential relationship of the dream to the dreamer. Unlike interpretive dreamwork, the dream is re-experienced on a heart and soul level, where the subconscious mind reveals real dramas being played out in life. Connecting with the dreamer's own innate wisdom, Randal skillfully combines an eclectic array of techniques with gifted intuition to lead the dreamer to profound insights and personal transformation."

- Cheryl Canfield, CHT, author of *Steps Toward Profound Healing*

"In *Become the Dream* Randal Churchill provides innovative approaches to combining hypnosis and dreamwork in support of therapeutic goals, which simultaneously encourages integration of conscious and unconscious processes in service of honoring the whole person. The generous inclusion of verbatim case history transcripts vividly underscores the significance of the client/therapist relationship in any counseling situation. The dialogues are particularly interesting and valuable in illustrating how much the client (and the client's unconscious resources) contributes to the therapeutic process."

- Dr. Joseph P. Reel, Director, Hypnosis Career Institute, NM

Catharsis in Regression Therapy
Transcripts of Transformation, Volume II

To be published April 2004: Companion volume to
Regression Hypnotherapy, Transcripts of Transformation

Catharsis in Regression Therapy further expands Randal Churchill's comprehensive strategies in working effectively with the strong emotions that frequently arise when using the affect bridge and Gestalt methods in regression work.

Rather than avoiding emotions, this powerful therapy uses abreaction, when appropriate, as a golden opportunity to work powerfully with and transform emotions, giving even greater opportunity for profound growth.

Catharsis in Regression Therapy integrates many modalities into a clearly written and much needed guide to the complex and often misunderstood therapeutic exploration of the subconscious mind.

Techniques and principles include:
- checking for subconscious permission to work with the strong emotions that arise when regressing to traumatic experiences
- the potential value of catharsis in regression work
- helping to prepare for potential abreaction
- encouraging vs discouraging emotions
- explorations to determine when to avoid or enhance emotional expression
- grounding and centering techniques for the therapist
- further aspects of developing careful neutrality when working with past trauma, including possible sexual abuse
- demonstrating the value of past life recall, even from a symbolic perspective

The impact of this powerful therapy and the giant leaps forward that can often be made in a single session, is demonstrated in the generous use of dramatic transcripts of actual sessions with exceptionally strong emotional expression. There are various forms of commentary and follow-up interviews. Some examples:

- in *Rose's Pervading Sadness: The Tragic Attempted Escape from Hungary*, Rose is regressed to her early childhood in Hungary when she was imprisoned, beaten, and watched people dying around her.
- in *Bob's Emotional Blocking: The Shock of the Sudden Divorce*, an emotional breakthrough leads him back to an early traumatic incident as a baby.
- in *Paul's Shame: The Felon Who Didn't Fit In*, Paul's regression uncovers painful emotions that trigger early memories of loneliness and alienation.
- in *Sandy's Road Rage: The Explosive Driver*, Sandy's struggle with the intense anger that has dramatically affected her life takes her back to a teenage trauma
- in *Virginia's Panic Attacks: Smothered by Her Disturbed Brother*, intensifying emotion through the affect bridge takes Virginia back to terrifying childhood memories

Direct inquiries to Transforming Press, **www.transformingpress.com**
phone & fax: 209/962-6403 • email: info@transformingpress.com

Here are Comments from HTI Graduates
please see the ad on the next page

"You certainly covered a broad range of modalities in your classes, but I was most impressed by your depth, especially during the therapy demonstrations. You are both masters of reaching the underlying issues and working through profoundly challenging problems. You are so skillful, sensitive and supportive, I would send anyone in the world to you."
                      Dr. Victoria West, Chiropractor, Fremont, CA

"When I saw your brilliant work in New Zealand last year I was so impressed I knew I certainly had to come and learn more. The month here has simply flown, full of real gems in terms of therapy, and in terms of getting to know myself better. The depth of the excellent therapy demonstrations and the personal knowledge, commitment and sincerity of each instructor is truly remarkable."
          Dr. David Page, Registered Psychologist, Palmerston North, New Zealand

"In my blind assumption that this was merely a fine school for the training of hypnotherapists, I found myself walking willingly into a sage and loving cocoon. In this place, I experienced and witnessed spiritual transformation and personal growth unparalleled in any other single event of my life. The depth and breadth of the wisdom and knowledge offered to your students far exceeded my wildest expectations, and the deep bonding I accomplished with the class I will carry in my heart forever."
        Catherine Hershon, Certified Hypnotherapist, Marketing Researcher, Sausalito, CA

"It's very hard to find the words to express my profound gratitude and appreciation for everything I was privileged to witness in class - it was almost like a fairytale where miracles can be worked easily, effortlessly, and joyful. Everything was performed with great skill, experience, feeling, respect, and deep love."
                Tanya Konyukhova, Hypnotherapist, Translator, Moscow, Russia

"The level of training and support I received from HTI, and you both, has been unsurpassed by any training I've received in any graduate school. The deep understanding of the importance of the subconscious mind that you provided me has had a profound impact on my ability to meet my client's needs."
                   Gayle Passaretti, M.A., Licensed Counselor, Shepard, MI

"Thanks to your excellent training and continuing support, my practice has become more successful every year since I began in 1989. I love my work, my clients are getting great results, and all five hypnotherapy books I've written have gotten rave reviews. The quality of your program is unsurpassed in the field."
      Katherine Zimmerman, CHT, Author of many hypnotherapy books, Davis, CA

Providing innovation and leadership in an emerging healing field...

HYPNOTHERAPY CERTIFICATION

Serving the world with accelerated programs up to four weeks long
Serving Northern California with programs on weekend days

Classes with **Randal Churchill & Marleen Mulder**
"The Teachers of the Teachers" ™

In-depth teaching of the most effective forms of hypnotherapy
with lectures, demonstrations and practice in the most valuable aspects of

TRANSPERSONAL HYPNOTHERAPY ✦ EMOTIONAL CLEARING ✦ INNER CHILD PROCESS
HYPNOTIC DREAMWORK™ ✦ QUANTUM HYPNOTHERAPY ✦ TRANSFORMING THERAPY
PARTS THERAPY ✦ ADVANCED DESENSITIZATION ✦ ANALYTICAL HYPNOTHERAPY
ADVANCED IDEOMOTOR METHODS ✦ VARIOUS FORMS OF REGRESSION

✦ PLUS THE INTEGRATION OF MANY EFFECTIVE MODALITIES INTO HYPNOSIS, INCLUDING
GESTALT, PSYCHOSYNTHESIS, BIOENERGETICS, HOLOTROPIC BREATHWORK,
INTUITION, AND SHAMANISM INCLUDING HUNA ✦ AND MORE

- **Become a Certified Hypnotherapist – Hypnosis as a Career**
  School Licensed – State of California. Approved – American Council of Hypnotist Examiners

- **Professionals: Expand Skills in the Health & Counseling Fields**
  All major approvals for CEU's, including Board of Behavioral Sciences and BRN

- **Hypnotherapists: Deepen Your Mastery of Therapy**
  Advanced courses approved for upgrading or renewing your Certification

Originality, Integrity, Leadership... As the 21st Century unfolds, hypnotherapy is transforming many aspects of the health professions and truly revolutionizing the counseling professions. We are honored to have a significant role in this, in leading the way for three decades with powerful, innovative therapy methods and in using the insights and therapy modalitites of ourselves and others to train many of the leaders in the field.

Free Brochure: call **800/256-6448** or email **info@hypnoschool.com**

HYPNOTHERAPY TRAINING INSTITUTE
www.hypnoschool.com

4730 Alta Vista Ave., Santa Rosa, CA 95404   Classes in Corte Madera, near San Francisco